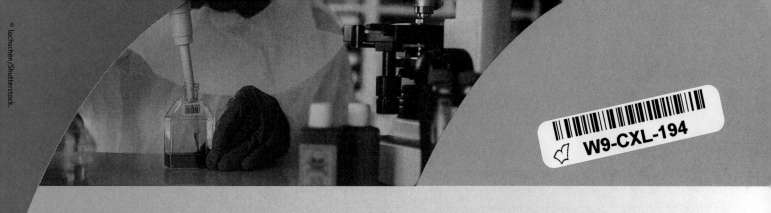

Essentials of Public Health

THIRD EDITION

Bernard J. Turnock, MD, MPH

Clinical Professor
Division of Community Health Sciences
School of Public Health
University of Illinois at Chicago
Chicago, Illinois

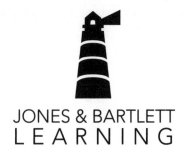

JONES & BARTLETT
LEARNING

World Headquarters
Jones & Bartlett Learning
5 Wall Street
Burlington, MA 01803
978-443-5000
info@jblearning.com
www.jblearning.com

Jones & Bartlett Learning books and products are available through most bookstores and online booksellers. To contact Jones & Bartlett Learning directly, call 800-832-0034, fax 978-443-8000, or visit our website, www.jblearning.com.

Substantial discounts on bulk quantities of Jones & Bartlett Learning publications are available to corporations, professional associations, and other qualified organizations. For details and specific discount information, contact the special sales department at Jones & Bartlett Learning via the above contact information or send an email to specialsales@jblearning.com.

08591-4

Production Credits

VP, Executive Publisher: David Cella
Publisher: Michael Brown
Associate Editor: Lindsey Mawhiney
Editorial Assistant: Nicholas Alakel
Production Manager: Tracey McCrea
Senior Marketing Manager: Sophie Fleck Teague
Art Development Editor: Joanna Lundeen
Art Development Assistant: Shannon Sheehan
Manufacturing and Inventory Control Supervisor: Amy Bacus
Composition: Cenveo Publisher Services
Cover Design: Kristin E. Parker
Manager of Photo Research, Rights & Permissions: Amy Rathburn
Cover Image: © luchschen/Shutterstock
Printing and Binding: LSC Communications
Cover Printing: LSC Communications

Library of Congress Cataloging-in-Publication Data
Turnock, Bernard J., author.
  Essentials of public health / Bernard J. Turnock.—Third edition.
    p. ; cm.
  Includes bibliographical references and index.
  ISBN 978-1-284-06935-8 (pbk.)
  I. Title.
  [DNLM: 1. Public Health Administration—United States. 2. Public Health Practice—United States. WA 540 AA1]
  RA445
  362.1—dc23
                              2014036062
6048

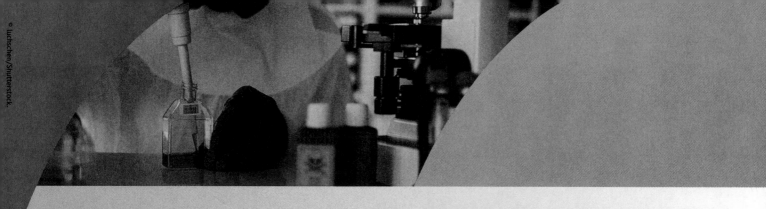

Dedication

To Terry, Scott, and Linda—my dearly missed siblings.

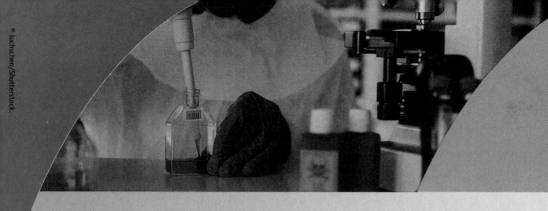

Contents

New to This Edition

The *Third Edition* offers a number of new features and incorporates information on a variety of recent developments in public health practice and the health sector. Implementation of the Affordable Care Act, strategic planning, accreditation of public health organizations, and credentialing of public health workers are among the recent developments covered in this revision. Extensive information on state and local public health practice derived from national surveys conducted since 2012 is included throughout the book. Community public health practice and emergency preparedness topics have been expanded into two separate chapters. New conceptual frameworks for the public health system, overall health system, and public health workforce have been added. The number of public health occupations examined in this edition has been increased from 23 to 39. More than 60 new or revised charts and tables are incorporated into the new edition, and a series of "outside-the-book thinking" exercises appears in each chapter.

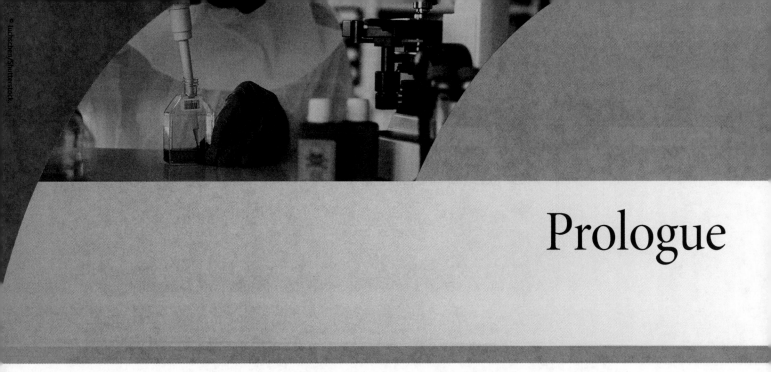

Prologue

Essentials of Public Health by Bernard Turnock has made important contributions to the *Essential Public Health* series. It was an early text in the series and set the stage for the long list of books that followed. Professor Turnock's text, now in its third edition, continues to be an important part of the *Essential Public Health* series.

The *Third Edition*, like previous editions, takes advantage of Professor Turnock's extensive experience working in governmental public health. His in-depth knowledge of health departments and the changes that are occurring in delivery of public health services is apparent throughout the book. He has a special interest and knowledge of careers in public health, which is highlighted throughout the text.

The text follows the same framework and style used in the earlier editions including a large number of examples, charts, graphs, and discussion questions. The *Third Edition* updates and expands on the second edition, providing a state of the art approach to public health and public health careers.

For those who want an introduction to public health with a special focus on public health careers and the workings of public health agencies, this is the perfect introductory text. Bernard Turnock writes with an approachable style and a depth of knowledge. We are pleased to have the third edition of *Essentials of Public Health* as a continuing part of the *Essential Public Health* series.

Richard Riegelman MD, MPH, PhD
Series Editor, *Essential Public Health* series

Preface

Blending basic public health practice concepts with the nuts and bolts of public health careers is both a unique approach and a formidable challenge for a public health text. This book addresses that challenge by focusing on basic concepts as well as career opportunities, topics that are often of interest for students seeking undergraduate or graduate degrees. This approach is especially useful in courses that provide an introduction to public health, either as a stand-alone survey course or as an introductory course for a concentration or major. Students are exposed to key concepts underlying public health as a system and social enterprise, as well as to careers in the field. As a result, students will take away an understanding of what public health is and how various occupations and professions contribute to its mission and success.

The first six chapters cover important concepts and information on what public health is in 21st-century America. Basic concepts underlying public health are presented in Chapter 1, including definitions, historical highlights, and unique features of public health. This and subsequent chapters focus largely on public health in the United States, although information on global public health and comparisons among nations appear in several chapters. Health and illness and the various factors that influence health and quality of life are discussed in Chapter 2. This chapter also presents data and information on health status and risk factors in the United States and introduces a method for analyzing health problems to identify their precursors. Chapter 3 examines the overall health system and its various intervention strategies, with special emphasis on trends and developments that are important to public health. It highlights interfaces between public health and a rapidly changing health system and examines the implementation status of key provisions of the Affordable Care Act. Chapter 4 examines the organization of public health responsibilities in the United States by reviewing their legal basis and the current structure of public health agencies at the federal, state, and local levels. Chapters 5 and 6 focus on the community health improvement and emergency preparedness and response roles of public health, including the opportunities afforded by increased public expectations and a substantial influx of federal funding. Together, these six chapters serve as a primer on what public health is and how it relates to health interests in modern America.

But public health is more than concepts and organizations. Its important work is carried out by a diverse and committed workforce. Chapters 7 through 13 examine key aspects of the work of different public health occupations and professionals in order to provide an understanding of the basic underpinnings of public health jobs and careers. Despite an increasing recognition of its importance, there is little information available on the public health workforce in terms of its size, distribution, composition, skills, and impact on health goals. Chapter 7 examines overall trends affecting the public health workforce. Key characteristics for occupations and careers in public health practice are defined and explained in this chapter. This framework of career characteristics becomes the lens through which the major occupational categories and career pathways available to public health workers are examined. Chapters 8 through 13 provide basic information on 40 occupational categories and disciplines. The concluding chapter focuses on future implications for public health workers and those considering a career in public health.

Each chapter includes a variety of figures and tables that illustrate key concepts and provide useful resources for public health practitioners. New with this edition is a series of "outside-the-book" thinking exercises incorporated into each chapter. These exercises allow the book to serve as a foundation for acquiring and integrating information from other sources and personal experience into issues introduced in the book. An extensive glossary of public health terminology is provided for the benefit of those unfamiliar with some of the commonly used terms, as well as to convey the intended meaning for terms that may have several different connotations in practice.

The story of public health is not a simple one to tell, in part because public health is broadly involved with the biologic, environmental, social, cultural, behavioral, and service utilization factors associated with health. Still, we all share in the successes and failures of our collective decisions and actions, making us all accountable to each other for the results of our efforts. My hope is that this book will present a broad view of the public health system and those who work within it in order to deter current and future public health workers from narrowly defining public health in terms of only what they do. At its core, the purpose of this book is to describe public health simply and clearly in terms of what it is, what it does, and why this work is important to all of us and fulfilling to those who do it on a daily basis.

![luchschen/Shutterstock.]

Acknowledgments

Whatever insights and wisdom might be found in this book have filtered through to me from my mentors, colleagues, coworkers, and friends after more than three decades in the field. So many people have shaped the concepts and insights provided in this book that it would be foolhardy for me to try to acknowledge them all here. This book blends information and material from two other works published by Jones & Bartlett Learning—*Public Health: What It Is and How It Works, Sixth Edition* (2015) and *Public Health: Career Opportunities That Make a Difference* (2006). Mike Brown at Jones & Bartlett Learning was instrumental in providing guidance and suggestions for the development of this book. Production Manager, Tracey McCrea, and Associate Editor, Lindsey Mawhiney, also at Jones & Bartlett Learning, helped make it a reality. I am grateful for their many and varied contributions.

About the Author

Bernard J. (Barney) Turnock, MD, MPH, is currently Clinical Professor of Community Health Sciences at the School of Public Health, University of Illinois at Chicago (UIC). Since he joined UIC School of Public Health in 1990, he has also served as Acting Dean, Associate Dean for Public Health Practice, Director of the Division of Community Health Sciences, as well as Director of the Center for Public Health Practice and Illinois Public Health Preparedness Center. His major areas of interest involve performance measurement, capacity building, and workforce development within the public health system. He is board certified in Preventive Medicine and Public Health, and he has extensive practice experience, having served as Director of the Illinois Department of Public Health from 1985 through 1990, Deputy Commissioner and Acting Commissioner of the Chicago Department of Health, and State Program Director for Maternal and Child Health and Emergency Medical Services during his distinguished career. He has played major roles in a wide variety of public policy and public health issues in Illinois since 1978. He frequently consults on a variety of public health and healthcare issues and has served as a member of the Illinois State Board of Health and as President of the Illinois Public Health Association. He is also the author of two other recently published works: *Public Health: Career Choices That Make a Difference* and *Public Health: What It Is and How It Works*. He has received two prestigious awards from the American Public Health Association—one for Excellence in Health Planning and Practice and another for Excellence in Health Administration. He is also a recipient of the UIC School of Public Health's "Golden Apple" award for excellence in teaching, and he was the developer and instructor for UIC's first completely online course.

CHAPTER **1**

What Is Public Health?

LEARNING OBJECTIVES

Given the historical phenomena that have shaped the development of public health, formulate a working definition and logic model for public health in the 21st century. Key aspects of this competency expectation include being able to

- Articulate several different definitions of public health
- Describe the origins and content of public health responses over history
- Trace the development of the public health system in the United States
- Broadly characterize the contributions and value of public health
- Identify three or more distinguishing features of public health
- Describe public health as a system using a logic model with inputs, processes, outputs, and results, emphasizing the role of core functions and essential public health services
- Identify five or more Internet web sites that provide useful information on the public health system in the United States

The passing of one century and the early decades of the next afford a rare opportunity to look back at where public health has been and forward to the challenges that lie ahead. Imagine a world 100 years from now where life expectancy is 30 years more and infant mortality rates are 95% lower than they are today. The average human life span would be more than 107 years, and less than one of every 2,000 infants would die before their first birthday. These seem like unrealistic expectations and unlikely achievements; yet, they are no greater than the gains realized during the 20th century in the United States. In 1900, few envisioned the century of progress in public health that lay ahead. Yet by 1925 public health leaders such as C.E.A. Winslow were noting a nearly 50% increase in life expectancy (from 36 years to 53 years) for residents of New York City between the years 1880 and 1920.[1] Accomplishments such as these caused Winslow to speculate what might be possible through widespread application of scientific knowledge. With the even more spectacular achievements over the rest of the 20th century, we all should wonder what is possible in the century that has just begun.

This year may be remembered for many things, but it is unlikely that many people will remember it as a spectacular year for public health in the United States. No major discoveries, innovations, or triumphs set this year apart from other years in recent memory. Yet, on closer examination, maybe there were! Like the story of the wise man who invented the game of chess for his king and asked for payment by having the king place one grain of wheat on the first square of the chessboard, two on the second, four on the third, eight on the fourth, and so on, the small victories of public health over the past century have resulted in cumulative gains so vast in scope that they are difficult to comprehend.

This year, there will be nearly 900,000 fewer cases of measles reported than in 1941, 200,000 fewer cases of diphtheria than in 1921, more than 250,000 fewer cases of whooping cough than in 1934, and 21,000 fewer cases of polio than in 1951.[2] The early decades of the new century witnessed 50 million fewer smokers than would have been expected, given trends in tobacco use through 1965. More than 2 million Americans were alive who otherwise would have died from heart disease and stroke, and nearly 100,000 Americans were alive as a result of automobile seat belt use. Protection of the U.S. blood supply had prevented more than 1.5 million hepatitis B and hepatitis C infections and more than 50,000 human immunodeficiency virus (HIV) infections, as well as more than $5 billion in medical costs associated with these three diseases.[3] Today, average blood lead levels in children are less than one-third of what they were a quarter century ago. This catalog of accomplishments could be expanded many times over. **Figure 1-1** summarizes this progress, including two of the most widely followed measures of a population's health status—life expectancy and infant mortality.

These results did not occur by themselves. They came about through decisions and actions that represent the essence of what is public health. It is the story of public health and its immense value and importance in our lives that is the focus of this text. With this impressive litany of accomplishments, it would seem that public health's story would be easily told. For many reasons, however, it is not. As a result, public health remains poorly understood by its prime beneficiary—the public—as well as many of its dedicated practitioners. Although public health's results, as measured in terms of improved health status, diseases prevented, scarce resources saved, and improved quality of life, are more apparent today than ever before, society seldom links the activities of public health with its results. This suggests that the public health community must more effectively

communicate what public health is and what it does, so that its results can be readily traced to their source.

This chapter is an introduction to public health that links basic concepts to practice. It considers three questions:

- What is public health?
- Where did it come from?
- Why is it important in the United States today?

To address these questions, this chapter begins with a sketch of the historical development of public health activities in the United States. It then examines several definitions and characterizations of what public health is and explores some of its unique features. Finally, it offers insight into the value of public health in biologic, economic, and human terms.

Taken together, these topics provide a foundation for understanding what public health is and why it is important. A conceptual framework that approaches public health from a systems perspective is introduced to identify the dimensions of the public health system and facilitate an understanding of the various images of public health that coexist in the United States today. We will see that, as in the story of the blind men examining the elephant, various sectors of our

FIGURE 1-1 Percentage Improvement in Selected Measures of Life Expectancy and Age-Adjusted, Cause-Specific Mortality for the Time Periods 1900–2000 and 1950–2000, United States

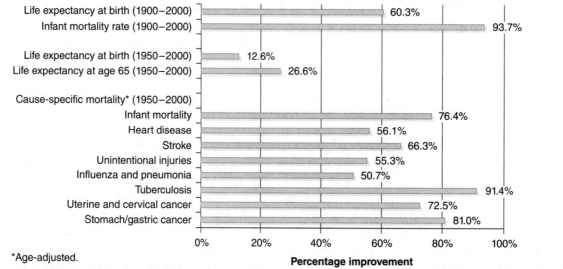

*Age-adjusted.

Data from Centers for Disease Control and Prevention, National Center for Health Statistics. *Health, United States* 2009. Hyattsville, MD: NCHS; 2009 and Rust G, Satcher D, Fryer GE, Levine RS, Blumenthal DS. Triangulating on success: innovation, public health, medical care, and cause-specific US mortality over a half century (1950–2000). *Am J Public Health*. 2010: 100: S95–S104.

society have mistaken separate components of public health for the entire system.

A BRIEF HISTORY OF PUBLIC HEALTH IN THE UNITED STATES

Early Influences on American Public Health

Although the complete history of public health is a fascinating saga in its own right, this section presents only selected highlights. When ancient cultures perceived illness as the manifestation of supernatural forces, they felt that little in the way of either personal or collective action was possible. For many centuries, disease was synonymous with epidemic. Diseases, including horrific epidemics of infectious diseases such as the Black Death (plague), leprosy, and cholera, were phenomena to be accepted. It was not until the so-called Age of Reason and the Enlightenment that scholarly inquiry began to challenge the "givens" or accepted realities of the time. Eventually expansion of the science and knowledge base would reap substantial rewards.

With the advent of industrialism and imperialism, the stage was set for epidemic diseases to increase their terrible toll. As populations shifted to urban centers for the purpose of commerce and industry, public health conditions worsened. The mixing of dense populations living in unsanitary conditions and working long hours in unsafe and exploitative industries with wave after wave of cholera, smallpox, typhoid, tuberculosis, yellow fever, and other diseases was a formula for disaster. Such disaster struck again and again across the globe, but most seriously and most often at the industrialized seaport cities that provided the portal of entry for diseases transported as stowaways alongside commercial cargo. The experience, and subsequent susceptibility, of different cultures to these diseases partly explains how relatively small bands of Europeans were able to overcome and subjugate vast Native American cultures. Seeing the Europeans unaffected by scourges such as smallpox served to reinforce beliefs that these light-skinned visitors were supernatural figures, unaffected by natural forces.[4]

The British colonies in North America and the new American republic certainly bore their share of the burden. American diaries of the 17th and 18th centuries chronicle one infectious disease onslaught after another. These epidemics left their mark on families, communities, and even history. For example, the national capital had to be moved out of Philadelphia because of a devastating yellow fever epidemic in 1793. This epidemic also prompted the city to develop its first board of health in that same year.

The formation of local boards of distinguished citizens, the first boards of health, was one of the earliest organized responses to epidemics. This response was revealing in that it represented an attempt to confront disease collectively. Because science had not yet determined that specific microorganisms were the causes of epidemics, avoidance had long been the primary tactic used. Avoidance meant evacuating the general location of the epidemic until it subsided or isolating diseased individuals or those recently exposed to diseases on the basis of a mix of fear, tradition, and scientific speculation. Several developments, however, were swinging the pendulum ever closer to more effective counteractions.

The work of public health pioneers such as Edward Jenner, John Snow, and Edwin Chadwick illustrates the value of public health, even when its methods are applied amidst scientific uncertainty. Well before Koch's postulates established scientific methods for linking bacteria with specific diseases and before Pasteur's experiments helped to establish the germ theory, both Jenner and Snow used deductive logic and common sense to do battle with smallpox and cholera, respectively. In 1796, Jenner successfully used vaccination for a disease that ran rampant through communities across the globe. This was the initial shot in a long and arduous campaign that, by the year 1977, had totally eradicated smallpox from all of its human hiding places in every country in the world. The potential for its reemergence through the actions of terrorists is a topic left to a fuller discussion of public health emergency preparedness and response.

Snow's accomplishments even further advanced the art and science of public health. In 1854, Snow traced an outbreak of cholera to the well water drawn from the pump at Broad Street and helped to prevent hundreds, perhaps thousands, of cholera cases. In that same year, he demonstrated that another large outbreak could be traced to one particular water company that drew its water from the Thames River, downstream from London, and that another company that drew its water upstream from London was not linked with cholera cases. In both efforts, Snow's ability to collect and analyze data allowed him to determine causation, which, in turn, allowed him to implement corrective actions that prevented additional cases. All of this occurred without benefit of the knowledge that there was an odd-shaped little bacterium that was carried in water and spread from person to person by hand-to-mouth contact!

England's General Board of Health conducted its own investigations of these outbreaks and concluded that air, rather than contaminated water, was the cause.[5] Its approach, however, was one of collecting a vast amount of information and accepting only that which supported its view of disease causation.

Snow, on the other hand, systematically tested his hypothesis by exploring evidence that ran contrary to his initial expectations.

Chadwick was a more official leader of what has become known as the sanitary movement of the latter half of the 19th century. In a variety of official capacities, he played a major part in structuring government's role and responsibilities for protecting the public's health. Because of the growing concern over the social and sanitary conditions in England, a National Vaccination Board was established in 1837. Shortly thereafter, Chadwick's *Report on an Inquiry into the Sanitary Conditions of the Laboring Population of Great Britain* articulated a framework for broad public actions that served as a blueprint for the growing sanitary movement. One result was the establishment in 1848 of a General Board of Health. Interestingly, Chadwick's interest in public health had its roots in Jeremy Bentham's utilitarian movement. For Chadwick, disease was viewed as causing poverty, and poverty was responsible for the great social ills of the time, including societal disorder and high taxation to provide for the general welfare.[6] Public health efforts were necessary to reduce poverty and its wider social effects. This view recognizes a link between poverty and health, although in an opposite direction to current thinking as to the social determinants of health and role of fundamental causes of societal ills. Today, it is more common to consider poor health as a result of poverty, rather than as its cause.

Chadwick was also a key participant in the partly scientific, partly political debate that took place in British government as to whether deaths should be attributed to pathological conditions or to their underlying factors, such as hunger and poverty. It was Chadwick's view that pathologic, as opposed to less proximal social and behavioral, factors should be the basis for classifying deaths.[6] Chadwick's arguments prevailed, although aspects of this debate continue to the present day. William Farr, sometimes called the father of modern vital statistics, championed the opposing view.

OUTSIDE-THE-BOOK THINKING 1-1

© Alfred Bondarenko/Shutterstock.

Access the website of the national honorary society for public health (www.deltaomega.org) and select one of the classic documents available there. Then describe the significance of this classic in the history of public health and its relevance for public health practitioners today.

In the latter half of the 19th century, as sanitation and environmental engineering methods evolved, more effective interventions became available against epidemic diseases. Further, the scientific advances of this period paved the way for modern disease control efforts targeting specific microorganisms.

Growth of Local and State Public Health Activities in the United States

Lemuel Shattuck's *Report of the Sanitary Commission of Massachusetts* in 1850 outlined existing and future public health needs for that state and became America's roadmap for development of a public health system. Shattuck called for the establishment of state and local health departments to organize public efforts aimed at sanitary inspections, communicable disease control, food sanitation, vital statistics, and services for infants and children. Although Shattuck's report closely paralleled Chadwick's efforts in Great Britain, acceptance of his recommendations did not occur for several decades. In the latter part of the century, his farsighted and far-reaching recommendations came to be widely implemented. With greater understanding of the value of environmental controls for water and sewage and of the role of specific control measures for specific diseases (including quarantine, isolation, and vaccination), the creation of local health agencies to carry out these activities supplemented—and, in some cases, supplanted—local boards of health. These local health departments developed rapidly in the seaports and other industrial urban centers, beginning with a health department in Baltimore in 1798, because these were the settings where the problems were reaching unacceptable levels.

Because infectious and environmental hazards are no respecters of local jurisdictional boundaries, states began to develop their own boards and agencies after 1870. These agencies often had very broad powers to protect the health and lives of state residents, although the clear intent at the time was that these powers be used to battle epidemics of infectious diseases. In examining how law impacts governmental public health roles, we will revisit these powers and duties because they serve as both a stimulus and a limitation for what can be done to address many contemporary public health issues and problems.

Federal Public Health Activities in the United States

This sketch of the development of public health in the United States would be incomplete without a brief introduction to the roles and powers of the federal government. Federal health powers, at least as enumerated in the U.S. Constitution, are minimal. It is surprising to some to learn that the word "health" does not even appear in the Constitution. As a result of not being a power explicitly granted to the federal government (such as defense, foreign diplomacy, international and interstate commerce, or printing money), health was a power to be exercised by states or reserved to the people themselves.

Two sections of the Constitution have been interpreted over time to allow for federal roles in health, in concert with the concept of the so-called implied powers necessary to carry out explicit powers. These are the ability to tax in order to provide for the "general welfare" (a phrase appearing in both the preamble and body of the Constitution) and the specific power to regulate commerce, both international and interstate. These provisions allowed the federal government to establish a beachhead in health, initially through the Marine Hospital Service (eventually to become the Public Health Service). After the ratification of the 16th Amendment in 1916, authorizing a national income tax, the federal government acquired the ability to raise substantial sums of money, which could then be directed toward promoting the general welfare. The specific means to this end were a variety of grants-in-aid to state and local governments. Beginning in the 1960s, federal grant-in-aid programs designed to fill gaps in the medical care system nudged state and local governments further and further into the business of medical service provision. Federal grant programs for other social, substance abuse, mental health, and community prevention services soon followed. The expansion of federal involvement into these areas, however, was not accomplished by these means alone.

Prior to 1900, and perhaps not until the Great Depression, Americans did not believe that the federal government should intervene in their social circumstances. Social values shifted dramatically during the Depression, a period of such great social insecurity and need that the federal government was now permitted—indeed, expected—to intercede. Other chapters will expand on the growth of the federal government's influence on public health activities and its impact on the activities of state and local governments.

OUTSIDE-THE-BOOK THINKING 1-2

© Alfred Bondarenko/Shutterstock.

Research the history of public health in your state or locality and then describe how public health strategies and responses have changed over time. What influences were most responsible for these changes? Does this suggest that public health roles and functions have changed over time, as well?

TABLE 1-1 Major Eras in Public Health History in the United States

Prior to 1850	Battling epidemics
1850–1949	Building state and local infrastructure
1950–1999	Filling gaps in medical care delivery
After 1999	Preparing for and responding to community health threats

To explain more easily the broad trends of public health in the United States, it is useful to delineate distinct eras in its history. One simple scheme, outlined in **Table 1-1**, uses the years 1850, 1950, and 2000 as approximate dividers. Prior to 1850, the system was characterized by recurrent epidemics of infectious diseases, with little in the way of collective response possible. During the sanitary movement in the second half of the 19th and first half of the 20th century, science-based control measures were organized and deployed through a public health infrastructure that was developing in the form of local and state health departments. After 1950, gaps in the medical care system and federal grant dollars acted together to increase public provision of a wide range of medical services. That increase set the stage for the current reexamination of the links between medical and public health practice. Some retrenchment from the direct service provision role has occurred since about 1990. As chronicled throughout this text, a new era for public health that seeks to balance community-driven public health practice with preparedness and response for public health emergencies is underway.

IMAGES AND DEFINITIONS OF PUBLIC HEALTH

The historical development of public health activities in the United States provides a case study for understanding what public health is today. Nonetheless, the term public health evokes several different images among the general public and those dedicated to its improvement. To only a relatively small number, the term describes a broad social enterprise or system.

To others, the term describes the professionals and workforce whose job it is to solve certain important health problems. At a meeting in the early 1980s to plan a community-wide education and outreach campaign in order to reduce infant mortality, a community relations director of a large television station made some comments that reflected this view. When asked whether his station had been involved in infant mortality reduction efforts in the past, he responded, "Yes, but that's not our job. If you people in public health had been doing your job properly, we wouldn't be called on to bail you out!" Obviously, this man viewed public health as an effort of which he was not a part.

Still another image of public health is that of a body of knowledge and techniques that can be applied to health-related problems. Here, public health is seen as what public health does. Snow's investigations exemplify this perspective.

Similarly, many people perceive public health primarily as the activities ascribed to governmental public health agencies. For the majority of the public, this latter image represents public health in the United States, resulting in the common view that public health primarily involves the provision of medical care to indigent populations. Since 2001, however, public health has also emerged as a front line defense against bioterrorism and other threats to personal security and safety.

A final image of public health is that of the intended results of these endeavors. In this image, public health is literally the health of the public, as measured in terms of health and illness in a population. The term population health, often defined as health outcomes and their distribution in a population, is increasingly used for this image of public health.[7]

This chapter will focus primarily on the first of these images, public health as a social enterprise or system. It is important to understand what people mean when they speak of public health. As summarized in **Table 1-2**, the profession, the methods, the governmental services, the ultimate outcomes, and even the broad social enterprise itself are all commonly encountered images of what public health is today.

With varying images of what public health is, we would expect no shortage of definitions. There have been many, but three definitions, each separated by a generation, provide especially important insights into what public health is. These are highlighted in **Table 1-3**.

TABLE 1-2   Images of Public Health

- Public health: the system and social enterprise
- Public health: the profession
- Public health: the methods (knowledge and techniques)
- Public health: governmental services (especially medical care for the poor)
- Public health: the health of the public

TABLE 1-3   Selected Definitions of Public Health

- "the science and art of preventing disease, prolonging life, and promoting health and efficiency through organized community effort"[9]
- "Successive re-definings of the unacceptable"[10]
- "fulfilling society's interest in assuring conditions in which people can be healthy"[8]

Data from Institute of Medicine, National Academy of Sciences. *The Future of Public Health*. Washington, DC: National Academy Press: 1988; Winslow CEA. The untilled field of public health. *Mod Med*. 1920; 2:183–191, and Vickers G., What sets the goals of public health? *Lancet*. 1958;1:599–604.

In 1988 the prestigious Institute of Medicine (IOM) provided a useful definition in its landmark study of public health in the United States, *The Future of Public Health*. The IOM report characterized public health's mission as "fulfilling society's interest in assuring conditions in which people can be healthy."[8] This definition directs attention to the many conditions that influence health and wellness, underscoring the broad scope of public health and legitimizing its interest in social, environmental, economic, political, and medical care factors that affect health and illness. The definition's premise that society has an interest in the health of its members implies that improving conditions and health status for others is acting in our own self-interest. The assertion that improving the health status of others provides benefits to all is a core value of public health.

Another core value of public health is reflected in the IOM definition's use of the term *assuring*. Assuring conditions in which people can be healthy means vigilantly promoting and protecting everyone's interests in health and well-being. This value echoes the wisdom in the often-quoted African aphorism that "it takes a village to raise a child." Former Surgeon General David Satcher, the first African American to head this country's most respected federal public health agency, the Centers for Disease Control and Prevention (CDC), once described a visit to Africa in which he met with African teenagers to learn firsthand of their personal health attitudes and behaviors. Satcher was struck by their concerns over the rapid urbanization of the various African nations and the changes that were threatening their culture and sense of community. These young people felt lost and abandoned; they questioned Satcher as to what America and the world community were willing to do to help them survive these changes. As one young man put it, "Where will we find our village?" In many respects, public health serves as everyone's village, whether we are teens in Africa or adults in the United States. The IOM report's characterization of public health advocated for just such a social enterprise and stands as a bold philosophical statement of mission and purpose.

The IOM report also sought to define the boundaries of public health by identifying three core functions of public health: assessment, policy development, and assurance. In one sense, these functions are comparable to those generally ascribed to the medical care system involving diagnosis and treatment. Assessment is the analogue of diagnosis, except that the diagnosis, or problem identification, is made for a group or population of individuals. Similarly, assurance is analogous to treatment and implies that the necessary remedies or interventions are put into place. Finally, policy development is an intermediate role of collectively deciding which remedies or interventions are most appropriate for the problems identified (the formulation of a treatment plan is the medical system's analogue). These core functions broadly describe what public health does— as opposed to what it is.

The concepts embedded in the IOM definition are also reflected in Winslow's definition, developed nearly a century ago. His definition describes both what public health does and how this gets done. It is a comprehensive definition that has stood the test of time in characterizing public health as

> … the science and art of preventing disease, prolonging life, and promoting health and efficiency through organized community effort for the sanitation of the environment, the control of communicable infections, the education of the individual in personal hygiene, the organization of medical and nursing services for the early diagnosis and preventive treatment of disease, and for the development of the social machinery to insure everyone a standard of living adequate for the maintenance of health, so organizing these benefits as to enable every citizen to realize his birthright of health and longevity.[9]

There is much to consider in Winslow's definition. The phrases, "science and art," "organized community effort," and "birthright of health and longevity" capture the substance and aims of public health. Winslow's catalog of methods illuminates the scope of the endeavor, embracing public health's initial targeting of infectious and environmental risks, as well as current activities related to the organization, financing, and accountability of medical care services. His allusion to the "social machinery to insure everyone a standard of living adequate for the maintenance of health" speaks to the relationship between social conditions and health in all societies.

There have been many other attempts to define public health, although these have received less attention than either the Winslow or IOM definitions. Several build on the observation that, over time, public health activities reflect the interaction of disease with two other phenomena that can be roughly characterized as science and social values: (1) what do we know, and (2) what do we choose to do with that knowledge?

A prominent British industrialist, Geoffrey Vickers, provided an interesting addition to this mix more than a half century ago while serving as Secretary of the Medical Research Council. In identifying the forces that set the agenda for public health, Vickers noted, "The landmarks of political, economic, and social history are the moments when some condition passed from the category of the given into the category of the intolerable. I believe that the history of public health might well be written as a record of successive re-definings of the unacceptable."[10]

The essence of Vickers' formulation lies in its focus on social justice and the delicate and shifting interface between science and social values. Through this lens, we can view a tracing of public health over history, facilitating an understanding of why and how different societies have reacted to health risks differently at various points in time and space. In this light, the history of public health is one of harnessing scientific knowledge to shape responses to problems that have crossed the boundary into social unacceptability.

OUTSIDE-THE-BOOK THINKING 1-3

© Alfred Bondarenko/Shutterstock.

Which of the definitions of public health presented in this chapter best describes public health in the 21st century? Why?

Each of these definitions offers important insights into what public health is and what it does. Individually and collectively, they describe a social enterprise and system that is both important and unique, as we will see in the sections that follow.

FIGURE 1-2 Population Health System

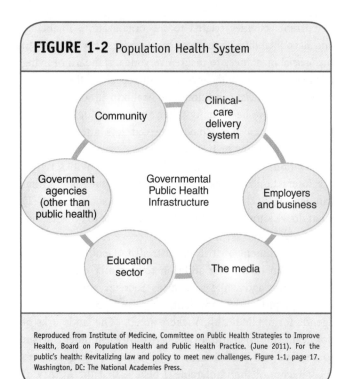

Reproduced from Institute of Medicine, Committee on Public Health Strategies to Improve Health, Board on Population Health and Public Health Practice. (June 2011). For the public's health: Revitalizing law and policy to meet new challenges, Figure 1-1, page 17. Washington, DC: The National Academies Press.

PUBLIC HEALTH AS A SYSTEM

So what is public health? Maybe no single answer will satisfy everyone. There are, in fact, several dimensions of public health that must be considered. Viewing public health as a system of interconnected components, such as the population health system illustrated in **Figure 1-2**, is one approach. Yet, the public health system described in this chapter is more complex than the simple network of participants presented in this figure. The public health described in this chapter is a broad social enterprise, more akin to a movement, that seeks to extend the benefits of current knowledge in ways that will have the maximum impact on the health status of a population. It does so by identifying problems that call for collective action to protect, promote, and improve health, primarily through preventive strategies. This public health is unique in its interdisciplinary approach and methods, its emphasis on preventive strategies, its linkage with government and political decision making, and its dynamic adaptation to new problems placed on its agenda. Above all else, it is a collective effort to identify and address the unacceptable realities that result in preventable and avoidable health and quality of life outcomes, and it is the composite of efforts and activities that are carried out by people and organizations committed to these ends.

With this broad view of public health as a social enterprise, the question shifts from what public health is to what these other images of public health represent and how they relate to each other. Logic models are widely used in modern public health practice to illustrate how the various dimensions of a program relate to each other and achieve their intended results. Basically, logic models indicate what occurs as a result of the preceding step using a basic "if…then" rationale. Programs have structural elements, sometimes referred to as input or capacity, (e.g., workers, information, relationships, facilities, funding, etc.) that are blended to carry out specific activities or processes which then produce certain outputs that lead in turn to various effects or outcomes. The underlying logic for programs is that inputs → processes → outputs → outcomes. Logic models are also useful in characterizing and analyzing more complex entities, including organizations and systems.

Figure 1-3 characterizes the public health system in

OUTSIDE-THE-BOOK THINKING 1-4

© Alfred Bondarenko/Shutterstock.

Develop a map or some other graphic representation of the national public health system. Your map can take any form you choose. Which components or dimensions of the public health system are most important to capture in such a map?

the form of such a logic model, demonstrating the utility of this approach. For example, it is useful to consider inputs as resource investments. The efficiency of a program or system reflects the ratio of outputs to inputs. The effectiveness of a program or system reflects the degree to which intended outcomes are achieved. Equity reflects the degree to which outcomes are distributed fairly or proportionally. Overall satisfaction with results in terms of effectiveness, efficiency and equity) contributes to whether a program or system is valued by its stakeholders which in turn contributes to the level of resources made available. This important feedback loop is apparent in the lower part of this logic model.

This logic model framework integrates the mission and functions of public health in relation to the inputs, processes, outputs, and outcomes of the system. Although descriptions for these system components are offered in **Table 1-4**, it is sometimes easier to appreciate this model when a more familiar industry, such as the automobile industry, is used as an example. The mission or purpose might be expressed as

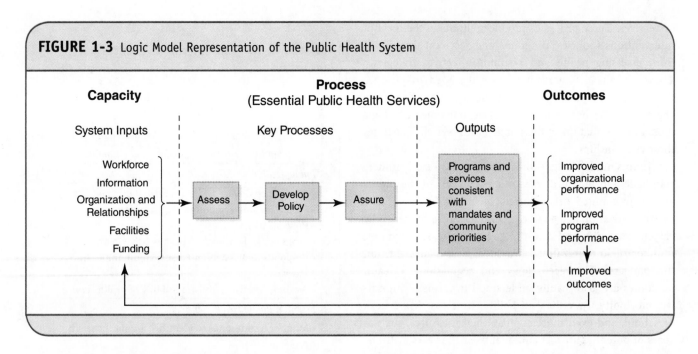

FIGURE 1-3 Logic Model Representation of the Public Health System

meeting the personal transportation needs of the population. This industry carries out its mission by providing appropriate vehicles to its customers; this characterizes its function.

TABLE 1-4 Dimensions of the Public Health System

Capacity (Inputs):
• The resources and relationships necessary to carry out the core functions and essential services of public health (e.g., human resources, information resources, fiscal and physical resources, appropriate relationships among the system components)

Process (Practices and Outputs):
• Those collective practices or processes that are necessary and sufficient to ensure that the core functions and essential services of public health are being carried out effectively, including the key processes that identify and address health problems and their causative factors and the interventions intended to prevent death, disease, and disability, and to promote quality of life

Outcomes (Results):
• Indicators of health status, risk reduction, and quality-of-life enhancement outcomes are long-term objectives that define optimal, measurable future levels of health status; maximum acceptable levels of disease, injury, or dysfunction; or prevalence of risk factors

Data from Centers for Disease Control and Prevention, Public Health Program Office, 1990.

In this light, we can now examine the inputs, processes, outputs, and outcomes of the system set up to carry out this function. Inputs would include steel, rubber, plastic, and so forth, as well as the workers, know-how, technology, facilities, machinery, and support services necessary to allow the raw materials to become cars and trucks. The key processes necessary to carry out the primary function might be characterized as designing vehicles, making or acquiring parts, assembling parts into vehicles, moving vehicles to dealers, and selling and servicing vehicles after purchase. No doubt this is an incomplete listing of this industry's processes; it is oversimplified here to make the point. In any event, these processes translate the abstract concept of getting vehicles to people into the operational steps necessary to carry out this basic function. The outputs of these processes are vehicles located where people can purchase them. The outcomes include satisfied customers and company profits.

Applying this same general framework to the public health system is also possible but may not be so obvious. The mission and functions of public health are well described in the IOM report's framework. The core functions of assessment, policy development, and assurance are somewhat more abstract functions than making vehicles but still can be made operational through descriptions of their key steps or processes.[11,12] The inputs of the public health system include its human, organizational, informational, fiscal, and other resources. These resources and relationships are structured to carry out public health's core functions through a variety of processes that are termed essential public health practices or services. These processes produce outputs in the form of interventions (policies, programs and services) that derive from assessing health and planning effective strategies.[13] These outputs or interventions are designed to produce the desired results, which, with public health, might well be characterized as health or quality-of-life outcomes. The logic model representation of the public health system illustrates these relationships.

In this model, not all components are as readily understandable and measurable as others. Several of the inputs are easily counted or measured, including human, fiscal, and organizational resources. Outputs are also generally easy to recognize and count (e.g., prenatal care programs, number of immunizations provided, health messages on the dangers of tobacco, laws and regulations). Health outcomes are also readily understood in terms of mortality, morbidity, functional disability, time lost from work or school, and even more sophisticated measures, such as years of potential life lost and quality-of-life years lost. The elements that are most difficult to understand and visualize are the processes or essential services of the public health system. Identifying these operational aspects of the public health system allow us to better understand public health practice, measure it, and relate it to its outputs and outcomes. A national work group assembled by the U.S. Public Health Service in 1994 developed a consensus statement of what public health is and does in language understandable to those both inside and outside the field of public health. **Table 1-5** presents the result of that effort, a statement entitled "Public Health in America."[14] The conceptual framework identified in the logic model representation of the public health system and the narrative representation in the "Public Health in America" statement are useful models for understanding the public health system and how it works. **Figure 1-4** demonstrates how the 10 essential public health services operationalize the three core public health functions identified in the 1988 IOM report.

This framework attempts to bridge the gap between what public health is, what it does, and how it does what it does (through its capacity, processes, and outcomes). It also allows us to examine the various components of the system so that we can better appreciate how the pieces fit together.

UNIQUE FEATURES OF PUBLIC HEALTH

Several unique features are apparent in the public health system. These are spotlighted in **Table 1-6** and include the underlying social justice philosophy of public health; its

TABLE 1-5 Public Health in America

Vision:
Healthy People in Healthy Communities
Mission:
Promote Physical and Mental Health and Prevent Disease, Injury, and Disability

Public Health
- Prevents epidemics and the spread of disease
- Protects against environmental hazards
- Prevents injuries
- Promotes and encourages healthy behaviors
- Responds to disasters and assists communities in recovery
- Assures the quality and accessibility of health services

Essential Public Health Services
- Monitor health status to identify community health problems
- Diagnose and investigate health problems and health hazards in the community
- Inform, educate, and empower people about health issues
- Mobilize community partnerships to identify and solve health problems
- Develop policies and plans that support individual and community health efforts
- Enforce laws and regulations that protect health and ensure safety
- Link people with needed personal health services and assure the provision of health care when otherwise unavailable
- Assure a competent public health and personal health care workforce
- Evaluate effectiveness, accessibility, and quality of personal and population-based health services
- Research for new insights and innovative solutions to health problems

Reproduced from Essential Public Health Services Working Group of the Core Public Health Functions Steering Committee, U.S. Public Health Service, 1994.

inherently political nature; its ever-expanding agenda, with new problems and issues being assigned over time; its link with government; its grounding in a broad base of evidence-based biologic, physical, quantitative, social, and behavioral sciences; its focus on prevention as a prime intervention strategy; and the unique bond and sense of mission that links its key stakeholders.

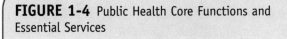

FIGURE 1-4 Public Health Core Functions and Essential Services

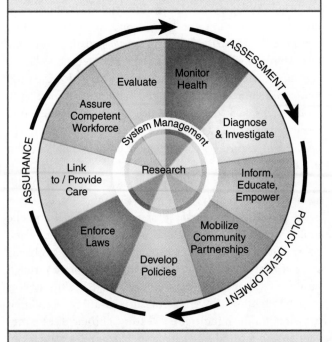

Reproduced from Centers for Disease Control and Prevention, National Public Health Performance Standards. Available at http://www.health.gov/phfunctions/public.htm. Accessed June 17, 2014.

Social Justice Philosophy

It is vital to recognize the social justice orientation of public health and even more critical to understand the potential for conflict and confrontation that it generates. Social justice is the foundation of public health. The concept first emerged around 1848, a time that might be considered the birth of modern public health. Social justice argues that public health is properly a public matter and that its results in terms of death, disease, health, and well-being reflect

TABLE 1-6 Selected Unique Features of Public Health

- Basis in social justice philosophy
- Inherently political nature
- Dynamic, ever-expanding agenda
- Link with government
- Grounding in the sciences
- Use of prevention as a prime strategy
- Uncommon culture and bond

the decisions and actions that a society makes, for good or for ill.[15] Justice is an abstract concept that determines how each member of a society is allocated his or her fair share of collective burdens and benefits. Societal benefits to be distributed may include happiness, income, or social status. Burdens include restrictions of individual action and taxation. Justice dictates that there is fairness in the distribution of benefits and burdens; injustices occur when persons are denied some benefit to which they are entitled or when some burden is imposed unduly. If access to health services, or even health itself, is considered to be a societal benefit (or if poor health is considered to be a burden), the links between the concepts of justice and public health become clear. Market justice and social justice represent two forms of modern justice.

Market justice emphasizes personal responsibility as the basis for distributing burdens and benefits. Other than respecting the basic rights of others, individuals are responsible primarily for their own actions and are free from collective obligations. Individual rights are highly valued, whereas collective responsibilities are minimized. In terms of health, individuals assume primary responsibility for their own health. There is little expectation that society should act to protect or promote the health of its members beyond addressing risks that cannot be controlled through individual action.

Social justice argues that significant factors within the society can impede the fair distribution of benefits and burdens.[16] Examples of such impediments include social class distinctions, heredity, and discrimination on the basis of race, ethnicity, gender, or sexual preference. Collective action, often leading to the assumption of additional burdens, is necessary to neutralize or overcome those impediments. In the case of public health, the goal of extending the potential benefits of the physical and behavioral sciences to all groups in the society, especially when the burden of disease and ill health within that society is unequally distributed, is largely based on principles of social justice. It is clear that many modern public health (and other public policy) problems disproportionately affect some groups, usually a minority of the population, more than others. As a result, their resolution requires collective actions in which those less affected take on greater burdens, while not commensurately benefiting from those actions. When the necessary collective actions are not taken, even the most important public policy problems remain unsolved, despite periodically becoming highly visible.[16] This scenario explains our inadequate responses to such intractable American problems as inadequate housing, poor public education systems, unemployment, racial discrimination, and poverty. However, it is also true for public health problems such as tobacco-related illnesses, infant mortality, substance abuse, mental health services, long-term care, and environmental pollution. The failure to effect comprehensive national health reform in 1994 is an example of this phenomenon. At that time, middle-class Americans deemed the modest price tag of health reform to be excessive, refusing to pay more out of their own pockets when they perceived that their own access and services were not likely to improve. The bitter political conflict accompanying the enactment of national health reform legislation in the form of the Affordable Care Act of 2010 reflected these same themes.

These and similar examples suggest that a critical challenge for public health as a social enterprise lies in overcoming the social and ethical barriers that prevent us from doing more with the knowledge and tools already available to us.[16] Extending the frontiers of science and knowledge may not be as effective for improving public health as shifting the collective values of our society to act on what we already know. Recent public health successes, such as public attitudes toward smoking in both public and private locations and operating motor vehicles after alcohol consumption, provide evidence in support of this assertion. These advances came through changes in social norms, rather than through bigger and better science.

Inherently Political Nature

The social justice underpinnings of public health serve to stimulate political conflict. Public health is both public and political in nature. It serves populations, which are composites of many different communities, cultures, and values. Politics allows for issues to be considered, negotiated, and finally determined within societies. At the core of political processes are differing values and perspectives as to both the ends to be achieved and the means for achieving those ends. Advocating causes and agitating various segments of society to identify and address unacceptable conditions that adversely affect health status often lead to increased expectations and demands on society, generally through government. As a result, public health advocates appear at times as antigovernment and anti-institutional. Governmental public health agencies seeking to serve the interests of both government and public health are frequently caught in the middle. This creates tensions and conflict that can put these public health professionals at odds with governmental leaders on the one hand and external public health advocates on the other.

Expanding Agenda

A third unique feature of public health is its broad and ever-increasing scope. Traditional domains of public health interest include biology, environment, lifestyle, and health service organization. Within each of these domains are many factors that affect health status; in recent decades, many new public policy problems have been moved onto the public health agenda as their predisposing factors have been identified and found to fall into one or more of these domains. A multilevel, multidimensional view of the determinants of population health, often termed a social-ecological model of health, represented in **Figure 1-5**, has emerged to guide public health practice.

The assignment of new problems to the public health agenda is an ever-evolving phenomenon. For example, prior to 1900, the primary problems addressed by public health were infectious diseases and related environmental risks. After 1900, the focus expanded to include problems and needs of children and mothers to be addressed through health education and maternal and child health services as public sentiment over the health and safety of children increased. In the middle of the century, chronic disease prevention and medical care fell into public health's realm as an epidemiologic revolution began to identify causative agents for chronic diseases and links between use of health services and health outcomes. Later, substance abuse, mental illness, teen pregnancy, long-term care, and other issues fell to public health, as did several emerging problems, most notably the epidemics of violence and HIV infections. The public health agenda expanded even further as a result of the recent national dialogue over health reform and how health services will be organized and managed. Bioterrorism preparedness is an even more recent addition to this agenda amidst heightened concerns and expectations after the events of September 11, 2001, and the anthrax attacks the following month.

Link with Government

A fourth unique facet of public health is its link with government. Although public health is far more than the aggregate activities of federal, state, and local health agencies, many people think only of governmental public health agencies when they think of public health. Government does play a unique role in seeing that the key elements are in place and that public health's mission gets addressed. Only government can exercise the enforcement provisions of our public policies that limit the personal and property rights of individuals and corporations in areas such as retail food establishments,

FIGURE 1-5 A Social-Ecological Framework for Thinking about the Determinants of Population Health

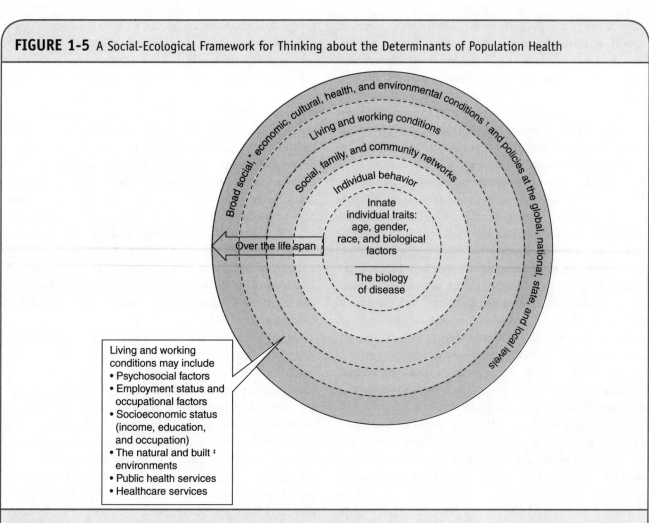

Living and working conditions may include
- Psychosocial factors
- Employment status and occupational factors
- Socioeconomic status (income, education, and occupation)
- The natural and built ‡ environments
- Public health services
- Healthcare services

Notes:
Adapted from Whitehead M and Dahlgren G. What can be done about inequalities in health? *Lancet.* 1991;338(8774):1059–63. The dashed lines between levels of the model denote interaction effects between and among the various levels of health determinants (Worthman, CM. Epidemiology of human development. In *Hormones, Health and Behavior: A Socio-Ecological and Lifespan Perspective.* Panter-Brink C and Worthman CM (eds), 47–104. Cambridge: Cambridge University Press.).
*Social conditions include, but are not limited to, economic inequality, urbanization, mobility, cultural values, attitudes, and policies related to discrimination and intolerance on the basis of race, gender, and other differences.
†Other conditions at the national level might include major sociopolitical shifts, such as recession, war, and governmental collapse.
‡The built environment includes transportation, water and sanitation, housing, and other dimensions of urban planning.
Reproduced from The Committee on Assuring the Health of the Public in the 21st Century, Institute of Medicine. *The Future of the Public's Health in the 21st Century.* Washington, DC: National Academy Press; 2003. Reprinted with permission, copyright 2003, National Academy of Sciences.

sewage and water systems, occupational health and safety, consumer product safety, infectious disease control, and drug efficacy and safety. Government also can play the convener and facilitator role for identifying and prioritizing health problems that might be addressed through public resources and actions. These roles derive from the underlying principle of beneficence, in that government exists to improve the well-being of its members. Beneficence often involves a balance between maximizing benefits and minimizing harms on the one hand and doing no harm on the other.

Two general strategies are available for governmental efforts to influence public health. At the broadest level, governments can modify public policies that influence health through social and environmental conditions, such as policies for education, employment, housing, public safety, child welfare, pollution control, workplace safety, and family support. In line with the IOM report's definition of public health, these actions seek to ensure conditions in which people can be healthy. Another strategy of government is to directly provide programs and services that are designed to meet the health needs of the population. It is often easier to garner support for relatively small-scale programs directed toward a specific problem (such as tuberculosis or HIV infections) than to achieve consensus around broader health and social issues. This strategy is basically a "command-and-control" approach, in which government attempts to increase access to and utilization of services largely through deployment of its own resources rather than through working with others. A variation of this strategy for government is to ensure access to healthcare services through public financing approaches (Medicare and Medicaid are prime examples) or through specialized delivery systems (such as the Veterans Administration facilities, the Indian Health Service, and federally funded community health centers).

Whereas the United States has largely opted for the latter of these strategies, other countries have acted to place greater emphasis on broader social policies. Both the overall level of investment for and relative emphasis between these strategies contribute to the widely varying results achieved in terms of health status indicators among different nations.

Many factors dictate the approaches used by a specific government at any point in time. These factors include history, culture, the structure of the government in question, and current social circumstances. There are also several underlying motivations that support government intervention. For paternalistic reasons, governments may act to control or restrict the liberties of individuals to benefit a group, whether or not that group seeks these benefits. For utilitarian reasons, governments intervene because of the perception that the state as a whole will benefit in some important way. For equality considerations, governments act to ensure that benefits and burdens are equally distributed among individuals. For equity considerations, governments justify interventions in order to distribute the benefits of society in proportion to need. These motivations reflect the views of each society as to whether health itself or merely access to health services is to be considered a right of individuals and populations within that society. Many societies, including the United States, act through government to ensure equal access to a broad array of preventive and treatment services. Equity in health status for all groups within the society may not be an explicit aspiration however, even where efforts are in place to ensure equality in access. Even more important for achieving equity in health status are concerted efforts to improve health status in population groups with the greatest disadvantage, mechanisms to monitor health status and contributing factors across all population groups, and participation of disadvantaged population groups in the key political decision-making processes within the society.[17] To the extent that equity in health status among all population groups does not guide actions of a society's government, these other elements will be only marginally effective.

As noted previously, the link between government and public health makes for a particularly precarious situation for governmental public health agencies. The conflicting value systems of public health and the wider community generally translate into public health agencies having to document their failure in order to make progress. It is said that only the squeaky wheel gets the grease; in public health, it often takes an outbreak, disaster, or other tragedy to demonstrate public health's value. Since 1985, increased funding for basic public health protection programs quickly followed outbreaks related to bacteria-contaminated milk in Illinois, tainted hamburgers in Washington State, and contaminated public water supplies in Milwaukee. Following concerns over preparedness of public health agencies to deal with bioterrorism and other public health threats, a massive infusion of federal funding occurred.

The assumption and delegation of public health responsibilities are quite complex in the United States, with different patterns in each of the 50 states. Over recent decades, the concept of a governmental presence in health has emerged and gained widespread acceptance within the public health community. This concept characterizes the role of local government, often, but not necessarily always, operating through its official health agencies, which serve as the residual guarantors that needed services will actually be there when needed. In practice it means that, no matter how duties are assigned locally, there is a presence that ensures that health needs are identified and considered for collective action. How this concept is operationalized will become apparent in chapters focusing on the role that government plays in carrying out the core functions of public health.

Grounded in Science

One of the most unique aspects of public health—and one that continues to separate public health from many other social movements—is its grounding in science. This relationship is clear for the medical and physical sciences that govern our understanding of the biologic aspects of humans, microorganisms, and vectors, as well as the risks present in our physical environments. However, it is also true for the social sciences of anthropology, sociology, psychology, and economics that affect our understanding of human culture and behaviors influencing health and illness. The quantitative sciences of epidemiology and biostatistics remain essential tools and methods of public health practice. Often five basic sciences of public health are identified: epidemiology, biostatistics, environmental science, management sciences, and behavioral sciences. These constitute the core education of public health professionals.

The importance of a solid and diverse scientific base is both a strength and weakness of public health. Surely there is no substitute for evidence-based science in the modern world. The public remains curiously attracted to scientific advances, at least in the physical and biologic sciences, and this base is important to market and promote public health interventions. For many years, epidemiology has been touted as the basic science of public health practice, suggesting that public health itself is applied epidemiology. Modern public health thinking views epidemiology less as the basic science of public health than as one of many contributors to a complex undertaking. In recent decades, knowledge from the social sciences has greatly enriched and supplemented the physical and biologic sciences. Yet these are areas less familiar to and perhaps less well appreciated by the public, making it difficult to garner public support for newer, more socially and behaviorally mediated public health interventions. The old image of public health based on the hard sciences underlying environmental sanitation and communicable disease control is being superseded by a new image of public health approaches more grounded in what the public perceives to be "softer" science. This transition, at least temporarily, lessens public understanding and confidence in public health and its methods.

Focus on Prevention

If public health professionals were pressed to provide a one-word synonym for public health, the most frequent response would probably be prevention. In general, prevention characterizes actions that are taken to reduce the possibility that something will happen or in hopes of minimizing the damage that may occur if it does happen. Prevention is a widely appreciated and valued concept that is best understood when its object is identified. Although prevention is considered by many to be the purpose of public health, the specific intentions of prevention can vary greatly. Prevention can target deaths, hospital admissions, days lost from school, consumption of human and fiscal resources, and many other ends. There are as many targets for prevention as there are various health outcomes and effects to be avoided.

Prevention efforts often lack a clear constituency because success results in unseen consequences. Because these consequences are unseen, people are less likely to develop an attachment for or support the efforts preventing them. Advocates for such causes as mental health services, care for individuals with developmental disabilities, and organ transplants often make

their presence felt. However, few state capitols have seen candlelight demonstrations by thousands of people who did not get diphtheria. This invisible constituency for prevention is partly a result of the interdisciplinary nature of public health. With no predominant discipline, it is even more difficult for people to understand and appreciate the work of public health. From one perspective, the undervaluation of public health is understandable; the majority of the beneficiaries of recent and current public health prevention efforts have not yet been born! Despite its lack of recognition, prevention as a strategy has been remarkably successful and appears to offer great potential for future success, as well.

Uncommon Culture

The final unique feature of public health to be discussed here appears to be both a strength and weakness. The tie that binds public health professionals is neither a common preparation through education and training nor a common set of work experiences and work settings. Public health is unique in that the common link is a set of intended outcomes toward which many different sciences, arts, and methods can contribute. As a result, public health professionals include anthropologists, sociologists, psychologists, physicians, nurses, nutritionists, lawyers, economists, political scientists, social workers, laboratory workers, managers, sanitarians, engineers, epidemiologists, biostatisticians, gerontologists, disability specialists, and dozens of other professions and disciplines. All are bound to common ends, and all employ somewhat different perspectives from their diverse education, training, and work experiences. "Whatever it takes to get the job done" is the theme, suggesting that the basic task is one of problem solving around health issues. This aspect of public health is the foundation for strategies and methods that rely heavily on collaborations and partnerships.

This multidisciplinary and interdisciplinary approach is unique among professions, calling into question whether public health is really a unified profession at all. An argument can be made that public health is not a profession. There is no minimum credential or training that distinguishes public health professionals from either other professionals or nonprofessionals. Only a tiny proportion of those who work in organizations dedicated to improving the health of the public possess one of the academic public health degrees (the master's of public health degree and several other master's and doctoral degrees granted by schools of public health and other institutions). With the vast majority of public health workers not formally trained in public health, it is difficult to characterize its workforce as a profession.

OUTSIDE-THE-BOOK THINKING 1-5

Which of its unique features distinguish public health from medicine as a profession? Which distinguish it from social work? From law?

Until only recently, public health has lacked key characteristics that distinguish professions from occupations. Significant progress has been made such that public health now meets several of these defining criteria, including: (1) a distinct body of knowledge, (2) an educational credential offered by schools and programs accredited by a specialized accrediting body, (3) career paths that include autonomous practice, and (4) a separate credential, Certified in Public Health (CPH), indicative of self-regulation based on the newly launched examination of the National Board of Public Health Examiners.[18]

Nonetheless, several obstacles will continue to challenge independent professional status, including the viability of the new credential and variability in the content of graduate training programs. The impact of complete professionalization could be considerable in terms of recruitment into the field, autonomy of practice, ultimate strengthening of the public health infrastructure, and impact on public health policy and outcomes.

VALUE OF PUBLIC HEALTH

How can we measure the value of public health efforts? This question is addressed both directly and indirectly throughout this text. Later chapters will examine the dimensions of public health's value in terms of lives saved and diseases prevented, as well as in dollars and cents. Nonetheless, some initial information will set the stage for greater detail later.

Public opinion polls conducted in recent years suggest that public health is already highly valued in the United States.[19] The overwhelming majority of the public rate a variety of key public health services as "very important." Substantially more Americans believe that "public health/protecting populations from disease" is more important than "medicine/treating people who are sick." Public opinion surveys such as these suggest that public health's contributions to health and quality of life have not gone unnoticed. Other assessments of the value of public health support this contention.

In 1965, McKeown concluded, "health has advanced significantly only since the late 18th century and until recently owed little to medical advances."[20] This conclusion is bolstered by more recent studies concluding that public health's prevention efforts are responsible for 25 years of the nearly 30-year improvement in life expectancy at birth in the United States since 1900. This bold claim is based on evidence that only 5 years of the 30-year improvement were the result of medical care.[21] Even for these 5 years, medical treatment accounted for 3.7 years, and clinical preventive services (such as immunizations and screening tests) accounted for 1.5 years. The remaining 25 years have resulted largely from prevention efforts in the form of social policies, community actions, and personal decisions. Many of these decisions and actions targeted infectious diseases affecting infants and children early in the 20th century. The dramatic reduction in deaths due to infectious diseases between 1900 and 1950 is evident in **Figure 1-6**. Later in that century, gains in life expectancy were largely achieved through reductions in chronic diseases affecting adults, including cardiovascular disease as demonstrated in Figure 1-1. A study of life years gained from modern health disease treatments and changes in population risk factors in England and Wales from 1981 to 2000 concluded that 79% of the increase in life years gained was attributed to reductions in major risk factors. Only 21% of the life years gained could be attributed to medical and surgical treatments of coronary heart disease.[22]

The value of public health is further reflected in **Table 1-7,** which identifies ten great public health achievements that occurred during the 20th century. These may appear to be distant and sterile accomplishments, but they tell also tell the story of public health in very human terms. A poignant example dates from the 1950s, when the United States was in the midst of a terrorizing polio epidemic. Few communities were spared during the periodic onslaughts of this serious disease during the first half of the 20th century in America. Public fear was so great that public libraries, community swimming pools, and other group activities were closed during the summers when the disease was most feared. Biomedical research had discovered a possible weapon against epidemic polio in the form of the Salk vaccine, however, which was developed in 1954 and licensed for use one year later. A massive and unprecedented campaign to immunize the public was quickly undertaken, setting the stage for a triumph of public health. The real triumph came in a way that might not have been expected,

FIGURE 1-6 Crude Death Rate (per 100,000) for Infectious Diseases United States, 1900–1996

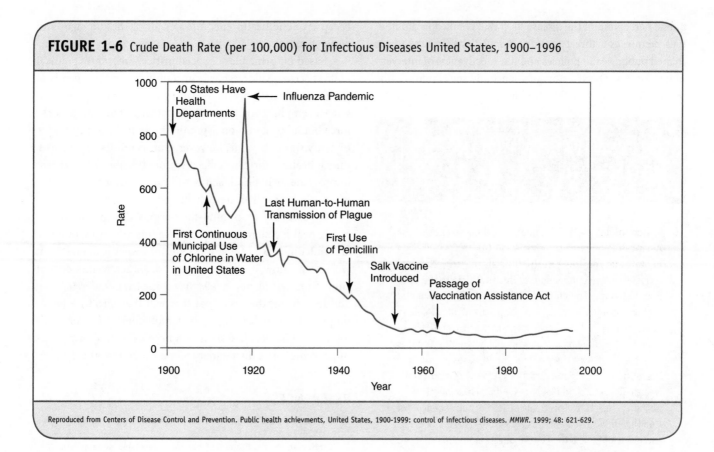

Reproduced from Centers of Disease Control and Prevention. Public health achievments, United States, 1900-1999: control of infectious diseases. *MMWR*. 1999; 48: 621-629.

TABLE 1-7 Ten Great Public Health Achievements—United States, 1900–1999

- Vaccination
- Motor-vehicle safety
- Safer workplaces
- Control of infectious diseases
- Decline in deaths from coronary heart disease and stroke
- Safer and healthier foods
- Healthier mothers and babies
- Family planning
- Fluoridation of drinking water
- Recognition of tobacco use as a health hazard

Data from Centers for Disease Control and Prevention. Ten great public health achievements—United States, 1900–1999. *MMWR*. 1999; 48(12): 241–243.

however, because soon into the campaign, isolated reports of vaccine-induced polio were identified in Chicago and California. Within two days of the initial case reports, action by governmental public health organizations at all levels resulted in the determination that these cases could be traced to one particular manufacturer. This conclusion was reached only a few hours before the same vaccine was to be provided to hundreds of thousands of California children. The result was prevention of a disaster and rescue of the credibility of an immunization campaign that has virtually cut this disease off at its knees. The campaign proceeded on schedule and, five decades later, wild poliovirus has been eradicated from the western hemisphere.

Similar examples have occurred throughout history. The battle against diphtheria is a case in point. A major cause of death in 1900, diphtheria infections are virtually unheard of today. This achievement cannot be traced solely to advances in bacteriology and the antitoxins and immunizations that were deployed against this disease. Neither was this disease defeated by brilliant political and programmatic initiatives led by public health experts. It was the confluence of scientific advances and public perception of the disease itself that resulted in diphtheria's demise as a threat to entire populations.[23] These forces shaped public health policies and the effectiveness of intervention strategies. This is a story of science and social values as the major forces shaping public health.

OUTSIDE-THE-BOOK THINKING 1-6

© Alfred Bondarenko/Shutterstock.

Search for and become familiar with the web sites of the American Public Health Association (APHA), Association of State and Territorial Health Officials (ASTHO), National Association of County and City Health Officials (NACCHO, Public Health Foundation (PHF), U.S. Environmental Protection Agency (EPA), U.S. Department of Homeland Security (DHS), U.S. Department of Health and Human Services (DHHS) and its various Public Health Services Agencies, such as the Centers for Disease Control and Prevention (CDC), Food and Drug Administration (FDA), Health Resources and Services Administration (HRSA), National Institutes of Health (HIH), and Agency for Healthcare Research and Quality (AHRQ). Each site offers useful insights into the central question for this chapter, "What Is Public Health?"

CONCLUSION

Public health evokes different images for different people, and, even to the same people, it can mean different things in different contexts. The intent of this chapter has been to describe some of the common perceptions of public health in the United States. Is it a complex, dynamic, social enterprise, akin to a movement? Or is it best characterized as a goal of the improved health outcomes and health status that can be achieved by the work of all of us, individually and collectively? Or is public health some collection of activities that move us ever closer toward our aspirations? Or is it the profession that includes all of those dedicated to its cause? Or is public health merely what we see coming out of our official governmental health agencies—a strange mix of safety-net medical services for the poor and a variety of often-invisible community prevention services?

Although it is tempting to consider expunging the term public health from our vocabularies because of the baggage associated with these various images, this would do little to address the obstacles to accomplishing our central task,

because public health encompasses all of these images and perhaps more!

Based on principles of social justice, inherently political in its processes, addressing a constantly expanding agenda of problems, inextricably linked with government, grounded in science, emphasizing preventive strategies, and with a workforce bound by common aspirations, public health is unique in many ways. Its value, however, transcends its uniqueness. Public health efforts have been major contributors to recent improvements in health status and can contribute even more in a new century with new challenges.

By carefully examining the various dimensions of the public health system in terms of its inputs, practices, outputs, and outcomes, we can gain insight into what it does, how it works, and how it can be improved. Better results do not come from setting new goals; they come from understanding and improving the processes that will then produce better outputs, in turn leading to better outcomes. Understanding the public health system as a necessary step towards its improvement is a theme that recurs throughout this text.

REFERENCES

1. Winslow CEA. Public health at the crossroads. *Am J Public Health.* 1926; *16*: 1075–1085.
2. Hinman A. Eradication of vaccine-preventable diseases. *Ann Rev Public Health.* 1999; *20*: 211–229.
3. U.S. Public Health Service. *For a Healthy Nation: Returns on Investment in Public Health.* Washington, DC: PHS; 1994.
4. McNeil WH. *Plagues and Peoples.* New York: Doubleday; 1977.
5. Paneth N, Vinten-Johansen P, Brody H. A rivalry of foulness: official and unofficial investigations of the London cholera epidemic of 1854. *Am J Public Health.* 1998; *88*: 1545–1553.
6. Hamlin C. Could you starve to death in England in 1839? The Chadwick-Farr controversy and the loss of the "social" in public health. *Am J Public Health.* 1995; *85*: 856–866.
7. Kindig DA. Understanding population health terminology. *Milbank Q.* 2007; *85*: 139–161.
8. Institute of Medicine, National Academy of Sciences. *The Future of Public Health.* Washington, DC: National Academy Press; 1988.
9. Winslow CEA. The untilled field of public health. *Mod Med.* 1920; *2*: 183–191.
10. Vickers G. What sets the goals of public health? *Lancet.* 1958; *1*: 599–604.
11. Baker EL, Melton RJ, Stange PV, et al. Health reform and the health of the public. *JAMA.* 1994; *272*: 1276–1282.
12. Harrell JA, Baker EL. The essential services of public health. *Leadership Public Health.* 1994; *3*: 27–30.
13. Handler A, Issel LM, Turnock BJ. A conceptual framework to measure performance of the public health system. *Am J Public Health.* 2001; *91*: 1235–1239.
14. Public Health Functions Steering Committee. *Public Health in America.* Washington, DC: U.S. Public Health Service; 1995.
15. Krieger N, Brin AE. A vision of social justice as the foundation of public health: commemorating 150 years of the spirit of 1848. *Am J Public Health.* 1998; *88*: 1603–1606.

16. Beauchamp DE. Public health as social justice. *Inquiry.* 1976; *13*: 3–14.

17. Susser M. Health as a human right: an epidemiologist's perspective on public health. *Am J Public Health.* 1993; *83*: 418–426.

18. Evashwick CJ, Begun JW, Finnegan JR. Public health as a distinct profession: has it arrived? *J Public Health Management Practice.* 2013; *19*(5): 412–419.

19. Harris Polls. Public Opinion about Public Health, United States. 1999.

20. McKeown T. *Medicine in Modern Society.* London, England: Allen & Unwin; 1965.

21. Bunker JP, Frazier HS, Mosteller F. Improving health: measuring effects of medical care. *Milbank Q.* 1994; *72*: 225–258.

22. Unal B, Critchley JA, Fidan D, Capewell S. Life-years gained from modern cardiological treatments and population risk factor changes in England and Wales, 1981–2000. *Am J Public Health.* 2005; *95*: 103–108.

23. Hammonds EM. *Childhood's Deadly Scourge: The Campaign to Control Diphtheria in New York City, 1880–1930.* Baltimore, MD: Johns Hopkins University Press; 1999.

CHAPTER **2**

Measuring Population Health

LEARNING OBJECTIVES

Given an ecological perspective of the varied influences on the health status of populations, incorporate appropriate measures of health and illness (including risk factors) into a population or community health needs assessment activity. Key aspects of this competency expectation include being able to

- Articulate a definition of health consistent with that of the World Health Organization
- Identify four or more categories of factors that influence health
- For each of these categories, specify three or more specific factors that influence health
- Identify several categories of commonly used measures of health status
- For each of these categories, identify three or more commonly used measures
- Describe major trends in health status for the United States over the past 100 years
- Access and utilize comprehensive and current national data on health status and factors influencing health in the United States
- Utilize information on factors that influence health and measures of health to develop community health priorities and effective interventions for improving community health status

The 21st century began much as its predecessor did, with immense opportunities to advance the health of the public through actions that ensure conditions favorable for health and quality of life. All systems direct their efforts toward certain outcomes; they track progress by ensuring that these outcomes are clearly defined and measurable. In public health, this calls for clear definitions and measures of health and quality of life in populations. That task is the focus of this chapter. Key questions to be addressed are:

- What is health?
- What factors influence health and illness?
- How can health status and quality of life be measured?
- What do current measures tell us about the health status and quality of life of Americans in the early decades of the 21st century?
- How can this information be used to assess population and community health status and develop effective public health interventions and public policy?

The relevance of these questions resides in their focus on factors that cause or influence particular health outcomes. Efforts to identify and measure key aspects of health and factors influencing health have relied largely on traditional approaches over the past century, although there are signs that this pattern may be changing. The key questions identified above will be addressed slightly out of order, for reasons that should become apparent as this chapter unfolds.

HEALTH IN THE UNITED STATES

Many important indicators of health status in the United States have improved considerably over the past century, although there is evidence that health status could be even better than it is. At the turn of the 20th century, nearly 2% of the U.S. population died each year. The crude mortality rate in 1900 was about 1,700 deaths per 100,000 population. Life expectancy at birth was 47 years. Additional life expectancy at age 65 was another 12 years. Medicine and health care were largely proprietary in 1900 and of questionable benefit to health. More extensive information on the health status of the population at that time would be useful, but very little exists.

Indicators of health status improved in the United States throughout the 20th century.[1] Between the years 1900 and 2000, the crude mortality rate was cut in half to 872 per 100,000. By the year 2000, life expectancy at birth was nearly 77 years and life expectancy at age 65 was another 18 years.

The leading causes of death also changed dramatically over the 20th century, as demonstrated in **Figure 2-1** depicting causes of death in 1900 and 2000. In 1900, the 10 leading causes of death were influenza and pneumonia, tuberculosis, diarrhea and related diseases, heart disease, stroke, chronic nephritis, accidents, cancer, perinatal conditions, and diphtheria. By the year 2000, tuberculosis, gastroenteritis, and diphtheria dropped off the list of the top 10 killers, and deaths from influenza and pneumonia fell from first to seventh position on the list. Diseases of aging and other chronic conditions superseded these infectious disease processes as changes in the age structure of the population, especially the increase in persons over age 65, resulted in higher overall crude rates for heart disease and cancer and the appearance of diabetes, Alzheimer's disease, chronic kidney conditions, and septicemia on the modern list of the top 10 killers.

Changes in crude death rates substantially understate the gains in life expectancy realized for all age groups over the 20th century. On an age-adjusted basis, improvements were even more impressive. Age-adjusted mortality rates fell about 75% between 1900 and 2000, with infant and child mortality rates 95% lower, adolescent and young adult mortality rates 80% lower, rates for 25–64 year-old adults lower by 60%, and rates for adults older than age 65 falling 35%.

These gains were not solely the result of better prevention and control of infectious diseases and advances in antibiotics and vaccinations in the first half of the century. During the second half of the 20th century, overall age-adjusted mortality rates fell about 50%, while infant mortality rates declined more than 75%. During that period, mortality rates among children and young adults (ages 1–24 years) and adults 45–64 years were reduced by more than one-half. Mortality rates among adults 25–44 years fell more than 40%, and rates for elderly persons (age 65 and older) fell about one-third. **Figure 2-2** demonstrates that age-adjusted mortality rates continued to fall faster than overall crude mortality rates through the first decade of the 21st century.

Gains for adult age groups in recent decades have outstripped those for younger age groups, a trend that began about 1960 as progress accelerated toward reduction of mortality from injuries and certain major chronic diseases that largely affected adults. Over the second half of the 20th century, dramatic reductions in the death rates for heart disease, stroke, unintentional injuries, influenza and pneumonia, and infant mortality have been joined by more recent reductions in rates for human immunodeficiency virus (HIV) infections, liver diseases, and suicide. On the other hand, death rates have increased for diabetes, Alzheimer's disease, and chronic lung and kidney conditions, signaling the new morbidities associated with longer life spans. Homicide rates have improved somewhat over the past decade but still reflect a substantial increase since 1950.[1]

Despite this progress, considerable disparities persist for many of the major causes of death. Differences among races are notable, but there are also significant differences by gender for the various causes of death. These differences are often dramatic and run from top to bottom through the chain of causation. Disparities are found not only in indicators of poor health outcomes, such as mortality, but also in the levels of risk factors in the population groups most severely affected. A sobering example of these disparities is reflected in the 12-year difference in life expectancy between white females and black males.

OUTSIDE-THE-BOOK THINKING 2-1

© Alfred Bondarenko/Shutterstock.

Examine each of these Web sites. Which ones are most useful for the major topics examined in this chapter? Why?

- Healthfinder (www.healthfinder.gov), a Department of Health and Human Services (DHHS)-sponsored gateway site that provides links to more than 550 Web sites (including more than 200 federal sites and 350 state, local, not-for-profit, university, and other consumer health sources), nearly 500 selected online documents, frequently asked questions on health issues, and databases and Web search engines by topic and agency
- Fedstats (fedstats.sites.usa.gov/), a gateway to a variety of federal agency data and information, including health statistics
- National Center for Health Statistics (NCHS) (www.cdc.gov/nchs/index.htm), an invaluable resource for data and information, especially "Health, United States," which can be downloaded from this site
- Centers for Disease Control and Prevention (CDC) Mortality and Morbidity Weekly Report (www.cdc.gov/mmwr/) and MMWR morbidity and mortality data by time and place (www.cdc.gov/mmwr/distrnds.html)
- U.S. Census data (www.census.gov), the best general denominator data anywhere

FIGURE 2-1 The 10 Leading Causes of Death as a Percentage of All Deaths in the United States, 1990 and 2000

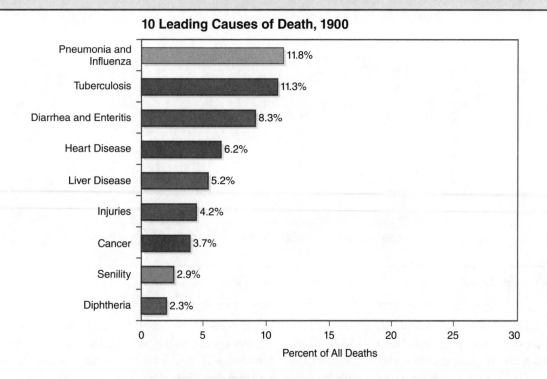

10 Leading Causes of Death, 1900

Cause	Percent
Pneumonia and Influenza	11.8%
Tuberculosis	11.3%
Diarrhea and Enteritis	8.3%
Heart Disease	6.2%
Liver Disease	5.2%
Injuries	4.2%
Cancer	3.7%
Senility	2.9%
Diphtheria	2.3%

Percent of All Deaths

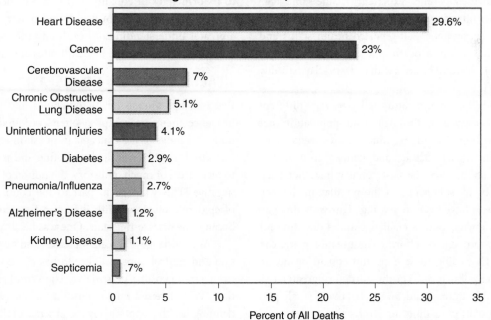

10 Leading Causes of Death, 2000

Cause	Percent
Heart Disease	29.6%
Cancer	23%
Cerebrovascular Disease	7%
Chronic Obstructive Lung Disease	5.1%
Unintentional Injuries	4.1%
Diabetes	2.9%
Pneumonia/Influenza	2.7%
Alzheimer's Disease	1.2%
Kidney Disease	1.1%
Septicemia	.7%

Percent of All Deaths

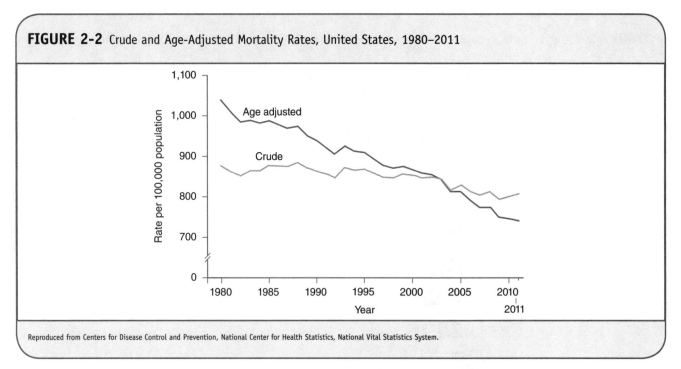

FIGURE 2-2 Crude and Age-Adjusted Mortality Rates, United States, 1980–2011

Reproduced from Centers for Disease Control and Prevention, National Center for Health Statistics, National Vital Statistics System.

There is also evidence that disability levels are declining in the general population over time. Disability levels among individuals aged 55–70 years who were offspring of the famous Framingham Heart Study cohort were substantially lower, in comparison with their parents' experience at the same age.[2] In addition, fewer offspring had chronic diseases or perceived their health as fair or poor. Self-reported health status and activity limitations because of chronic conditions changed little during the 1990s, and injuries with lost workdays steadily declined during the 1990s.

In sum, U.S. health indicators tell two very different tales. By many measures, the American population has never been healthier. By others, much more needs to be done for specific racial, ethnic, and gender groups. The gains in health status over the past century have not been shared equally by all subgroups of the population. In fact, relative differences have been increasing. This widening gap in health status creates both a challenge and a dilemma for future health improvement efforts. The greatest gains can be made through closing these gaps and equalizing health status within the population. Yet the burden of greater risk and poorer health status resides in a relatively small part of the total population, calling for efforts that target those minorities with increased resources. An alternative approach is to continue current strategies and resource deployment levels in order to sustain steady overall improvement among all groups in the population. This strategy, however, is likely to continue or worsen existing gaps. In the early years of the

new century, the major health challenge facing the United States appears to be less related to the need to improve population-wide health outcomes than the need to eliminate or reduce disparities. This challenges the nation's commitment to its principles of equality and social justice as addressing inequities in measures of health and quality of life requires a greater understanding of health and the measures used to describe it than afforded by death rates and life expectancies.

HEALTH, ILLNESS, AND DISEASE

Relationships among health outcomes and the factors that influence them are complex, often confounded by different understandings of the concepts in question and how they are measured. Health is difficult to define and more difficult yet to measure. For much of history, the notion of health has been negative. This was due in part to the continuous onslaught of epidemic diseases. With disease a frequent visitor, health became the disease-free state. One was healthy by exclusion.

As knowledge of disease increased and methods of prevention and control improved, health has come to be considered from a more positive perspective. The World Health Organization (WHO) seized this opportunity in its 1946 constitution, defining health as not merely the absence of disease but a state of complete physical, mental, and social well-being.[3] This definition of health emphasizes that there are different, complexly related forms of wellness and illness, and suggests that a wide range of factors can influence the health of individuals and groups. It also suggests that health is not an absolute concept.

Although health and well-being may be synonyms, health and disease are not necessarily opposites. Most people view health and illness as existing along a continuum and as opposite and mutually exclusive states. However, this simplistic, one-dimensional model of health and illness does not comport very well with the real world. A person can have a condition or injury and still be healthy and feel well. There are many examples, but certainly Olympic wheelchair racers would fit into this category. It is also possible for someone without a specific disease or injury to feel ill or not well. If health and illness are not mutually exclusive, then they exist in separate dimensions, with wellness and illness in one dimension and the presence or absence of disease or injury in another.

These distinctions are important because disease is a relatively objective, pathologic phenomenon, whereas wellness and illness represent subjective experiences. This allows for several different states to exist: wellness without disease or injury, wellness with disease or injury, illness with disease or injury, and illness without physical disease or injury. This multidimensional view of health states is consistent with the WHO delineation of physical, mental, and social dimensions of health or well-being. Health or wellness is more than the absence of disease alone. Furthermore, one can be physically but not mentally and socially well.

With health measurable in several different dimensions, the question arises as to whether there is some maximum or optimal end point of health or well-being or whether health is something that can always be improved through changes in its physical, mental, and social facets. This suggests that the goal should be a minimal acceptable level of health, rather than a state of complete and absolute health. Due in part to these considerations, WHO revised its definition in 1978, calling for a level of health that permits people to lead socially and economically productive lives.[4] This shifts the focus of health from an end in itself to a resource for everyday life, linking physical to personal and social capacities. It also suggests that it will be easier to identify measures of illness than of health.

Disease and injury are often viewed as phenomena that may lead to significant loss or disability in social functioning, making one unable to carry out one's main personal or social functions in life, such as parenting, schooling, or employment. In this perspective, health is equivalent to the absence of disability; individuals able to carry out their basic functions in life are healthy. This characterization of health as the absence of significant functional disabilities is perhaps the most common one for this highly sought state. Still, this definition is a negative one in that it defines health as the absence of disability.

The concept of well-being advanced in the WHO definition goes beyond the physical aspects of health that are the usual focus of measurements and comparisons. Including the mental and social aspects of well-being or health legitimizes the examination of factors that affect mental and social health. Together, these themes underscore the need to consider carefully what is being measured in order to understand what these measures tell us about health, illness, and disease states in a population and the factors that influence these outcomes.

MEASURING HEALTH

The plethora of information on health outcomes suggests that measuring the health status of populations is a simple task. However, although often interesting and sometimes even dramatic, the commonly used measures of health status fail to paint a complete picture of health. Many of the reasons are obvious. The commonly used measures actually reflect disease and mortality, rather than health itself. The long-standing misperception that health is the absence of disease is reinforced by the relative ease of measuring disease states, in comparison with states of health. Actually, the most commonly used indicators focus on a state that is neither health nor disease—namely, death.

Despite the many problems with using mortality as a proxy for health, mortality data are generally available and widely used to describe the health status of populations. This is ironic because such data only indirectly describe the health status of living populations. Unfortunately, data on morbidity (illnesses, injuries, and functional limitations of the population) are neither as available nor as readily understood as are mortality data. This situation is improving, however, as new forms and sources of information on health conditions become more readily available. Sources for information on morbidities and disabilities now include medical records from hospitals, managed care organizations, and other providers, as well as information derived from surveys, businesses, schools, and other sources. Assessments of the health status of populations are increasingly utilizing measures from these sources. An excellent compilation of data and information on both health status and health services, *Health United States*, is published annually by the National Center for Health Statistics.[1] Much of the data used in this chapter is derived from this source.

Mortality-Based Measures

Although mortality-based indicators of health status are both widely used and useful, there are some important differences in their use and interpretation. The most commonly used are crude mortality, age-specific and age-adjusted mortality, life expectancy, and years of potential life lost (YPLL). Although all are based on the same events, each provides somewhat different information as to the health status of a population.

Crude mortality rates count deaths within the entire population and are not sensitive to differences in the age distribution of different populations. The mortality comparisons presented in Figure 2-2 comparing crude and age-adjusted death rates illustrate the limitations of using crude death rates to assess the mortality experience of the U.S. population. On the basis of these data, we might conclude that mortality rates in the United States had declined about 10% since 1980. However, because there has been an increasing proportion of population in the higher age categories over recent decades, these are not truly comparable populations. The 10% reduction actually understates the differences in mortality experience over this 30-year period after changes in the age structure of the population are controlled. The 10% reduction then becomes a 30% reduction! Because differences in the age characteristics of the two populations are a primary concern, we look for methods to correct or adjust for the age factor. Age-specific and age-adjusted rates do just that. The second half of the 20th century witnessed decreases of 50% or more for age-adjusted mortality rates for stroke, heart disease, infant deaths, tuberculosis, influenza and pneumonia, syphilis, unintentional injuries, HIV infections, and gastric, uterine and cervical cancers.[1] Improvements in age-adjusted mortality rates for the leading causes of death are continuing in the early years of the new century.[1]

Age-specific mortality rates relate the number of deaths to the number of persons in a specific age group. The infant mortality rate is probably the best-known example, describing the number of deaths of live-born infants occurring in the first year of life per 1,000 live births. Public health studies often use age-adjusted mortality rates to compensate for different mixes of age groups within a population (e.g., a high proportion of children or elderly). Age-adjusted rates are calculated by applying age-specific rates to a standard population (we now use the 2000 U.S. population). This adjustment permits more meaningful comparisons of mortality experience between populations with different age distribution patterns. Differences between crude and age-adjusted mortality rates can be substantial.

Life expectancy, also based on the mortality experience of a population, is a computation of the number of years between any given age (e.g., birth or age 65) and the average age of death for that population. **Figure 2-3** presents recent data and trends for life expectancy at birth in the United States; **Figure 2-4** provides international comparisons for life expectancy. Together with infant mortality rates, life expectancies are commonly used in comparisons of health status among nations. These two mortality-based indicators are often considered to be general indicators of the overall health status of a population. Infant mortality and life expectancy

---

FIGURE 2-3 Life Expectancy at Birth by Race and Gender, United States, 1980–2010

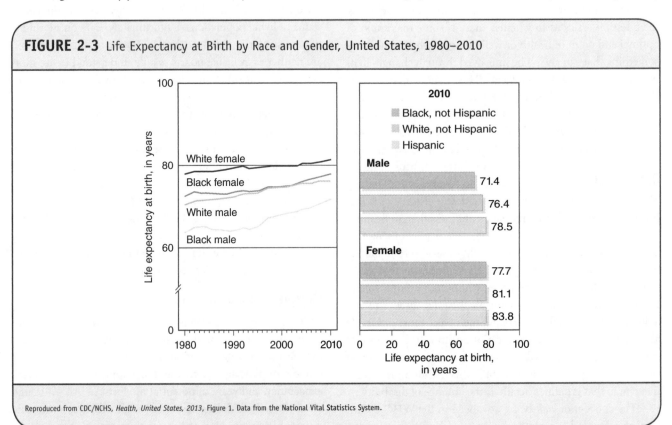

Reproduced from CDC/NCHS, *Health, United States, 2013*, Figure 1. Data from the National Vital Statistics System.

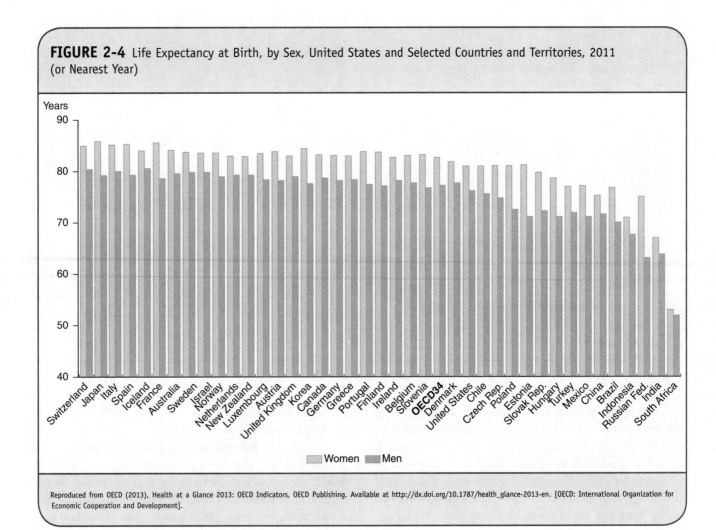

FIGURE 2-4 Life Expectancy at Birth, by Sex, United States and Selected Countries and Territories, 2011 (or Nearest Year)

measures for the United States are lackluster in comparison with those of other developed nations. The figure presenting international comparisons of life expectancy at birth by gender suggests that the United States is far from being the healthiest nation in the world.

YPLL is a mortality-based indicator that places greater weight on deaths that occur at younger ages. Years of life lost before some arbitrary age (often age 65 or 75) are computed and used to measure the relative impact on society of different causes of death. If age 65 is used as the threshold for calculating YPLL, an infant death would contribute 65 YPLL, and a homicide at age 25 would contribute 40 YPLL. A death due to stroke at age 70 would contribute no years of life lost before age 65, and so on. Until relatively recently, age 65 was widely used as the threshold age. With life expectancies now exceeding 75 years at birth, YPLL calculations using age 75 as the threshold have become more common. Data on YPLL before age 75 is presented in **Table 2-1**, illustrating the usefulness of this approach in providing a somewhat different perspective

as to which problems are most important in terms of their magnitude and impact. The use of YPLL ranks cancer, HIV infections, and various forms of injury-related deaths higher than does the use of crude numbers or rates. Conversely, the use of crude rates ranks heart disease, stroke, pneumonia, diabetes, and chronic lung and liver diseases higher than does the use of YPLL. Four of the top 10 causes of death, as determined by the number of deaths, do not appear in the list of the top 10 causes of YPLL. Each of these various mortality indicators can be examined for various racial and ethnic subpopulations to identify disparities among these groups.

Morbidity, Disability, and Quality Measures

Mortality indicators can also be combined with other health indicators that describe quality considerations to provide a measure of the span of healthy life. These indicators can be an especially meaningful measure of health status in a population because they also consider morbidity and

TABLE 2-1   Age-Adjusted Years of Potential Life Lost (YPLL) before Age 75 by Cause of Death and Ranks for YPLL and Number of Deaths, United States, 2000

Causes of Death	YPLL	Rank by YPLL	Rank by Number of Deaths
Cancer	1,698,500	1	2
Heart disease	1,270,700	2	1
Unintentional injuries	1,052,500	3	5
Suicide	343,300	4	11
Homicide	274,200	5	14
Cerebrovascular diseases	226,500	6	3
Chronic obstructive lung disease	190,700	7	4
Diabetes mellitus	181,200	8	6
HIV infections	178,900	9	18
Chronic liver disease and cirrhosis	141,700	10	12

Note: Years lost before age 75 per 100,000 population younger than 75 years of age.

Reproduced from National Center for Health Statistics. *Health, United States*, 2002. Hyattsville, MD: NCHS; 2002.

disability from conditions that impact on functioning but do not cause death (e.g., cerebral palsy, schizophrenia, arthritis). A commonly used measure of aggregate disease burden is the disability-adjusted life-year or DALY. Other variants on this theme are span-of-healthy-life indicators (called years of healthy life) that combine mortality data with self-reported health status and activity limitation data acquired through the National Health Interview Survey. Depending on the healthy life expectancy measure, Americans average about 10 years of poor health, 15 years of activity limitation, and 30 years of living with a chronic disease. Women have better health status than men, and whites do better than blacks on virtually all of these measures. For healthy life expectancies at age 65, a similar picture appears. The implication is that extending healthy life expectancy can be achieved through several pathways. One would be to extend life expectancy without increasing the measures of poor health, activity limitation, and chronic disease burden. Another would be to reduce the measures of poor health, activity limitation, and chronic disease burden within a constant life expectancy. The optimal approach would accomplish both by extending life expectancy and reducing the burden of poor health, activity limitation, and chronic disease.

Although less frequently encountered, indicators of morbidity and disability are also quite useful in measuring health status. Both prevalence (the number or rate of cases at a specific point or period in time) and incidence (the number

or rate of new cases occurring during a specific period) are widely used measures of morbidity.

Increasingly, information on self-reported health status and on days lost from work or school because of acute or chronic conditions is collected through surveys of the general population. The National Center for Health Statistics also conducts ongoing surveys of health providers on complaints and conditions requiring medical care in outpatient settings. These surveys provide direct information on self-reported health status and illuminate some of the factors, such as household income levels, that are associated with health status.

INFLUENCES ON HEALTH

In 1996, public health surveillance in the United States took a historic step. At that time, the Centers for Disease Control and Prevention (CDC) added prevalence of cigarette smoking to the list of diseases and conditions to be reported by states to CDC.[5] This action marked the first time that a health behavior, rather than an illness or disease, was considered nationally reportable—a groundbreaking step for surveillance efforts. How the focus of public health efforts shifted from conventional disease outcomes to reporting on underlying causes amenable to public health intervention is an important story.

Risk Factors

The recognition of tobacco use as a major health hazard was no simple achievement, partly because many factors directly or indirectly influence the level of a health outcome in a given population. For example, greater per capita tobacco use in a population is associated with higher rates of heart disease and lung cancer, and lower rates of early prenatal care are associated with higher infant mortality rates. Because these factors are part of the chain of causation for health outcomes, tracking their levels provides an early indication as to the direction in which the health outcome is likely to change. These factors increase the likelihood or risk of particular health outcomes occurring and can be characterized broadly as risk factors.

The types and number of risk factors are as varied as the influences themselves. Depending on how these factors are lumped or split, traditional categories include biologic factors (from genetic endowment to aging), environmental factors (from food, air, and water to communicable diseases), lifestyle factors (from diet to injury avoidance and sexual behaviors), psychosocial factors (from poverty to stress, personality, and cultural factors), and use of and access to health-related services. Refinements of this framework are

reflected in **Figure 2-5**, which differentiates several outcomes of interest, including disease, functional capacity, prosperity, and well-being that can be influenced by various risk factors. These various components are often interrelated (e.g., stress, a social environmental factor, may stimulate individual responses, such as tobacco or illicit drug use, which, in turn, influence the likelihood of disease, functional capacity, and well-being). In addition, variations in one outcome, such as disease, may influence changes in others, such as well-being, depending on the mix of other factors present. This complex set of interactions, consistent with the social-ecological model, draws attention to fundamental factors or causes that can result in many diseases, rather than focusing on specific factors that contribute little to population-wide health status.

Although many factors are causally related to health outcomes, some are more direct and proximal causes than others. Specific risk factors have been clearly linked to specific adverse health states through epidemiologic studies. For example, numerous studies have linked unintentional

FIGURE 2-5 Determinants of Health

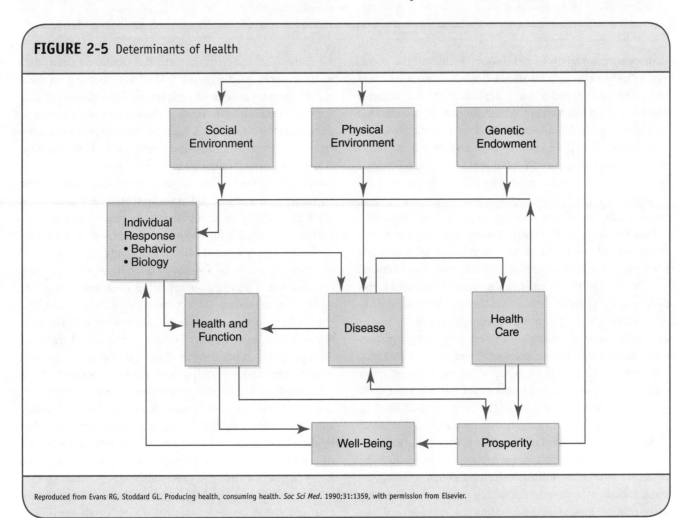

Reproduced from Evans RG, Stoddard GL. Producing health, consuming health. *Soc Sci Med.* 1990;31:1359, with permission from Elsevier.

TABLE 2-2   Selected Behavioral Risk Factors Related to Leading Causes of Deaths in the United States, 2000

Cause of Death and Percent of all Deaths	Smoking	High Fat/ Low Fiber	Sedentary Lifestyle	High Blood Pressure	Elevated Cholesterol	Obesity	Alcohol Use
Heart disease (30%)	X	X	X	X	X	X	X
Cancer (23%)	X	X	X			X	X
Stroke (7%)	X	X		X	X	X	
Chronic lung disease (5%)	X						
Unintentional injuries (4%)	X						X
Pneumonia & influenza (3%)	X						
Diabetes (3%)		X	X			X	
HIV infection (1%)							
Suicide (1%)							X
Chronic liver disease (1%)							X
Atherosclerosis (1%)	X	X	X		X		

Data for causes and percent deaths from National Center for Health Statistics. *Health United States 2002*. Hyattsville, MD: NCHS; 2002. Risk factors related to causes from Brownson RC, Remington PL, Davis JR, et al. *Chronic Disease Epidemiology and Control*. 2nd ed. Washington, DC; American Public Health Association; 1998 and U.S. Public Health Service. *The Surgeon General's Report on Nutrition and Health*. Washington, DC: PHS; 1988.

injuries with a variety of risk factors, including the accessibility to firearms and the use of alcohol, tobacco, and seat belts. Tobacco, hypertension, over-nutrition, and diabetes are well-known risk factors for heart disease. As documented in **Table 2-2**, epidemiologic research and studies over the past 50 years have linked numerous behavioral risk factors to many common diseases and conditions.[6] Ongoing behavioral risk factor surveys (often through telephone interviews) are conducted by governmental public health agencies to track trends in the prevalence of many important risk behaviors within the population. These surveys document that the health-related behaviors of tens of millions of Americans place them at risk for developing chronic disease and injuries.

Despite the recent emphasis on behavioral factors, risk factors in the physical environment remain important influences on health. Air pollution, for example, is directly related to a wide range of diseases, including lung cancer, pulmonary emphysema, chronic bronchitis, and bronchial asthma. National standards exist for many of the most important air pollutants and are tracked to determine the extent of these risks in the general population. The proportion of the U.S. population residing in counties that have exceeded national standards for these pollutants suggests that air pollution risks, like behavioral risks, affect tens of millions of Americans.[7] The physical environment influences health through several pathways, including facilitating risk-taking behaviors, influencing social relationships, and even exposing residents to visual cues that can arouse fear, anxiety, and depression.

Behavioral and environmental risk factors are clearly germane to public health interest and efforts. Focusing on these factors provides a different perspective of the enemies of personal and public health than that conveyed by disease-specific incidence or mortality data. Such a focus also promotes more rational policy development and interventions. Unfortunately, determining which underlying factors are most important is more difficult than it appears because of differences in the outcomes under study and measures used. For example, a study using 1980 data found tobacco, hypertension, and over-nutrition responsible for about three-fourths of deaths before age 65 and injury risks, alcohol, tobacco, and gaps in primary prevention accounting for about three-fourths of all YPLL before age 65.[8] Further complicating these analyses is the finding that individual risk factors may result in several different health outcomes. For example, alcohol use is linked with motor vehicle injuries, other injuries, cancer, and cirrhosis; tobacco use can result in heart disease, stroke, ulcers, fire and burn injuries, and low birth weight, as well as cancer.[6,8]

Despite problems with their measurement, the identification of antecedent causes is important for public health policy and interventions. **Table 2-3** compares deaths in the year 2000 by their listed causes of death and their actual causes (major risk factors).[9] The two lists provide contrasting views as to the major health problems and needs of the U.S. population.

Coroners and medical examiners report immediate and underlying causes of death through death certificates which have two parts, one for entering the immediate and

TABLE 2-3 Listed and Actual Causes of Death, United States, 2000

10 Leading Causes of Death	Number	Actual Causes of Death	Number
Heart disease	710,760	Tobacco	435,000
Malignant neoplasm	553,091	Poor diet and physical inactivity	400,000
Cerebrovascular disease	167,661	Alcohol consumption	85,000
Chronic lower respiratory tract diseases	122,009	Microbial agents	75,000
Unintentional injuries	97,900	Toxic agents	55,000
Diabetes mellitus	69,301	Motor vehicle	43,000
Influenza and pneumonia	65,313	Firearms	29,000
Alzheimer's disease	49,558	Sexual behavior	20,000
Nephritis, nephrotic syndrome, and nephrosis	37,251	Illicit drug use	17,000
Septicemia	31,224	**Total**	**1,159,000**
Other	499,283		
Total	**2,403,351**		

Data from Mokdad AM, Marks JS, Stoup DF, Gerberding JL. Actual causes of death in the United States, 2000. *JAMA*. 2004; 291: 1238–1245.

underlying conditions that caused the death and a second for identifying conditions or injuries that contributed to death but did not cause death. For example, a death attributed to cardiovascular disease might list cardiac tamponade as the immediate cause, due to or as a consequence of a ruptured myocardial infarction, which itself was due to or a consequence of coronary arteriosclerosis. For this death, hypertensive cardiovascular disease might be listed as a significant condition contributing to, but not causing, the immediate

OUTSIDE-THE-BOOK THINKING 2-2

© Alfred Bondarenko/Shutterstock.

Visit the Internet web site of several national print media and use the search features to identify articles on public health for a recent month. Catalog the health problems (both conditions and risks) from that search and compare this with the listing of health problems and issues on Table 2-3. Are the types of conditions and risks you encountered in the print media similar? Were some conditions and risks either overrepresented or underrepresented in the media, in comparison with their relative importance as suggested by Table 2-3? What are the implications for the role of the media in informing and educating the public regarding public health issues?

and underlying causes. So where do smoking, obesity, diet, and physical inactivity get identified as the real causes of such deaths? Perhaps the Chadwick-Farr debate of the mid-19th century continues today in terms of whether deaths in the year 2000 should be attributed to tobacco use, just as many of those in England in 1839 might have been attributed to starvation.

Social and Cultural Influences

Understanding the health effects of biologic, behavioral, and environmental risk factors is straightforward in comparison with understanding the effects of social, economic, and cultural factors on the health of populations. This is due in part to a lack of agreement as to what is being measured. Socioeconomic status and poverty are two factors that generally reflect position in society. There is considerable evidence that social position is an overarching fundamental determinant of health status, even though the indicators used to measure social standing are imprecise, at best.

Social standing affects lifestyle, environment, and the utilization of services; it remains an important predictor of good and poor health in our society. Social class differences in mortality have long been recognized around the world. In 1842, Chadwick reported that the average ages at death for occupationally stratified groups in England were as follows: "gentlemen and persons engaged in the professions, 45 years; tradesmen and their families, 26 years; mechanics, servants and laborers, and their families, 16 years."[10] Life expectancies and other health indicators have improved considerably in

England and elsewhere since 1842, but differences in mortality rates among the various social classes persist to the present day.

Several countries, including Great Britain and the United States, have identifiable social strata that permit comparisons of health status by social class. Britain conducts ongoing analyses of socioeconomic differences according to official categorizations based on general social standing within the community. For the United States, educational status, race, and family income are often used as indirect or proxy measures of social class. Despite the differences in approaches and indicators, there is little evidence of any real difference between Britain and the United States in terms of what is being measured. In both countries, explanations for the differences in mortality appear to relate primarily to inequalities in social position and material resources.[11,12] This effect operates all up and down the hierarchy of social standing; at each step improvements in social status are linked with improvements in measures of health status. For example, a study based on 1971 British census follow-up data found that a relatively affluent, home-owning group with two cars had a lower mortality risk than did a similar relatively privileged group with only one car.[11]

In the United States, epidemiologists have studied socioeconomic differences in mortality risk since the early 1900s. Infant mortality has been the subject of many studies that have consistently documented the effects of poverty. Findings from the National Maternal and Infant Health Survey, for example, demonstrated that the effects of poverty were greater for infants born to mothers with no other risk factors than for infants born to high-risk mothers.[13] Poverty status was associated with a 60% higher rate of neonatal mortality and a 200% higher rate for postneonatal mortality than for those infants of higher-income mothers.

Poverty affects many health outcomes. Low-income families in the United States have an increased likelihood (or relative risk) of a variety of adverse health outcomes, often two to five times greater than that of higher-income families. The percentage of persons reporting fair or poor health is about four times as high for persons living below the poverty level as for those with family income at least twice the poverty level.[1]

The implications of the consistent relationship between measures of social standing and health outcomes suggest that studies need to consider how and how well social class is categorized and measured. Imprecise measures may understate the actual differences that are the result of socioeconomic position in society. Importantly, if racial or ethnic differences are simply attributed to social class differences, factors that operate through race and ethnicity, such as racism or ethnic discrimination, will be overlooked. These additional factors also affect the difference between the social position one has and the position one would have attained, were it not for one's race or ethnicity. Race in the United States, independent of socioeconomic status, is linked to mortality, although these effects vary across age and disease categories.[14] Nevertheless, anthropologists concluded long ago that race is not an appropriate generic category for comparing health outcomes. Its usefulness does not derive from any biologic or genetic differences, but rather, it derives from its social, cultural, political, and historical meanings.

Studies of the effect of social factors on health status across nations add some interesting insights. In general, health appears to be closely associated with income differentials within countries, but there is only a weak link between national mortality rates and average income among the developed countries.[15] This pattern suggests that health is affected less by changes in absolute material standards across affluent populations than by relative income differences and the resulting disadvantage in each country. It is not the richest countries that have the greatest life expectancy. Rather, it is those developed nations with the narrowest income differentials between rich and poor. This finding argues that health in the developed world is less a matter of a population's absolute material wealth than of how the population's circumstances compare with those of other members of their society. A similar perspective views income to be related to health through two pathways: a direct effect on the material conditions necessary for survival, and an effect on social participation and the opportunity to control one's own life circumstances.[16] In settings or societies that provide little in the way of material conditions (e.g., clean water, sanitation services, ample food, adequate housing), income is more important for health. Where material conditions are conducive to good health, income acts through social participation.

The effects of culture on health and illness are also becoming better understood. To medical anthropologists, diseases are not purely independent phenomena. Rather, they are to be viewed and understood in relation to ecology and culture. Certainly, the type and severity of disease varies by age, sex, social class, and ethnic group. For example, Puerto Rican children overall have a higher prevalence of asthma than Mexican American, non-Hispanic white, and African American children.[17] Differences in poverty status do not explain the disparities for Puerto Rican and African American children, two populations that have higher asthma rates than non-Hispanic white and Mexican American children regardless of poverty status. The reason for the higher rate among Puerto Rican children overall is unknown, but the different distributions and social patterns suggest differences in culture-mediated behaviors. Such insights are essential to developing successful prevention and control programs. Culture serves to shape health-related behaviors, as well as human responses to diseases including changes in the environment, which, in turn, affect health. As a mechanism of adapting to the environment, culture has great potential for both positively and negatively affecting health.

There is evidence that different societies shape the ways in which diseases are experienced and that social patterns of disease persist, even after risk factors are identified and effective interventions become available.[18,19] For example, the link between poverty and various outcomes has been well established; yet even after advances in medicine and public health and significant improvement in general living and working conditions, the association persists. One explanation is that as some risks were addressed, others developed, such as health-related behaviors, including violent behavior and alcohol, tobacco, and drug use. In this way, societies create and shape the diseases that they experience. This makes sense, especially if we view the social context in which health and disease reside—the setting and social networks. For problems such as HIV infections, sexually transmitted diseases, and illicit drug use, spread is heavily influenced by the links between those at risk.[20] This also helps to explain why people in disorganized social structures are more likely to report their own health as poor than are similar persons with more social capital.[21,22]

Societal responses to diseases are also socially constructed. Efforts to prevent the spread of typhoid fever by limiting the rights of carriers (such as Typhoid Mary) differed greatly from those to reduce transmission risks from diphtheria carriers. Because many otherwise normal citizens would have been subjected to extreme measures in order to avoid the risk of transmission, it was not socially acceptable to invoke similar measures for these similar risks.

If these themes of social and cultural influences are on target, they place the study of health disparities and inequities at the top of the public health agenda. They also argue that health should be viewed as a social phenomenon. Rather than attempting to identify each and every risk factor that contributes only marginally to disparate health outcomes of the lower social classes, a more effective approach would be to directly address the broader social policies (distribution of wealth, education, employment, discrimination, and the like) that foster the social disparities that cause the observed differences in health outcomes.[19] This social-ecological view of health and its determinants is critical to understanding and improving health status in the United States and other nations.

Global Health Influences

Considerable variation exists among the world's nations on virtually every measure of health and illness currently in use. The principal factors responsible for observed trends and obvious inequities across the globe fall into the general categories of the social and physical environment, personal behavior, and health services. Given the considerable variation in social, economic, and health status among the developed, developing, and underdeveloped nations, it is naive to make broad generalizations. Countries with favorable health status indicators, however, generally have a well-developed health infrastructure, ample opportunities for education and training, relatively high status for women, and economic development that counterbalances population growth. Nonetheless, countries at all levels of development share some problems, including the escalating costs involved in providing a broad range of health, social, and economic development services to disadvantaged subgroups within the population. Social and cultural upheaval associated with urbanization is another problem common to countries at all levels of development. Over the course of the 20th century, the proportion of the world's population living in urban areas tripled—to about 40%; this trend is expected to continue throughout the new century.

The principal environmental hazards in the world today appear to be those associated with poverty. This is true for developed as well as developing and underdeveloped countries. Some international epidemiologists predict that, in the 21st century, the effects of overpopulation and production of greenhouse gases will join poverty as major threats to global health. These factors represent human effects on the world's climate and resources and are easily remembered as the "3 Ps" of global health (pollution, population, and poverty):

- Pollution of the atmosphere by greenhouse gases, which will result in significant global warming, affecting both climate and the occurrence of disease
- Worldwide population growth, which will result in a population of 10–12 billion people within the next century
- Poverty, which is always associated with ill health and disease [23,24]

It surprises many Americans that population is a major global health concern. Birth rates vary inversely with the level of economic development and the status of women among the nations of the world. Continuing high birth rates and declining death rates will mean even more rapid growth in population in developing countries. It has taken all of history to reach the world's current population level, but it will take less than half a century to double that. Many factors have influenced this growth, including public health, which has increased the chances of conception by improving the health status of adults, increasing infant and child survival, preventing premature deaths of adults in the most fertile age groups, and reducing the number of marriages dissolved by one partner's premature death.

Global warming represents yet another phenomenon with considerable potential for health effects. Climate change has direct temperature effects on humans and increases the likelihood of extreme weather events. A number of infectious diseases are also climate sensitive, some because of effects on mosquitoes, ticks, and other vectors in terms of their population size and density and changes in population movement, forest clearance and land use practices, surface water configurations, and human population density.[25] Global warming will also contribute to air quality-related health conditions and concerns.

In general, public health approaches to dealing with world health problems must overcome formidable obstacles, including the unequal and inefficient distribution of health services, lack of appropriate technology, poor management, poverty, and inadequate or inappropriate government programs to finance needed services. Much of the preventable disease in the world is concentrated in the developing and underdeveloped countries, where the most profound differences exist in terms of social and economic influences.

Although many of these factors appear to stem from low levels of national wealth, the link between national health status and national wealth is not firm, and comparisons across nations are seldom straightforward. Improved health status correlates more closely with changes in standards of living, advances in the politics of human relations, and a nation's literacy, education, and welfare policies than with specific preventive interventions. The complexities involved in identifying and understanding these forces and their interrelationships often confound comparisons of health status between the United States and other nations.

ANALYZING HEALTH PROBLEMS FOR CAUSATIVE FACTORS

The ability to identify risk factors and pathways for causation is essential for rational public health decisions and actions to address important health problems in a population. First, however, it is necessary to define what is meant by health problem. Here, health problem means a condition of humans that can be represented in terms of measurable health status or quality-of-life indicators. It is important to note that this basic definition must be modified for the purposes of community problem solving and the development of interventions. This characterization of a health problem as something measured only in terms of outcomes is difficult for some to accept. They point to important factors, such as access to care or poverty itself, and feel that these should rightfully be considered as health problems. Important problems they may be, but if they are truly important in the causation of some unacceptable health outcome, they can be dealt with as related factors rather than health problems.

The factors linked with specific health problems are often generically termed risk factors and can exist at one of three levels. Those risk factors most closely associated with the health outcome in question are often termed determinants. Risk factors that play a role further back in the chain of causation are called direct and indirect contributing factors. Risk factors can be described at either an individual or a population level. For example, tobacco use for an individual increases the chances of developing heart disease or lung cancer, and an increased prevalence of tobacco use in a population increases that population's incidence of (and mortality rates from) these conditions.

Determinants are scientifically established factors that relate directly to the level of a health problem. As the level of the determinant changes, the level of the health outcome changes. Determinants are the most proximal risk factors through which other levels of risk factors act. The link between the determinant and the health outcome should be well established through scientific or epidemiologic studies. For example, for neonatal mortality rates, two well-established determinants are the low birth weight rate (the number of infants born weighing less than 2,500 g, or about 5.5 pounds, per 100 live births) and weight-specific mortality rates. Improvement in the neonatal mortality rate cannot occur unless one of these determinants improves. Health outcomes can have one or many determinants.

Direct contributing factors are scientifically established factors that directly affect the level of a determinant. Again, there should be solid evidence that the level of the direct contributing factor affects the level of the determinant. For the neonatal mortality rate example, the prevalence of tobacco use among pregnant women has been associated with the risk of low birth weight. A determinant can have many direct contributing factors. For low birth weight, other direct contributing factors include low maternal weight gain and inadequate prenatal care.

Indirect contributing factors affect the level of the direct contributing factors. Although several steps distant from the health outcome in question, these factors are often proximal enough to be modified. The indirect contributing factor affects the level of the direct contributing factor, which, in turn, affects the level of the determinant. The level of the determinant then affects the level of the health outcome. Many indirect contributing factors can exist for each direct contributing factor. For prevalence of tobacco use among pregnant women, indirect contributing factors might include easy access to tobacco products for young women, lack of health education, and lack of smoking cessation programs.

OUTSIDE-THE-BOOK THINKING 2-4

© Alfred Bondarenko/Shutterstock.

Select a health outcome and analyze that outcome for its determinants and contributing factors, using the method described in the text. Identify at least two major determinants for the problem that you select. For each determinant, identify at least two direct contributing factors, and for each direct contributing factor, identify at least two indirect contributing factors.

The health problem analysis framework begins with the identification of a health problem (defined in terms of

TABLE 2-4 Risk Factors

Determinant	Scientifically established factor that relates directly to the level of the health problem. A health problem may have any number of determinants identified for it.	Example: Low birth weight is a prime determinant for the health problem of neonatal mortality.
Direct contributing factor	Scientifically established factor that directly affects the level of the determinant.	Example: Use of prenatal care is one factor that affects the low-birth-weight rate.
Indirect contributing factor	Community-specific factor that affects the level of a direct contributing factor. Such factors can vary considerably from one community to another.	Example: Availability of day care or transportation services within the community may affect the use of prenatal care services.

Data from Centers for Disease Control and Prevention, Public Health Practice Program Office, 1991.

health status indicators) and proceeds to establish one or more determinants; for each determinant, one or more direct contributing factors; and for each direct contributing factor, one or more indirect contributing factors. Intervention strategies at the community level generally involve addressing these indirect contributing factors. When completed, an analysis identifies as many of the causal pathways as possible to determine which contributing factors exist in the setting in which an intervention strategy is planned. The framework for this approach is presented in **Table 2-4** and **Figure 2-6**. This framework forms the basis for developing meaningful interventions; it is used in several of the processes and instruments to assess community health needs that are currently in wide use at the local level. Community health improvement processes and tools are topics for another chapter.

FIGURE 2-6 Health Problem Analysis Worksheet

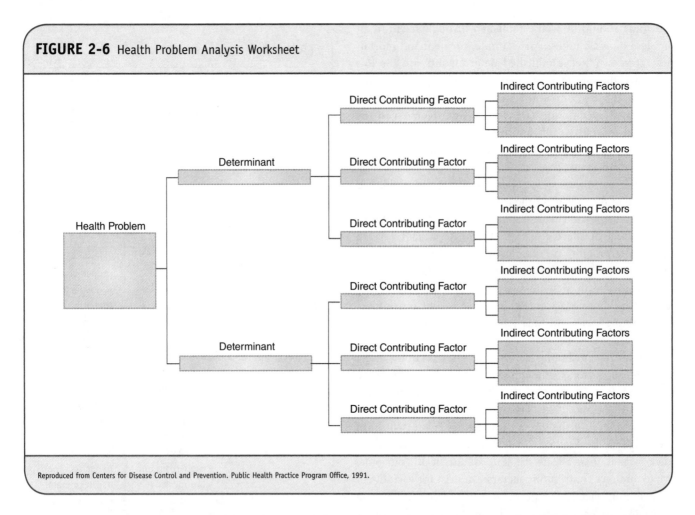

Although this framework is useful, it does not fully account for the relationships among the various levels of risk factors. Some direct contributing factors may affect more than one determinant, and some indirect contributing factors may influence more than one direct contributing factor. For example, illicit drug use during pregnancy influences both the likelihood of low birth weight and birth weight-specific survival rates. To account fully for these interactions, some direct and indirect contributing factors may need to be included in several different locations on the worksheet. Despite the advancement of epidemiologic methods, many studies ignore the contributing factors that affect the level of these major risk factors, leading to simplistic formulations of multiple risk factors for health problems that exist at the community level.[26]

ECONOMIC DIMENSIONS OF HEALTH OUTCOMES

The ability to measure and quantify outcomes and risks is essential for rational decisions and actions. Specific indicators, as well as methods of economic analysis, are available to provide both objective and subjective valuations. Several health indicators attempt to value differentially health status; outcomes, including age-adjusted rates; span of healthy life; and YPLL. For example, YPLL represents a method of weighting or valuing health outcomes by placing a higher value on deaths that occur at earlier ages. Years of life lost thus become a common denominator or, in one sense, a common currency. Health outcomes can be translated into this currency or into an actual currency, such as dollars. This translation allows for comparisons to be made among outcomes in terms of which costs more per person, per episode, or per another reference point. Cost comparisons of health outcomes and health events have become common in public health. Approaches include cost-benefit, cost-effectiveness, and cost-utility studies.

Cost-benefit analyses provide comprehensive information on both the costs and the benefits of an intervention. All health outcomes and other relevant impacts are included in the determination of benefits. The results are expressed in terms of net costs, net benefits, and time required to recoup an initial investment. If the benefits are expressed in health outcome terms, years of life gained or quality-adjusted life-years (QALYs) may be calculated. This provides a framework for comparing disparate interventions. QALYs are calculated from a particular perspective that determines which costs and consequences are included in the analysis. For public health analyses, societal perspectives are necessary. When comprehensively performed, cost-benefit analyses are considered the gold standard of economic evaluations.

Cost-effectiveness analyses focus on one outcome to determine the most cost-effective intervention when several options are possible. Cost-effectiveness examines a specific option's costs to achieve a particular outcome. Results are often specified as the cost per case prevented or cost per life saved. For example, screening an entire town for a specific disease might identify cases at a cost of $150 per new case, whereas a screening program directed only at high-risk groups within that town might identify cases at a cost of $50 per new case. Although useful for evaluating different strategies for achieving the same result, cost-effectiveness approaches are not very helpful in evaluating interventions intended for different health conditions.

Cost-utility analyses are similar to cost-effectiveness studies, except that the results are characterized as cost per QALY. These are most useful when the intervention affects both morbidity and mortality, and there are a variety of possible outcomes that include quality of life.

These approaches are especially important for interventions based on preventive strategies. The argument is frequently made that "an ounce of prevention is worth a pound of cure." If this wisdom is true, preventive interventions should result in savings equal to 16 times their actual cost. Not many preventive interventions measure up to this standard, but even crude information on the costs of many health outcomes suggests that prevention has economic as well as human savings. The U.S. Public Health Service has estimated that as much as 11% of health expenditures for the year 2000 could have been averted through investments in public health for six conditions: motor vehicle injuries, occupationally related injuries, stroke, coronary heart disease, firearms-related injuries, and low-birth-weight infants.[27] Beyond the direct medical effects, there are often nonmedical costs related to lost wages, taxes, and productivity.

Economists assert that the future costs for care and services that result from prevention of mortality must be considered a negative benefit of prevention. For example, the costs of preventing a death from motor vehicle injuries should include all subsequent medical care costs for that individual over his or her lifetime, because these costs would not have occurred otherwise. They also argue that it is unfair to compare future savings to the costs of current prevention programs and that those savings must be discounted to their current value. If a preventive program will save $10 million 20 years from now, that $10 million must be translated into its current value in computing cost benefits, cost-effectiveness, or cost utility. It may be that the value of $10 million 20 years from now is only $4 million now. If the program costs $1 million, its benefit/cost ratio would be 4:1 instead of 10:1 before we even added any additional costs associated with medical care for the lives that were saved. These economic considerations contribute to the difficulty of marketing preventive interventions.

Two additional economic considerations are important for public health policy and practice. The first of these is what is known as opportunity costs, which represents the costs involved in choosing one course of action over another. Resources spent for one purpose are not available to be spent for another. As a result, there is a need to consider the costs of not realizing the benefits or gains from paths not chosen. A second economic consideration important for public health is related to the heavy emphasis of public health on preventive strategies. The savings or gains from successful prevention efforts are generally not reinvested in public health or even other health purposes. These savings or gains from investments in prevention are lost. Maybe this is proper, because the overall benefits accrue more broadly to society, and public health remains, above all else, a social enterprise. However, imagine the situation for American industry and businesses if they could not reinvest their gains to grow their businesses. This is often the situation faced by public health, further exacerbating the difficulty of arguing for and securing needed resources.

HEALTHY PEOPLE 2020

The data and discussion in this chapter only broadly describe health status measures in the United States in the early decades of the new century. Several common themes emerge, however, that form the basis for national health objectives focusing on the year 2020.[28] **Figure 2-7** (consistent with the social-ecological model described earlier) presents a *Healthy People* process grounded in a broad view of the many factors influencing health. The year 2020 objectives build on the nation's experience with three previous panels of health objectives established for the years 1990, 2000, and 2010.

Assessments of the *Healthy People 2000* and *Healthy People 2010* efforts yielded similar findings. In general, progress was apparent for many of the broader goals, especially the age-adjusted mortality targets for age groups under

FIGURE 2-7 The *Healthy People 2020* Model

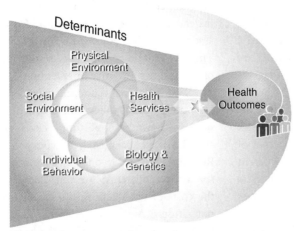

Healthy People 2020
A society in which all people live long, healthy lives

Overarching Goals:

- Attain high-quality longer lives free of preventable disease, disability, injury, and premature death.
- Achieve health equity, eliminate disparities, and improve the health of all groups.
- Create social and physical environments that promote good health for all.
- Promote quality of life, healthy development, and healthy behaviors across all life stages.

Reproduced from U.S. Department of Health and Human Services, *Healthy People 2020* Framework, available at www.healthypeople.gov website. Accessed March 15, 2014.

age 70. Nonetheless, a substantial proportion of the objectives targeting special populations, especially African Americans and Native Americans, were found to be moving in the wrong direction. These findings fueled concerns that health inequities and disparities were persisting, if not increasing, in the United States. In addition, with nearly 500 objectives established in both the 2000 and 2010 efforts, tracking became a complex undertaking. Many objectives could not be tracked because of the unavailability of or lack of consensus for the tracking measures.

Healthy People 2020 (HP2020), summarized in **Table 2-5**, provides a comprehensive set of 10-year, national goals and objectives for improving the health of all Americans. HP2020 contains 42 topic areas with over 1,200 objectives. A smaller set of objectives, called Leading Health Indicators, is identified in **Table 2-6**; these were selected to communicate high-priority health issues and actions that can be taken to address them.

The graphic framework for HP2020 offered in Figure 2-5 illustrates the fundamental interrelationships among the social determinants of health and emphasizes their collective impact and influence on health outcomes and conditions. The HP2020 framework also underscores a continued focus on population disparities, including those categorized by

race/ethnicity, socioeconomic status, gender, age, disability status, sexual orientation, and geographic location. Four foundational health measures serve as indicators of progress towards achieving these goals: general health status, health-related quality of life, determinants of health, and disparities. **Table 2-7** provides additional details on these measures.

Central to the *Healthy People 2020* effort are four overarching goals, two of which focus on:

1. Attaining high-quality, longer lives free of preventable disease, disability, injury, and premature death; and
2. Achieving health equity, eliminating disparities, and improving the health of all groups.

Although these two overarching goals appear appropriate, they are only arguably linked. From one perspective, they represent two very different approaches to improving outcomes for the population as a whole. If we view the health status of the entire population as a Gaussian curve, one approach would be to shift the entire curve further toward better outcomes, and a second approach would be to change the shape of the curve, reducing the difference between the extremes. These represent quite different strategies that would be associated with quite

TABLE 2-5 *Healthy People 2020* Vision, Mission, Goals, and Focus Areas

Vision

A society in which all people live long, healthy lives.

Mission

Healthy People 2020 strives to:
- Identify nationwide health improvement priorities.
- Increase public awareness and understanding of the determinants of health, disease, and disability and the opportunities for progress.
- Provide measurable objectives and goals that are applicable at the national, state, and local levels.
- Engage multiple sectors to take actions to strengthen policies and improve practices that are driven by the best available evidence and knowledge.
- Identify critical research, evaluation, and data collection needs.

Overarching Goals
- Attain high-quality, longer lives free of preventable disease, disability, injury, and premature death.
- Achieve health equity, eliminate disparities, and improve the health of all groups.
- Create social and physical environments that promote good health for all.
- Promote quality of life, healthy development, and healthy behaviors across all life stages.

Focus Areas
 1. Access to health services
 2. Adolescent health
 3. Arthritis, osteoporosis, and chronic back conditions
 4. Blood disorders and blood safety
 5. Cancer
 6. Chronic kidney diseases
 7. Dementia, including Alzheimer's disease
 8. Diabetes
 9. Disability and secondary conditions
10. Early and middle childhood
11. Educational and community-based programs
12. Environmental health
13. Family planning
14. Food safety
15. Genomics
16. Global health
17. Health communication and health information technology
18. Healthcare-associated infections
19. Hearing and other sensory or communication disorders (ear, nose, throat—voice, speech, and language)
20. Heart disease and stroke
21. HIV
22. Immunization and infectious diseases
23. Injury and violence prevention
24. Lesbian, gay, bisexual, and transgender health
25. Maternal, infant, and child health
26. Medical product safety
27. Mental health and mental disorders
28. Nutrition and weight status
29. Occupational safety and health
30. Older adults

(continues)

TABLE 2-5 *Healthy People 2020* Vision, Mission, Goals, and Focus Areas (*continued*)

31. Oral health
32. Physical activity
33. Preparedness
34. Public health infrastructure
35. Quality of life and well-being
36. Respiratory diseases
37. Sexually transmitted diseases
38. Sleep health
39. Social determinants of health
40. Substance abuse
41. Tobacco use
42. Vision

Reproduced from U.S. Department of Health and Human Services. *Healthy People 2020* Web site. www.healthypeople.gov. Accessed June 3, 2014.

different policies and interventions. Focusing on the tail end of the distribution of health requires investment in questionably effective attempts that benefit relatively few and fail to promote the health of the majority. On the other hand, even small improvements in overall society-wide health measures have provided greater gains for society than very perceptible improvements in the health of a few.[29] The choice is one that can be viewed as focusing on "epiphenomena," such as risk factors or on the larger context and social environment. *Healthy People 2020* ambitiously seeks to do both.

Monitoring all national health objectives is not considered feasible at the state and local level. Instead, only priorities linked to the national health objectives will likely be tracked. An Institute of Medicine committee in 1997 identified a basic set of indicators for use in community health improvement processes (**Table 2-8**). Together with the catalog of leading health indicators from the current Healthy People process, these measures provide a useful starting point for population-based community health assessment and improvement initiatives.

OUTSIDE-THE-BOOK THINKING 2-5

© Alfred Bondarenko/Shutterstock.

Projections call for a continuing increase in life expectancy through the first half of the 21st century. What effect will increased life expectancy have on the major goals of *Healthy People 2020*—increasing the quality and years of healthy life and eliminating health disparities?

OUTSIDE-THE-BOOK THINKING 2-6

© Alfred Bondarenko/Shutterstock.

Your community is about to undertake a community health assessment and you have been tasked to review and improve the list of community health profile indicators proposed for this process. These include the *Healthy People 2020* Leading Health Indicators (Table 2-6) and the basic community health indictors proposed by the IOM (Table 2-8). Identify and justify three indicators you would add to this list, based on what you know about the health status and needs of your community.

TABLE 2-6 *Healthy People 2020* Leading Health Indicators

Access to Health Services   • Persons with medical insurance   • Persons with a usual primary care provider
Clinical Preventive Services   • Adults who receive a colorectal cancer screening based on the most recent guidelines   • Adults with hypertension whose blood pressure is under control   • Adult diabetic population with an A1c value greater than 9 percent   • Children aged 19 to 35 months who receive the recommended doses of DTaP, polio, MMR, Hib, hepatitis B, varicella, and PCV vaccines
Environmental Quality   • Air Quality Index (AQI) exceeding 100   • Children aged 3 to 11 years exposed to secondhand smoke
Injury and Violence   • Fatal injuries   • Homicides
Maternal, Infant, and Child Health   • Infant deaths   • Preterm births
Mental Health   • Suicides   • Adolescents who experience major depressive episodes
Nutrition, Physical Activity, and Obesity   • Adults who meet current Federal physical activity guidelines for aerobic physical activity and muscle-strengthening activity   • Adults who are obese   • Children and adolescents who are considered obese   • Total vegetable intake for persons aged 2 years and older
Oral Health   • Persons aged 2 years and older who used the oral health care system in past 12 months
Reproductive and Sexual Health   • Sexually active females aged 15 to 44 years who received reproductive health services in the past 12 months   • Persons living with HIV who know their serostatus
Social Determinants   • Students who graduate with a regular diploma 4 years after starting 9th grade
Substance Abuse   • Adolescents using alcohol or any illicit drugs during the past 30 days   • Adults engaging in binge drinking during the past 30 days
Tobacco   • Adults who are current cigarette smokers   • Adolescents who smoked cigarettes in the past 30 days

Reproduced from U.S. Department of Health and Human Services. *Healthy People 2020* Web site. www.healthypeople.gov. Accessed June 3, 2014.

TABLE 2-7 Measures of Progress toward *Healthy People 2020* Goals

General Health Status   • Life expectancy (with international comparison)   • Healthy life expectancy   • Years of potential life lost (YPLL) (with international comparison)   • Physically and mentally unhealthy days   • Self-assessed health status   • Limitation of activity   • Chronic disease prevalence
Health-Related Quality of Life (HRQoL) and Well-Being   • Patient Reported Outcomes Measurement Information System (PROMIS) Global Health Measure – assesses global physical, mental and social HRQoL through questions on self-rated health, physical HRQoL, mental HRQoL, fatigue, pain, emotional distress, social activities, and roles.   • Well-Being Measures – assess the positive evaluations of people's daily lives – when they feel very healthy and satisfied or content with life, the quality of their relationships, their positive emotions, resilience, and realization of their potential.   • Participation Measures – reflect individuals' assessments of the impact of their health on their social participation within their current environment. Participation includes education, employment, civic, social and leisure activities. The principle behind participation measures is that a person with a functional limitation – for example, vision loss, mobility difficulty, or intellectual disability – can live a long and productive life and enjoy a good quality of life.
Determinants of Health   • Policymaking   • Social factors   • Health services   • Individual behavior   • Biology and genetics
Disparities   • Race and ethnicity   • Gender   • Sexual identity and orientation   • Disability status or special health care needs   • Geographic location (rural and urban)

Reproduced from U.S. Department of Health and Human Services. *Healthy People 2020* Web site. www.healthypeople.gov. Accessed June 3, 2014.

TABLE 2-8   Proposed Indicators for a Community Health Profile

Sociodemographic Characteristics

1. Distribution of the population by age and race/ethnicity
2. Number and proportion of persons in groups such as migrants, homeless, or the non-English speaking for whom access to community services and resources may be a concern
3. Number and proportion of persons aged 25 and older with less than a high school education
4. Ratio of the number of students graduating from high school to the number of students who entered ninth grade 3 years previously
5. Median household income
6. Proportion of children less than 15 years of age living in families at or below the poverty level
7. Unemployment rate
8. Number and proportion of single-parent families
9. Number and proportion of persons without health insurance

Health Status

10. Infant mortality rate by race/ethnicity
11. Numbers of deaths or age-adjusted death rates for motor vehicle crashes, work-related injuries, suicide, homicide, lung cancer, breast cancer, cardiovascular diseases, and all causes, by age, race, and gender, as appropriate
12. Reported incidence of AIDS, measles, tuberculosis, and primary and secondary syphilis, by age, race, and gender, as appropriate
13. Births to adolescents (ages 10–17) as proportion of total live births
14. Number and rate of confirmed abuse and neglect cases among children

Health Risk Factors

15. Proportion of 2-year-old children who have received all age-appropriate vaccines, as recommended by the Advisory Committee on Immunization Practices
16. Proportion of adults aged 65 and older who have ever been immunized for pneumococcal pneumonia; proportion who have been immunized in the past 12 months for influenza
17. Proportion of the population who smoke, by age, race, and gender, as appropriate
18. Proportion of the population aged 18 or older who are obese
19. Number and type of U.S. Environmental Protection Agency air quality standards not met
20. Proportion of assessed rivers, lakes, and estuaries that support beneficial uses (e.g., fishing- and swimming-approved)

Health Care Resource Consumption

21. Per-capita health care spending for Medicare beneficiaries (the Medicaid adjusted average per-capita cost)

Functional Status

22. Proportion of adults reporting that their general health is good to excellent
23. During the past 30 days, average number of days for which adults report that their physical or mental health was not good

Quality of Life

24. Proportion of adults satisfied with the healthcare system in the community
25. Proportion of persons satisfied with the quality of life in the community

Data from the Institute of Medicine. *Using Performance Monitoring to Improve Community Health: A Role for Performance Monitoring.* Washington, DC: National Academy Press; 1997.

CONCLUSION

From a social-ecological perspective, the health status of a population is influenced by many factors drawn from biology, behavior, the physical and social environment, and the use of health services. Social and cultural factors also play an important role in the disease patterns experienced by different populations, as well as in the responses of these populations to disease and illness. Globally, risks associated with population growth, pollution, and poverty result in mortality and morbidity that are still associated with infectious disease processes. In the United States, behaviorally mediated risks, including tobacco, diet, alcohol, and injury risks, rather than infectious disease processes, are the major contributors to health status, and the considerable gap between low-income minority populations and other Americans continues to widen. Public health activities strive to improve population health status (effectiveness) through cost-beneficial strategies and interventions (efficacy) and with equal benefits for all segments of the population (equity). Elimination and reduction of the disparities in health status among population groups have emerged as the most critical national health goal for the year 2020. With the increasing availability of data on health status, as well as on determinants and contributing factors, the potential for more rational policies and interventions has increased. Over the long term, public policies that narrow income disparities and increase access to education, jobs, and housing do far more to improve the health status of populations than do efforts to provide more healthcare services. Health improvement efforts require more than data on health problems and contributing factors, which view health from a negative perspective. Also needed is information from a positive perspective, in terms of community capacities, assets, and willingness. More important still, there must be recognition and acceptance that the right to health is a basic human right and one inextricably linked to all other human rights, lest quality of life be seriously compromised.[30] It is this right to health that energizes and challenges public health workers to measure health and quality of life in ways that promote its improvement.

REFERENCES

1. National Center for Health Statistics. *Health, United States, 2013.* Hyattsville, MD: NCHS; 2014.

2. Allaire SH, LaValley MP, Evans SR, et al. Evidence for decline in disability and improved health among persons aged 55 to 70 years: the Framingham heart study. *Am J Public Health.* 1999; 89: 1678–1683.

3. Constitution of World Health Organization. In: World Health Organization. Chronicle of World Health Organization. Geneva, Switzerland: WHO; 1947; 1: 29–43.

4. Whaley RF, Hashim TJ. *A Textbook of World Health.* New York: Parthenon; 1995.

5. Centers for Disease Control and Prevention. First reportable underlying cause of death. *MMWR.* 1996; 45: 537.

6. Brownson RC, Remington PL, Davis JR, eds. *Chronic Disease Epidemiology and Control.* 2nd ed. Washington, DC: American Public Health Association; 1998.

7. Seitz F, Plepys C. Monitoring air quality in *Healthy People 2000. Healthy People 2000 Statistical Notes.* Hyattsville, MD: National Center for Health Statistics; 1995:No. 9.

8. Amler RW, Eddins DL. Cross-sectional analysis: precursors of premature death in the U.S. In: Amler RW, Dull DL, eds. Closing the Gap. Atlanta, GA: Carter Center; 1985: 181–187.

9. Mokdad AM, Marks JS, Stroup DF, Gerberding JL. Actual causes of death in the United States, 2000. *JAMA.* 2004; 291: 1238–1245.

10. Chadwick E. *Report on the Sanitary Conditions of the Labouring Population of Great Britain 1842.* Edinburgh, Scotland: Edinburgh University Press; 1965.

11. Smith GD, Egger M. Socioeconomic differences in mortality in Britain and the United States. *Am J Public Health.* 1992; 82: 1079–1081.

12. Schrijvers CTM, Stronks K, van de Mheen HD, Mackenbach JP. Explaining educational differences in mortality: the role of behavioral and material factors. *Am J Public Health.* 1999; 89: 535–540.

13. Centers for Disease Control and Prevention. Poverty and infant mortality: United States, 1988. *MMWR.* 1996; 44: 922–927.

14. Ng-Mak DS, Dohrenwend BP, Abraido-Lanza AF, Turner JB. A further analysis of race differences in the national longitudinal mortality study. *Am J Public Health.* 1999; 89: 1748–1751.

15. Wilkenson RG. National mortality rates: the impact of inequality. *Am J Public Health.* 1992; 82: 1082–1084.

16. Marmot M. The influence of income on health: views of an epidemiologist. *Health Affairs.* 2002; 21: 31–46.

17. Centers for Disease Control and Prevention. Percentage of children <18 years who currently have asthma, by race/ethnicity and poverty status, United States, 2003–2005. MMWR. 2007; 56(5): 99.

18. Sargent CF, Johnson TM, eds. *Medical Anthropology: Contemporary Theory and Method.* Rev ed. Westport, CT: Praeger; 1996.

19. Link BG, Phelan JC. Understanding sociodemographic differences in health: the role of fundamental social causes. *Am J Public Health.* 1996; 86: 471–473.

20. Friedman SR, Curtis R, Neaigus A, Jose B, Des Jarlais DC. *Social Networks, Drug Injectors' Lives and HIV/AIDS.* New York: Kluwer; 1999.

21. Kawachi I, Kennedy BP, Glass R. Social capital and self-rated health: a contextual analysis. *Am J Public Health.* 1999; 89: 1187–1193.

22. Malmstom M, Sundquist J, Johansson SE. Neighborhood environment and self-reported health status: a multilevel analysis. *Am J Public Health.* 1999; 89: 1181–1186.

23. Doll R. Health and the environment in the 1990s. *Am J Public Health.* 1992; 82: 933–941.

24. Winkelstein W. Determinants of worldwide health. *Am J Public Health.* 1992; 82: 931–932.

25. Intergovernmental Panel on Climate Change. Impacts, adaptation, and vulnerability: contribution of Working Group II to the Third Assessment Report of the Intergovernmental Panel on Climate Change. In: McCarthy JJ, Canziani OF, Leary NA, Dokken DJ, White KS, eds. *Climate Change 2001.* Cambridge, UK: Cambridge University Press; 2001: 75–913.

26. Fielding JE. Public health in the twentieth century: advances and challenges. *Ann Rev Public Health.* 1999; 20: xiii–xxx.

27. U.S. Public Health Service. *For a Healthy Nation: Return on Investments in Public Health.* Washington, DC: PHS; 1994.

28. U.S. Department of Health and Human Services. *Healthy People 2020.* Available at www.healthypeople.gov. Accessed June 16, 2014.

29. McKinlay JB, Marceau LD. A tale of 3 tails. *Am J Public Health.* 1999; 89: 295–298.

30. Universal Declaration of Human Rights. GA res 217 A(iii), UN Doc A/810, art 25(1);1948.

CHAPTER **3**

Public Health and the Health System

LEARNING OBJECTIVES

Given a prevalent health problem (disease or condition), incorporate strategies of health-related and illness-related interventions impacting through each of the three levels of prevention in a plan to prevent further spread of the disease/condition and minimize its effects to the greatest extent possible. Key aspects of this competency expectation include being able to

- Describe three or more major issues that make the health system a public health concern
- Identify five intervention strategies directed toward health and illness
- Identify and describe three levels of preventive interventions
- Describe the approximate level of national expenditures for all health and medical services and for the population-based and public health activity components of this total
- Cite important economic, demographic, and utilization dimensions of the health sector
- Access and utilize current data and information resources available through the Internet's World Wide Web characterizing the roles and interests of key stakeholders in the health sector

More than five decades of discussion, debate, and inaction later, significant health reform finally came to the health system in the United States in the second decade of the 21st century. Some believe it was too much, too quickly. Others found it too little and too late. The Patient Protection and Affordable Care Act (P.L. 111-148, more commonly known as the Affordable Care Act or "Obamacare") was enacted in 2010 with its major provisions to be implemented piecemeal over the ensuing decade. The extent to which the Affordable Care Act addresses the major problems and issues facing the health system in the United States rests in large part on what those problems and issues were, are, and will be. This chapter picks up where the previous chapter left off—with influences on health. The influences to be examined in this chapter, however, are the interventions and services available through the health system.

The relationship between public health and other health-related activities has never been clear. Some of the lack of clarity may be the result of the several different images of public health described previously, but certainly not all. In addition to the health system remaining poorly understood by the American public, there are different views among health professionals and policymakers as to whether public health is part of the health system or whether it is a separate, parallel enterprise. Most agree that these entities serve the same ends but disagree as to the balance between the two and the locus for strategic decisions and actions. The issue of ownership—which entity's leadership and strategies will predominate— underlies these different perspectives. In this text, the term health system will refer to all aspects of the organization, financing, and provision of programs and services for the prevention and treatment of illness and injury. Public health activities are an important component of this larger health system and, indeed, the entire health system serves the health of the public. This view differs from the image that most people have of our health system; the public commonly perceives the health system to include only the medical care and treatment aspects of the overall system.

Although their relationship may not be clear, there is ample cause for public health interest in the health system. Perhaps most compelling is the sheer size and scope of the U.S. health system, characteristics that have made the health system as much an ethical as an economic issue. More than 15 million workers and $3.0 trillion in resources are devoted to health-related purposes.[1] However, this huge investment in fiscal and human resources may not be accomplishing what it can and should in terms of health outcomes. Lack of access to needed health services for an alarming number of Americans and inconsistent quality have been contributing to less than optimal health outcomes. Although access and quality have long been public health concerns, costs associated with excess capacity within the health system has emerged as another important issue for public health.

This chapter examines the U.S. health system from several perspectives that consider the public health implications of costs and affordability, as well as several other important public policy and public health questions:

- Does the United States have a rational strategy for investing its resources to maintain and improve people's health?
- Does the current strategy inequitably limit access to and benefit from needed services?
- Is the health system accountable to its end-users and ultimate payers for the quality and results of its services?
- Are the changes occurring from recent health reform legislation (Affordable Care Act) bringing meaningful reform to the U.S. health system?

It is these issues of health, excess, access, accountability, and quality that make the health system a public health concern.

Complementary, even synergistic, efforts involving medicine and public health are apparent in many of the important gains in health outcomes achieved during the 20th century. Underlying these synergies is an appreciation that a successful health system deploys and integrates a variety of strategies and activities that differ in terms of their strategic intent, level of prevention, relationship to medical and public health practice, and community or individual focus. Key economic, demographic, and resource trends will then be briefly presented as a prelude to understanding important themes and emerging paradigm shifts. New opportunities afforded by sweeping changes in the health system will be apparent in the review of these issues.

OUTSIDE-THE-BOOK THINKING 3-1

© Alfred Bondarenko/Shutterstock.

Great debate: This debate examines contributors to improvement in health status in the United States since 1900. There are two propositions to be considered. Proposition A: Public health interventions are responsible for these improvements. Proposition B: Medical care interventions are responsible for these improvements. Select one—and only one—of these positions and present a compelling argument.

PREVENTION AND HEALTH SERVICES

Improved health status in the United States over the past 100+ years is due to a variety of intervention strategies and services.[2] Key relationships among health, illness, and various interventions intended to maintain or restore health are illustrated in **Figure 3-1**. Wellness and illness are dynamic states that are influenced by a wide variety of biologic, environmental, behavioral, social, cultural, and health service factors that interact within a social-ecological framework. The complex interaction of these factors contributes to the occurrence or absence of disease or injury, which, in turn, contributes to the health status and well-being of individuals and populations.

Several different intervention points are possible, including two general strategies—health promotion and specific protection—that seek to maintain health by intervening prior to the development of disease or injury.[3] Each involves activities that alter the interaction of the various health-influencing factors in ways that either avert or alter the occurrence of disease or injury.

Health Promotion and Specific Protection

Health promotion activities attempt to modify human behaviors to reduce those known to affect adversely the ability to resist disease or injury-inducing factors, thereby eliminating exposures to harmful factors. Examples of health promotion activities include interventions such as nutrition counseling, genetic counseling, family counseling, and the myriad activities that constitute health education. However, health promotion also properly includes the provision of adequate housing, employment, and recreational conditions,

FIGURE 3-1 Public Health Intervention Strategies and Effects

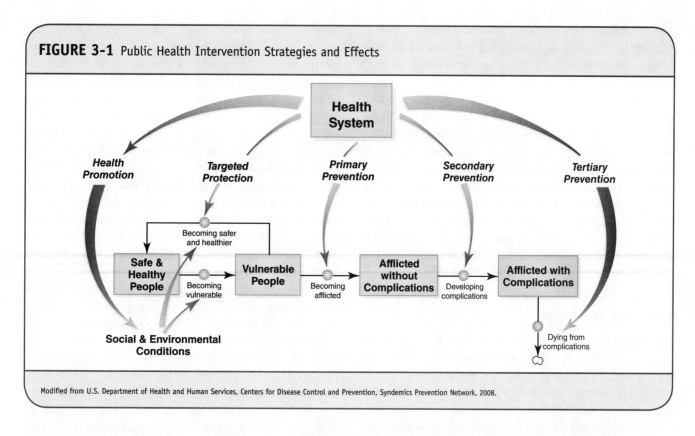

Modified from U.S. Department of Health and Human Services, Centers for Disease Control and Prevention, Syndemics Prevention Network, 2008.

as well as other forms of community development activities. What is clear from these examples is that many fall outside the common understanding of what constitutes health care. Several of these are viewed as the duty or responsibility of other societal institutions, including public safety, housing, education, and even business. It is somewhat ironic that activities that focus on the state of health and that seek to maintain and promote health are not commonly perceived to be "health services." To some extent, this is also true for the other category of health-maintaining strategies—specific protection activities.

Specific protection activities provide individuals with resistance to factors (such as microorganisms like viruses and bacteria) or modify environments to decrease potentially harmful interactions of health-influencing factors (such as toxic exposures in the workplace). Examples of specific protection include activities directed toward specific risks (e.g., the use of protective equipment for asbestos removal), immunizations, occupational and environmental engineering, and regulatory controls and activities to protect individuals from environmental carcinogens (such as exposure to secondhand or side-stream smoke) and toxins. Several of these are often identified with settings other than traditional healthcare settings. Many are implemented and enforced through governmental agencies.

Early Case Finding and Prompt Treatment, Disability Limitation, and Rehabilitation

Although health promotion and specific protection focus on the healthy state and seek to prevent disease, a different set of strategies and activities is necessary after disease or injury occurs. In such circumstances, the appropriate strategies are those facilitating early detection, prompt treatment, or rehabilitation, depending on the stage of development of the disease.

In general, early detection and prompt treatment reduce individual pain and suffering and are less costly to both the individual and society than treatment initiated after a condition has reached a more advanced state. Interventions to achieve early detection and prompt treatment include screening tests, case-finding efforts, and periodic physical exams. Screening tests are increasingly available to detect illnesses before they become symptomatic. Case-finding efforts for both infectious and noninfectious conditions are directed at populations at greater risk for the condition on the basis of criteria appropriate for that condition. Periodic physical exams and other screenings, such as those consistent with the age-specific recommendations of the U.S. Preventive Health Services Task Force, incorporate these practices and are best provided through an effective primary medical care system.[4] Primary care providers who are sensitive to disease patterns and predisposing factors can play substantial roles in the early identification and management of most medical conditions.

Another strategy targeting disease is disease management through effective and complete treatment. It is these activities that most Americans equate with the term health care, largely because this strategy constitutes the lion's share of the U.S. health system in terms of resource deployment. Quite appropriately, these efforts largely aim to arrest or eradicate disease and to limit disability and prevent death. The final intervention strategy focusing on disease—rehabilitation—is designed to return individuals who have experienced a condition to the maximum level of function consistent with their capacities.

Links with Prevention

An important aspect of this view of the health system is that it emphasizes the potential for prevention inherent in each of the five health intervention strategies. Prevention can be categorized in several ways. The best-known approach classifies prevention in relation to the stage of the disease or condition.

Preventive intervention strategies are considered primary, secondary, or tertiary. Primary prevention involves prevention of the disease or injury itself, generally through reducing exposure or risk factor levels. Secondary prevention attempts to identify and control disease processes in their early stages, often before signs and symptoms become apparent. In this case, prevention is akin to preemptive treatment. Tertiary prevention seeks to prevent disability through restoring individuals to their optimal level of functioning after damage is done.

The relationship of the five health intervention strategies to the three levels of prevention is also illustrated in Figure 3-1. Health promotion and specific protection are primary prevention strategies seeking to prevent the development of disease. Early case finding and prompt treatment represent secondary prevention, because they seek to interrupt the disease process before complications occur. Disease management and rehabilitation are considered tertiary-level prevention in that they seek to prevent or reduce disability associated with disease or injury. Although these are considered tertiary prevention, they receive primary attention under current policy and resource deployment.

Figure 3-2 further illustrates each of the three levels of prevention strategies in relation to population disease status and effect on disease incidence and prevalence. The various potential benefits from the three prevention levels derive from the basic epidemiologic concepts of incidence and prevalence. Prevalence (the rate of existing cases of illness, injury, or a health event) is a function of both incidence (the rate of new cases) and duration. Reducing either incidence or duration can lower prevalence. Primary prevention aims to reduce the incidence of conditions, whereas secondary and tertiary prevention seek to reduce prevalence by shortening duration and minimizing the effects of disease or injury. It should be apparent that there is a finite limit to how much a condition's duration can be reduced. As a result, approaches emphasizing primary prevention have greater potential benefit than do approaches emphasizing other levels of prevention. The importance of the differential impact of prevention and treatment approaches to a particular health problem or condition cannot be overstated.

These same considerations are pertinent to the concept of postponement of morbidity as a prevention strategy. Increased life expectancy without postponement of morbidity may actually increase the burden of illness within a population, as measured by prevalence. However, postponement may result in the development of a condition so late in life that it results in either no or less disability in functioning.

Within this framework for considering intervention strategies aimed at health or illness, the potential for prevention as an element of all strategies is clear. There are substantial opportunities to use primary and secondary prevention strategies to improve health in general and reduce the burden of illness for individuals and for society. As noted in the discussion of measuring population health, reducing the burden of illness carries the potential for substantial cost savings. These concepts serve to promote a more rational intervention and investment strategy for the U.S. health system.

OUTSIDE-THE-BOOK THINKING 3-2

© Alfred Bondarenko/Shutterstock.

Select an important health problem (disease or condition) and describe interventions for this problem across the five strategies of health-related and illness-related interventions (health promotion, specific protection, early detection, disability limitation, and rehabilitation) discussed in this chapter.

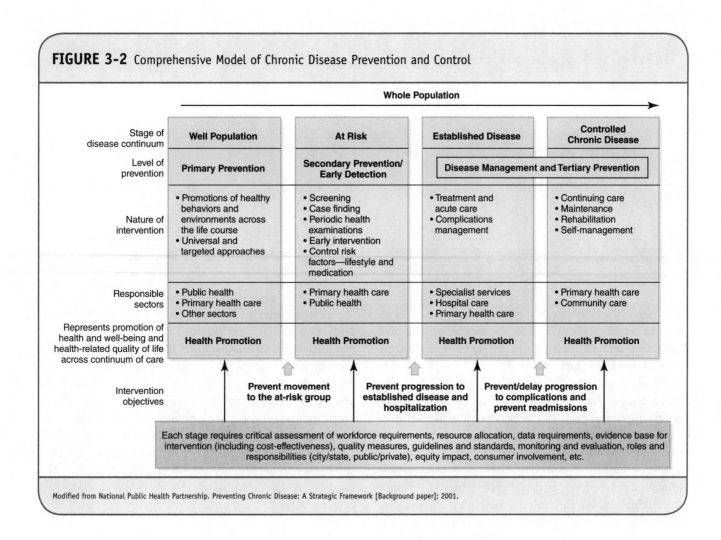

FIGURE 3-2 Comprehensive Model of Chronic Disease Prevention and Control

Modified from National Public Health Partnership. Preventing Chronic Disease: A Strategic Framework [Background paper]; 2001.

Links with Public Health and Medical Practice

Another useful aspect of this view of the health system is in its allocation of responsibilities for carrying out the various interventions. Three practice domains can be roughly delineated: public health practice, medical practice, and long-term care practice.[3] This framework assigns public health practice primary responsibility for health promotion, specific protection, and a good share of early case finding. It is important to note that the concept of public health practice here is a broad one that accommodates the activities carried out by many different types of health professionals and workers, not only those working in public health agencies. Although many of these activities are carried out in public health agencies of the federal, state, or local government, many are not. Public health practice occurs in voluntary health agencies, as well as in settings such as schools, social service agencies, industry, and even traditional medical care settings. In terms of prevention, public health practice embraces all of the primary

prevention activities in the model, as well as some of the activities for early diagnosis and prompt treatment.

The demarcations between public health and medical practice are neither clear nor absolute. In recent decades, public health practice has been extensively involved in screening and has become an important source of primary medical care for populations with diminished access to care.

The mix of population-based and personal health services considered to represent public health practice varies over time and by location and history. The essential public health services framework largely focuses on population-based activities, including monitoring health status, investigating health problems and hazards, informing and educating people about health issues, mobilizing community partnerships, developing policies and plans, enforcing laws and regulations, ensuring a competent workforce, evaluating effectiveness and quality of services, and researching for new insights and solutions. One of

TABLE 3-1   Healthcare Pyramid Levels

- Tertiary Medical Care
  - Subspecialty referral care requiring highly specialized personnel and facilities
  - Secondary Medical Care
  - Specialized attention and ongoing management for common and less frequently encountered medical conditions, including support services for people with special challenges due to chronic or long-term conditions
- Primary Medical Care
  - Clinical preventive services, first-contact treatment services, and ongoing care for commonly encountered medical conditions
  - Population-Based Public Health Services
  - Interventions aimed at disease prevention and health promotion that shape a community's overall health profile

Reproduced from U.S. Public Health Service. *For a Healthy Nation: Return on Investments in Public Health*. Hyattsville, MD: PHS; 1994.

these essential public health services, however, focuses on personal health services by linking people with needed health services and ensuring the provision of health care when it is otherwise unavailable.

Even as public health practice has branched into personal health services, medical practice continues to provide the major share of primary care services to most segments of the population. Medical practice—those services usually provided by or under the supervision of a physician or other traditional healthcare provider—have long been viewed as including three levels as depicted in **Table 3-1**. Primary medical care has been variously defined but generally focuses on the basic health needs of individuals and families. It is first-contact health care in the view of the patient; provides at least 80% of necessary care; includes a comprehensive array of services, on site or through referral, including health promotion and disease prevention, as well as curative services; and is accessible and acceptable to the patient population. This comprehensive characterization of primary care differs substantially from what is commonly encountered as primary care in the U.S. health system. Often lacking from current so-called primary care services are those relating to health promotion and disease prevention.

Modern concepts of disease management have evolved from efforts to provide a more integrated approach to health care delivery in order to improve health outcomes and reduce costs, often for defined populations such as Medicaid enrollees. Disease management focuses on identifying and proactively monitoring high risk populations, assisting patients and providers to adhere to treatment plans that are based on proven interventions, promoting provider coordination, increasing patient education, and preventing avoidable medical complications.

Beyond primary medical care are two more specialized categories of care that are often termed secondary and tertiary care. Secondary care is specialized care serving the major share of the remaining 20% of the need that lies beyond the scope of primary care. Physicians or hospitals generally provide secondary care, ideally upon referral from a primary care source. Tertiary medical care is even more highly specialized and technologically sophisticated medical and surgical care for those with unusual or complex conditions (generally no more than a few percent of the need in any service category). Tertiary care is characteristically provided in large medical centers or academic health centers.

Long-term care is appropriately classified separately because of the special needs of the population requiring such services and the specialized settings where many of these services are offered. This, too, is changing as specialized long-term care services increasingly move out of long-term care facilities and into home and community settings.

These three levels of healthcare services are often portrayed as the upper tiers of a pyramid with population-based public health services included as a fourth tier, as illustrated in **Figure 3-3**. In this pyramid, primary prevention is largely represented by the bottom tier and secondary prevention activities are largely included in primary medical care. Tertiary prevention activities fall largely in the secondary and tertiary medical care components of the pyramid. The use of a pyramid to represent health services implies that each level serves a different proportion of the total population. Everyone should be served by population-wide public health services, and nearly everyone should be served by primary medical care. However, increasingly smaller proportions of the total population require secondary- and

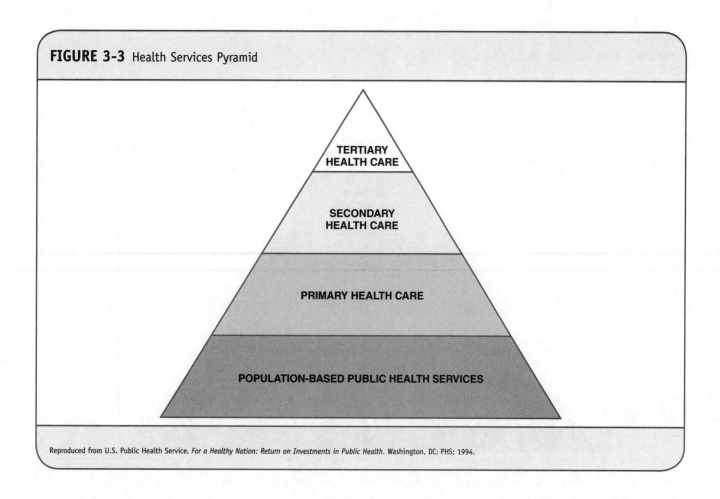

FIGURE 3-3 Health Services Pyramid

TERTIARY
HEALTH CARE

SECONDARY
HEALTH CARE

PRIMARY HEALTH CARE

POPULATION-BASED PUBLIC HEALTH SERVICES

Reproduced from U.S. Public Health Service. *For a Healthy Nation: Return on Investments in Public Health*. Washington, DC: PHS; 1994.

tertiary-level medical care services. This formulation suggests that the medical services should be built on a foundation of population-based services and that the system of services, like a pyramid, should be constructed from the bottom up. It would not be rational to build a pyramid or a health system from the top down; there might not be enough resources to address the lower levels that served the vast majority of the population. Nonetheless, there is ample evidence in later sections of this chapter that this is exactly what has occurred with the U.S. health system. An alternative perspective to the health services pyramid, the health impact pyramid presented in **Figure 3-4**, suggests a more rational design for a health system.

Targets of Health Service Strategies

A final facet of this health system framework characterizes the targets for the various strategies and activities. Generally, primary preventive services are community-based and targeted toward populations or groups rather than individuals. Early case-finding activities can be directed toward groups or toward individuals. For example, many screening activities

target groups at higher risk when these are provided through public health agencies. The same screening activities can also be provided for individuals through physicians' offices and hospital outpatient departments. Much of primary and virtually all of secondary and tertiary medical care is appropriately individually oriented. It should be noted that there is a concept, termed community-oriented primary care, in which primary care providers assume responsibility for all of the individuals in a community, rather than only those who seek out care from the provider. Even in this model, however, care is provided on an individual basis. Long-term care involves elements of both community-based service and individually oriented service. These services are tailored for individuals but often in a group setting or as part of a package of services for a defined number of recipients, as in a long-term care facility.

Public Health and Medical Practice Interfaces

This framework also sheds light on the potential conflicts between public health and medical practice. Although the two are described as separate domains of practice, there

FIGURE 3-4 Health Impact Pyramid

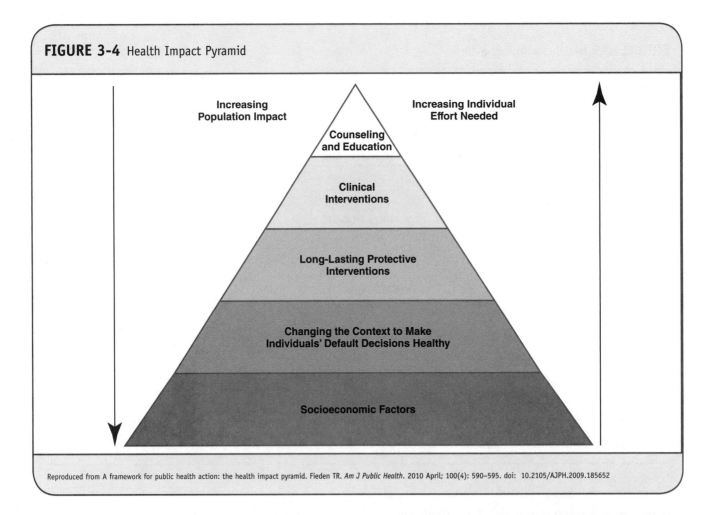

Increasing
Population Impact

Increasing Individual
Effort Needed

Counseling
and Education

Clinical
Interventions

Long-Lasting Protective
Interventions

Changing the Context to Make
Individuals' Default Decisions Healthy

Socioeconomic Factors

Reproduced from A framework for public health action: the health impact pyramid. Fieden TR. *Am J Public Health.* 2010 April; 100(4): 590–595. doi: 10.2105/AJPH.2009.185652

are many interfaces that provide a template for either collaboration or conflict. Both paths have been taken over the past century. Public health practitioners have traditionally deferred to medical practitioners for providing the broad spectrum of services for disease and injuries in individuals. Medical practitioners have generally acknowledged the need for public health practice for health promotion and specific protection strategies. The interfaces raise difficult issues. For example, for one specific protection activity—childhood immunizations—the extensive role of public health practice may actually have served to fragment health services for children. It would be logical to provide these services within a well-functioning primary care system, where they could be better integrated with other services for this population. Despite occasional differences as to roles, in most circumstances, medical practice has supported the role of public health to serve as the provider of last resort in ensuring medical care for persons who lack financial access to private health care. This, too, has varied over time and from place to place.

OUTSIDE-THE-BOOK THINKING 3-3

© Alfred Bondarenko/Shutterstock.

What are the most critical issues facing the healthcare system in the United States today? Before answering this question, see what insights you can find at the web sites of these major health organizations: American Medical Association (www.ama-assn.org), American Hospital Association (www.aha.org), American Nurses Association (www.ana.org), and the Association of American Medical Colleges (www.aamc.org).

Advances in bacteriologic diagnoses in public health laboratories, for example, fostered friction between medical practitioners and public health professionals for diseases such as tuberculosis and diphtheria that were often difficult for clinicians to identify from other common but less serious maladies. Clinicians feared that laboratory diagnoses would replace clinical diagnoses and that, in highly competitive medical markets, paying patients would abandon private physicians for public health agencies.

Some of the most serious conflicts have come in the area of primary care services, including early case-finding activities. Because of the increased yield of screening tests when these are applied to groups at higher risk, public health practice has sought to deploy more widely risk group or community case-finding methods (including outreach and linkage activities). This has, at times, been perceived by medical practitioners as encroachment on their practice domain for certain primary care services, such as prenatal care. Although there has been no rule that public health practice could not be provided within the medical practice domain and vice versa, the perception that these are separate, but perhaps unequal, territories has been widely held by both groups.

It is important to note that this territoriality is not based only on turf issues. There are significant differences in the world views and approaches of these two domains. Medical practice quite properly seeks to produce the best possible outcome through the development and execution of individualized treatment plans. Seeking the best possible outcome for an individual suggests that decisions are made primarily for the benefit of that individual. Costs and resource availability are secondary considerations. Public health practice, on the other hand, seeks to deploy its limited resources to avoid the worst outcomes at the group or population level. Some level of risk is tolerated at the collective level to prevent an unacceptable level of adverse outcomes from occurring. These are quite different approaches to practice: maximizing individual positive outcomes, as opposed to minimizing adverse collective outcomes. As a result, differences in perspective and philosophy often underlie differences in approaches that initially appear to be concerns over territoriality.

An example that illustrates these differences is apparent in approaches to widespread use of human immunodeficiency virus (HIV) antibody testing in the mid- and late 1980s. Medical practitioners perceived that HIV antibody testing would be very useful in clinical practice and that its widespread use would enhance case finding. As a result, medical practitioners generally opposed restrictions on use of these tests, such as specific written informed consent and additional confidentiality provisions. Public health practitioners perceived that widespread use of the test without safeguards and protections would actually result in fewer persons at risk being tested and decreased case finding in the community. With both groups focusing on the same science

in terms of the accuracy of the specific testing regimen, these differences in practice approaches may be difficult to understand. However, in view of their ultimate aims and concerns as to individual versus collective outcomes, the conflict is more understandable.

Perspectives and roles may differ for public health and medical practice, but both are important and necessary. The real question is how best to blend these approaches for purposes of improving health status throughout the population. There is sufficient cause to question current policy and investment strategies. **Table 3-2** examines the potential contributions of various strategies (personal responsibility, healthcare services, community action, and social policies) toward reducing the impact of the actual causes of death discussed previously. This table suggests that more medical care services are not as likely to reduce the toll from these causes as are public health approaches (community action and social policies). Yet, there are opportunities available through the current system and perhaps even greater opportunities in the near term as the system seeks to address the serious problems that have brought it to the brink of major reform.

Medicine and Public Health Collaborations

The need for a renewed partnership between medicine and public health generated several promising initiatives in the final years of the 20th century. Just as bacteriology brought together public health professionals and practicing physicians at the turn of the 20th century to battle diphtheria and other infectious diseases, technology and economics may become the driving forces for a renewed partnership at the dawn of the 21st century. In pursuit of this vision, the American Medical Association and the American Public Health Association established the Medicine/Public Health Initiative to provide an ongoing forum to define mutual interests and promote models for successful collaborations. As a result of this initiative, a variety of collaborations developed, foreshadowing several important components of the Affordable Care Act.[5]

Collaborations between public health and hospitals have also gained momentum. Even prior to the enactment of the Affordable Care Act in 2010, hospitals and managed care organizations had begun to pursue community health goals, at times in concert with public health organizations and at other times filling voids that exist at the community level. In many parts of the United States, hospitals play a leading role in organizing community health planning activities. More frequently, however, they participate as major community stakeholders in health planning efforts organized through the local public health agency. A variety of positive interfaces with managed care organizations have been documented.

TABLE 3-2   Actual Causes of Death in the United States and Potential Contribution to Reduction

	Deaths		Potential Contribution to Reduction*			
Causes	Estimated No.	%	Personal	Healthcare System	Community Action	Social Policy
Tobacco	435,000	19	++++	+	+	++
Diet/activity patterns	400,000	14	+++	+	+	++
Alcohol	85,000	5	+++	+	+	+
Microbial agents	75,000	4	+	++	++	++
Toxic agents	55,000	3	+	+	++	++++
Motor vehicles	43,000	1	++	+	+	++
Firearms	29,000	2	++	+	+++	+++
Sexual behavior	20,000	1	++++	+	+	+
Illicit use of drugs	20,000	<1	+++	+	++	++

*Plus sign indicates relative magnitude (4+ scale).

Data from Fielding J, Halfon L. Where is the health in health system reform? *JAMA*. 1994;272:1292–1296 and Mokdad AH, Marks JS, Stroup DF, Gerberding JL. Actual causes of death in the United States, 2000. *JAMA*. 2004;291:1238–1245.

Hospital boards and executives now commonly include community benefit objectives in their annual performance evaluations. Examples of community health strategies include:

- Establishing "boundary spanner" positions that report to the chief executive officer but focus on community-wide, rather than institutional, interests
- Changing reward systems in terms of salaries and bonuses that executives and board members linked to the achievement of community health goals
- Educating staff on the mission, vision, and values of the institution, and linking these with community health outcomes
- Exposing board to the work of community partners
- Engaging board members with the staff and community
- Reporting on community health performance (report cards)[6]

THE HEALTH SYSTEM IN THE UNITED STATES

This section does not attempt to provide a comprehensive view of the health system in the United States. The intent here is to examine those aspects of the health industry and health system that interface with public health or raise issues of public health significance, with a special focus on the problems of the system that are fueling reform and change.

Data from the *Health United States* series, published annually by the National Center for Health Statistics, will be used throughout these sections to describe the economic, demographic, and resource aspects of the American health system.

Economic Dimensions

The health system in the United States is immense and growing steadily, as illustrated in **Figure 3-5**. Total national health expenditures in the United States doubled in the first dozen years of the 21st century to over $2.8 trillion, four times the sum expended in 1990 and 10 times more than in 1980. Health expenditures are on a pace to reach $4.5 trillion by the year 2020. In order to understand how public health interfaces with other components of the health system in the United States, it is important to consider the context in which these interactions take place—the health sector of modern America. The first decade of the new century witnessed weak economic growth and employment in the United States until the economy deteriorated even further into the recession of 2008–2009. Nonetheless, through periods of both economic prosperity and retrenchment, the health sector has remained a powerful component of the overall U.S. economy accounting for more than one-sixth of the total national gross domestic product (GDP) in 2012. **Figure 3-6** traces the growth in health expenditures as a proportion of GDP.

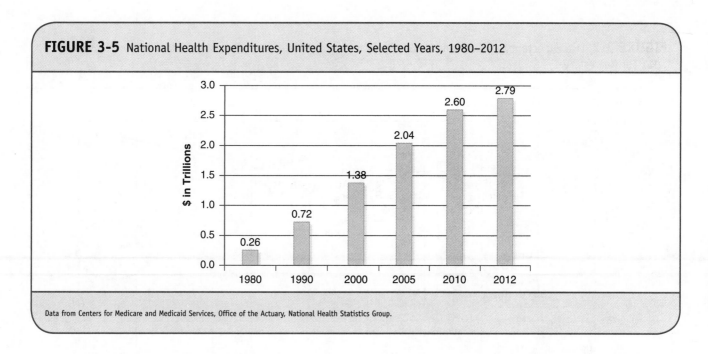

FIGURE 3-5 National Health Expenditures, United States, Selected Years, 1980–2012

Data from Centers for Medicare and Medicaid Services, Office of the Actuary, National Health Statistics Group.

The United States spends a greater share of its GDP on health care than any other industrialized nation. Health expenditures in the United Kingdom and Japan are about one-half and in Germany and Canada about two-thirds the United States figure. Per capita expenditures on health show the same pattern, with United States per capita spending on health more than twice that of Germany, Canada, Japan, and the United Kingdom. Several factors, illustrated in **Figure 3-7**, suggest that this is too much; such as (1) the current system is reaching the point of no longer being affordable; (2) the U.S. population is no healthier than other nations that spend far less; and (3) the opportunity costs are considerable.

Figures 3-8 and **3-9** trace where the money comes from and what it purchases in the U.S. health system.

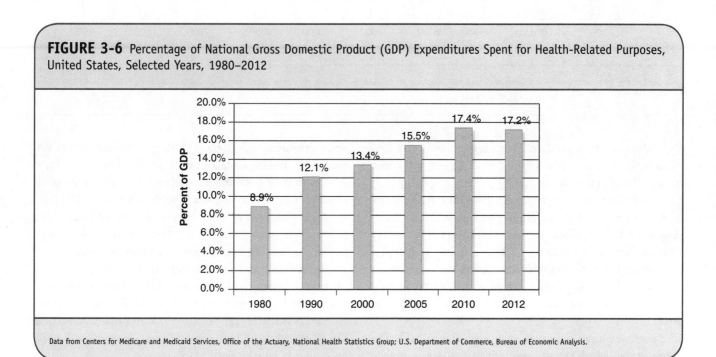

FIGURE 3-6 Percentage of National Gross Domestic Product (GDP) Expenditures Spent for Health-Related Purposes, United States, Selected Years, 1980–2012

Data from Centers for Medicare and Medicaid Services, Office of the Actuary, National Health Statistics Group; U.S. Department of Commerce, Bureau of Economic Analysis.

FIGURE 3-7 Life Expectancy at Birth and Health Spending per Capita, United States and Other OECD Countries, 2011 (or Nearest Year)

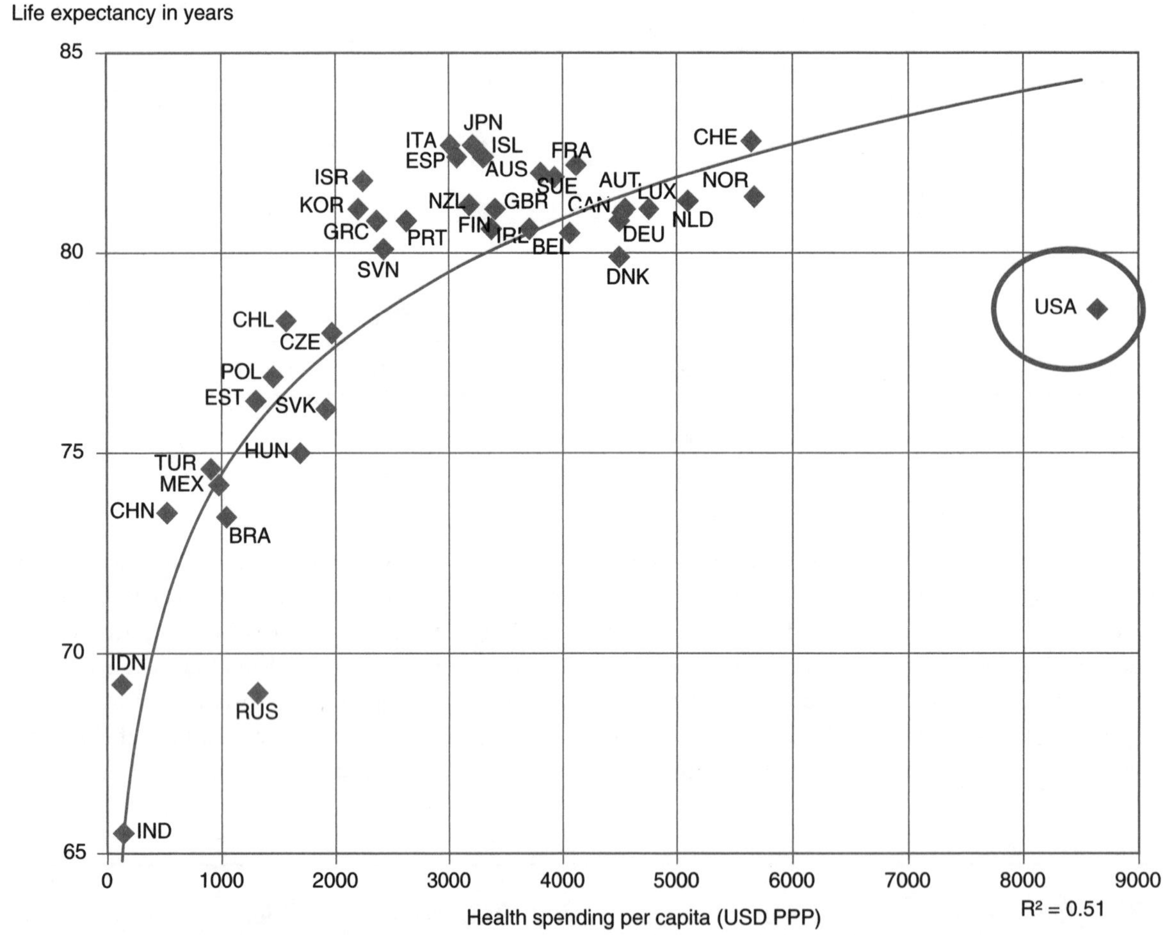

Reproduced from OECD (2013), Health at a Glance 2013: OECD Indicators, OECD Publishing. http://dx.doi.org/10.1787/health_glance-2013-en. [OECD: International Organization for Economic Cooperation and Development].

Expenditures for personal healthcare services comprise 85% of all health expenditures. A little more than one-half of the nation's health expenditures (52%) pay for hospital, physician, and other clinical services; 5% goes for nursing home care, 9% purchases prescription drugs, and 7% supports program administration. Another 24% covers a wide array of other services, including oral health, home health care, durable medical products, over-the-counter medicines, other personal care, research, and facilities, with only 3% devoted to government public health activities (about $75 billion in 2012).

There are three main sources for overall national health expenditures, which include government at all levels, private health insurance, and individuals paying out of pocket. Steadily increasing costs for health services have hit all three sources in their pocketbooks, and each is reaching the point at which further increases may not be affordable. The largest single purchaser of health care in the United States is the federal government, but for all three sources, the ultimate payers are individuals as taxpayers, employees, and consumers. Individuals and families covered by health insurance plans have been experiencing a steady increase in the triple burden of higher premiums, increased cost sharing, and reduced benefits. Health reform provisions of the Affordable Care Act seek to address some of these concerns as we will encounter in later sections of this chapter.

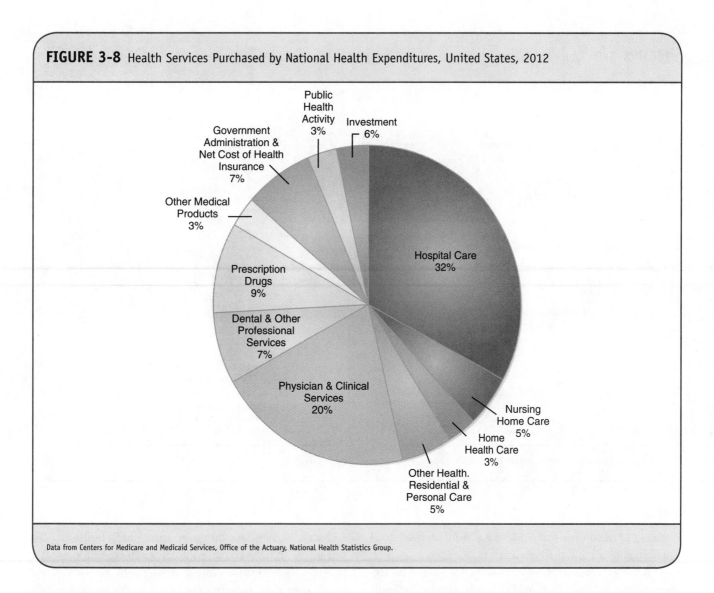

FIGURE 3-8 Health Services Purchased by National Health Expenditures, United States, 2012

Data from Centers for Medicare and Medicaid Services, Office of the Actuary, National Health Statistics Group.

Only limited historical information is available on expenditures for prevention and population-based public health services. A study using 1988 data estimated that total national expenditures for all forms of health-related prevention (including clinical preventive services provided to individuals and population-based public health programs, such as communicable disease control and environmental protection) amounted to $33 billion.[7] The analysis sought to include all activities directed toward health promotion, health protection, disease screening, and counseling. Included in this total, however, was $14 billion for activities not included in the calculation of national health expenditures (such as sewage systems, water purification, and air traffic safety). The remaining $18 billion in prevention-related health expenditures that was included in the calculation of total national health expenditures represented only

3.4% of all national health expenditures for that year. The share of these expenditures that represents population-based public health services cannot be determined precisely from this study but appears to be in the $6 billion to $7 billion range for 1988.

As part of the development of a national health reform proposal in 1994, federal officials developed an estimate of national health expenditures for population-based services.[8] On the basis of expenditures in 1993, this analysis concluded that about 1% of all national health expenditures ($8.4 billion) supported population-based programs and services. U.S. Public Health Service (PHS) agencies spent $4.3 billion for population-based services in 1993, and state and local health agencies expended another $4.1 billion. PHS officials estimated that achieving an "essential" level of population-based services nationwide would require doubling 1993 expenditure

FIGURE 3-9 Sources of Funding for National Health Expenditures, United States, 2012

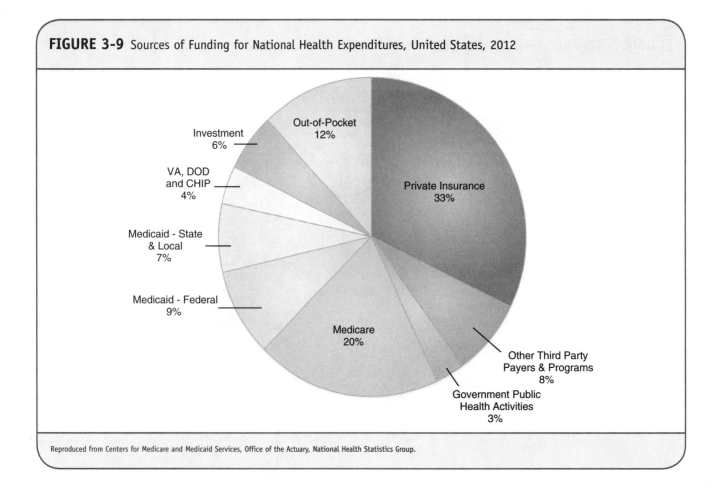

levels to $17 billion and that achieving a "fully effective" level would require tripling the 1993 levels to 25 billion.

The 1994 national health reform effort likely under-counted population-based public health activity expenditures by state and local governments. The results from a comprehensive examination of public health-related expenditures in nine states for 1994 and 1995, together with federal public health activity spending for 1995, suggest that national population-based public health spending totaled $13.8 billion in that year.

Data from the National Health Accounts identify government public health activity as a distinct category within total national health expenditures. The public health activity category captures the bulk of public health spending funded by government agencies, although it excludes spending for several personal services programs widely considered to be important public health services, such as maternal and child health, public hospitals, substance abuse prevention, and mental health services. Environmental health activities provided through environmental protection agencies are also

excluded. Nonetheless, the government public health activity category within the annual national health expenditures total provides useful insights into general public health funding trends over time. Government public health activity spending was $75 billion in 2012, $11 billion from the federal level, and $64 billion from state and local governments. **Figure 3-10** documents the tenfold increase in federal, state and local, and total government public health activity expenditures from 1980 through 2012.

Adjustments to public health activity expenditures are necessary in order to more accurately reflect the full array of activities included in the essential public health services framework, which includes the provision of personal health services when otherwise unavailable in addition to a battery of population-based activities. Figure 3-10 includes an estimate of total essential public health services expenditures developed by adding spending for mental health and substance abuse prevention, maternal and child health services, school health, and public hospitals to the public health activity category in the national health expenditures. For 2012,

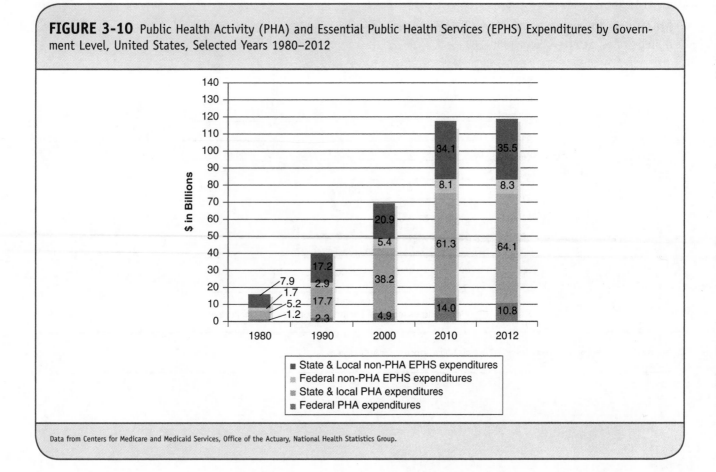

FIGURE 3-10 Public Health Activity (PHA) and Essential Public Health Services (EPHS) Expenditures by Government Level, United States, Selected Years 1980–2012

Data from Centers for Medicare and Medicaid Services, Office of the Actuary, National Health Statistics Group.

estimated essential public health services expenditures were $120 billion, about two times greater than in 2000 and three times more than in 1990.

A subset of overall public health activity expenditures supports population-based public health activities. Methods for estimating population-based public health expenditures, derived from studies completed in the mid-1990s, suggest that national population-based public health expenditures represent only about 1% of total national health expenditures.[9]

On a per capita basis, expenditures for essential public health services and overall governmental public health activities increased by 5–8 times between 1980 and 2012 (**Figure 3-11**). Nonetheless, per capita public health expenditures represented only a tiny fraction of total per capita health spending ($9,500 per person) in the United States in 2012. That share was only 4.3% ($380 per capita) for total essential public health services spending and 2.6% ($240 per capita) for governmental public health activity spending in that year (**Figure 3-12**).

OUTSIDE-THE-BOOK THINKING 3-4

© Alfred Bondarenko/Shutterstock.

Is an ounce of prevention still worth a pound of cure in the United States? If not, what is the relative value of prevention in comparison with treatment?

Macroeconomic trends, however, tell only part of the story. The disparities between rich and poor have also been growing, leaving an increasing number of Americans without financial access to many healthcare services. These and other important aspects will be examined as we review the demands on and resources of the U.S. health system.

FIGURE 3-11 Per Capita Governmental Public Health Activity and Essential Public Health Services Expenditures, United States, Selected Years 1980–2012

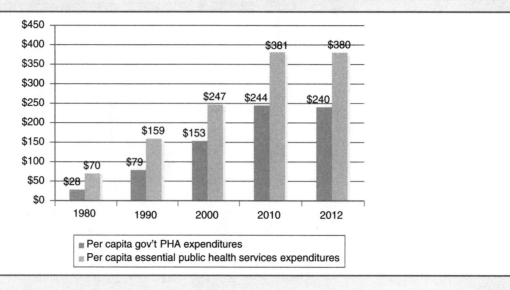

Legend:
■ Per capita gov't PHA expenditures
■ Per capita essential public health services expenditures

Data from Centers for Medicare and Medicaid Services, Office of the Actuary, National Health Statistics Group.

FIGURE 3-12 Expenditures for Essential Public Health Services and Government Public Health Activity as a Percentage of Total Health Spending, United States, Selected Years 1980–2012

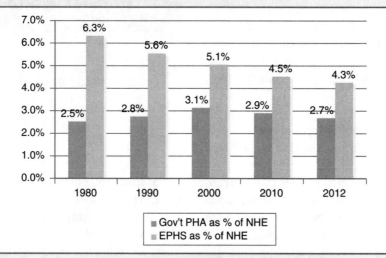

Legend:
■ Gov't PHA as % of NHE
■ EPHS as % of NHE

Data from Centers for Medicare and Medicaid Services, Office of the Actuary, National Health Statistics Group.

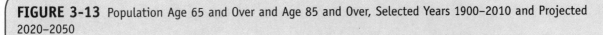

FIGURE 3-13 Population Age 65 and Over and Age 85 and Over, Selected Years 1900–2010 and Projected 2020–2050

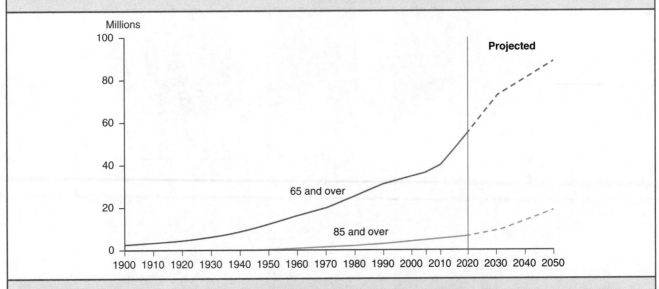

Reproduced from Federal Interagency Forum on Aging-Related Statistics. Available at www.agingstats.gov. Accessed June 28, 2014. Date from U.S. Census Bureau, 1900 to 1940, 1970, and 1980, U.S. Census Bureau, 1983, Table 42; 1950, U.S. Census Bureau, 1953, Table 38; 1960, U.S. Census Bureau, 1964, Table 155; 1990, U.S. Census Bureau, 1991, 1990 Summary Table File; 2000, U.S. Census Bureau, 2001, Census 2000 Summary File 1; U.S. Census Bureau, Table 1: Intercensal Estimates of the Resident Population by Sex and Age for the U.S.: April 1, 2000 to July 1, 2010 (US-EST00INT-01); U.S. Census Bureau, 2011. 2010 Census Summary File 1; U.S. Census Bureau, Table 2: Projections of the population by selected age groups and sex for the United States: 2010–2050 (NP2008-t2).

Demographic and Utilization Trends

Several important demographic trends affect the U.S. health-care system. These include the slowing population growth rate, the shift toward an older population, the increasing diversity of the population, changes in family structure, and persistent lack of access to needed health services for too many Americans. The relative prevalence of particular diseases is another demographic phenomenon but will not be addressed here, although recent history with diseases such as HIV infections and H1N1 influenza illustrates how specific conditions can place increasing demands on fragile health-care systems.

Census studies document that the growth of the U.S. population has been slowing, a trend that would be expected to restrain future growth in demand for healthcare services. However, this must be viewed in light of the projected changes in the age distribution of the U.S. population that are illustrated in **Figure 3-13**. Between 2000 and 2030, the population older than age 65 and older than 85 will double, whereas the younger age groups will grow little, if at all.

There is no evidence that excessive utilization or over-use of services contributes significantly to the high cost of health care in the United States. Underuse of care is actually a greater problem than overuse. Quality reviews consistently document that patients fail to receive recommended care almost half the time and that only about 10% of the time do they receive additional care that is not recommended for their specific health problem or condition.[10] Use of health-care services, in general, is closely correlated with the age distribution of the population. For example, adults age 75 years and older visit physicians three to four times as frequently as do children younger than age 17. Because older persons utilize more healthcare services than do younger people, their expenditures are higher. Obvious reasons for the higher utilization of healthcare resources by the elderly include the high prevalence of chronic conditions, such as arteriosclerosis, cerebrovascular disease, diabetes, senility, arthritis, and mental disorders. As the population ages, it is expected that the prevalence of chronic disorders and the treatment costs associated with them will also increase. This could be minimized through prevention efforts that either avert or postpone the onset of these chronic diseases. Nonetheless, these important demographic shifts portend greater demand for healthcare services in the future.

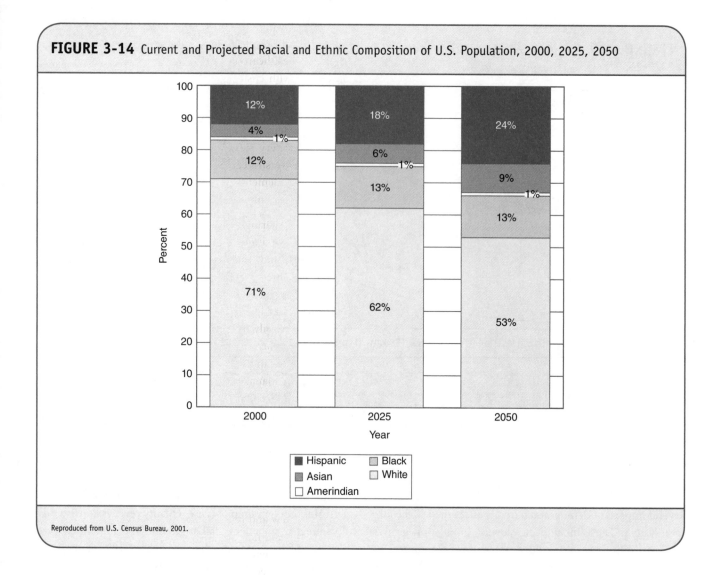

FIGURE 3-14 Current and Projected Racial and Ethnic Composition of U.S. Population, 2000, 2025, 2050

Another important demographic trend is the increasing diversity of the population. The nonwhite population is growing three times faster than the white population, and the Hispanic population is increasing at five times the rate for the entire U.S. population. Between 1980 and 2000, Hispanics increased from 6.4% to 12.5% of the U.S. population. African Americans increased from 11.5% to 14.5% of the total population, while the number of Asian/Pacific Islanders more than doubled from 1.6% to 3.7%. The white population declined from 79.7% to 69.1% of the total population over these two decades. **Figure 3-14** projects these trends forward through mid-century. Notably, these trends reflect differences in fertility and immigration patterns and disproportionately affect the younger age groups, suggesting that services for mothers and children will face considerable

challenges in their ability to provide culturally sensitive and acceptable services. This scenario also underscores the importance of cultural competence skills for health professionals. Cultural competence is a set of behaviors and attitudes, as well as a culture within an institution or system that respects and takes into account the cultural background, cultural beliefs, and values of those served and incorporates this into the way services are delivered. At the same time, the considerably less diverse baby boom generation will be increasing its ability to affect public policy decisions and resource allocations in the early decades of the 21st century.

Changes in family structure also represent a significant demographic trend in the United States. There is only a 50% chance that married partners will reach their 25th anniversary. One in three children live part of their lives in a one-parent household; for black children, the chances are two in three. Labor force participation for women has more than doubled over the past 50 years. Even more indicative of gender changes in the labor market, the proportion of married women in the workforce with children under age five has been increasing in recent decades. Many American households have maintained their economic status over the recent decades with the second paycheck from women in the workforce. As the structure of families diversifies, so do their needs for access, availability, and even types of services (such as substance abuse, family violence, and child welfare services).

Intermingled with many of these trends are the persistent inequalities in access to services for low-income populations, including blacks and Hispanics. For example, despite higher rates of self-reported fair or poor health and greater utilization of hospital inpatient services, low-income persons are substantially less likely to report physician contacts within the past 2 years than are persons in high-income households. Utilization rates for prenatal care and childhood immunizations are also lower for low-income populations.

Healthcare Resources

The supply of healthcare resources is another key dimension of the healthcare system. During the past quarter-century, the number of active U.S. physicians increased by more than two-thirds, with even greater increases among women physicians and international medical graduates. The specialty composition of the physician population also changed during this period, as a result of many factors, including changing employment opportunities, advances in medical technology, and the availability of residency positions. Suffice it to say that medical and surgical subspecialties grew more rapidly than did the primary care specialties. Projections suggest that the 21st century will see a substantial shortage of primary care physicians even while there will be a surplus of physicians trained in the surgical and medical specialties. A continuing shortage of registered nurses has reached crisis proportions in many regions of the United States.

Healthcare delivery models have also experienced major changes in recent years. For example, hospital-based resources have changed dramatically. Since the mid-1970s, the number of community hospitals has decreased, and the numbers of admissions, days of care, average occupancy rates, and average length of stay have all declined, as well. On the other hand, the number of hospital employees per 100 average daily patients has continued to increase. Hospital outpatient visits have also been increasing since the mid-1970s.

The growth in the number and types of healthcare delivery systems in recent years is another reflection of a rapidly changing healthcare environment. Increasing competition, combined with cost containment initiatives, has led to the proliferation of group medical practices, health maintenance organizations, preferred provider organizations, ambulatory surgery centers, and emergency centers. Common to many of these delivery systems since the early 1990s have been managed care strategies designed to control the utilization of services. Elements of managed care strategies generally include some combination of the following:

- Risk sharing with providers to discourage the provision of unnecessary diagnostic and treatment services and, to some degree, to encourage preventive measures
- To attract specific groups, designing of tailored benefit packages that include the most important (but not necessarily all) services for that group; cost sharing for some services through deductibles and copayments can be built into these packages
- Case management, especially for high-cost conditions, to encourage seeking out of less expensive treatments or settings
- Primary care gatekeepers, generally the enrollee's primary care physician, who control referrals to specialists
- Second opinions as to the need for expensive diagnostic or elective invasive procedures
- Review and certification for hospitalizations, in general, and hospital admissions through the emergency department, in particular
- Continued-stay review for hospitalized patients as they reach the expected number of days for their illness (as determined by diagnosis-related groupings)
- Discharge planning to move patients out of hospitals to less expensive care settings as quickly as possible[11]

The growth and expansion of these delivery systems has significant implications for the cost of, access to, and quality of health services. These, in turn, have substantial impact on public health organizations and their programs and services. The majority of the U.S. population is now served through a managed care organization, and that share continues to increase.

CHANGING ROLES, THEMES, AND PARADIGMS IN THE HEALTH SYSTEM

Even a cursory review of the health sector requires an examination of the key participants or key players in the health industry. The list of major stakeholders has been expanding as the system has grown and now includes government, business, third-party payers, healthcare providers, drug companies, and labor, as well as consumers. The federal government has become the largest purchaser of health care and, along with business, has attempted to become a more prudent buyer by exerting more control over payments for services. Government seeks to reduce rising costs by altering the economic performance of the health sector through stimulation of a more competitive healthcare market. At the same time, efforts to expand access through Medicaid and state child health insurance programs and isolated state initiatives toward universal coverage require more, not less, governmental spending. Still, budget problems at all levels make it increasingly difficult for government to fulfill commitments to provide healthcare services to the poor, the disadvantaged, and the elderly. Over recent years, new and expensive medical technology, inflation, and unexpected increases in utilization forced third parties to pay out more for health care than they anticipated when premiums were determined. As a result, insurers have joined government in becoming more aggressive in efforts to contain healthcare costs. Many commercial carriers deploy methods to anticipate utilization more accurately and to control outlays through managed care strategies. Business, labor, patients, hospitals, and professional organizations are all trying to restrain costs while maintaining access to health services.

Reducing the national deficit and balancing the federal budget rely in part on controlling costs within Medicare and Medicaid, as well as in discretionary federal health programs. Except for Medicare, such efforts are likely to be politically popular, even though the public has little understanding of the federal budget. For example, a 1994 poll found that Americans believe healthcare costs comprise 5% of the federal budget, although these costs actually constituted 16% at the time.[12] At the same time, Americans believed that foreign aid and welfare comprise 27% and 19%, respectively, of the federal budget when, in fact, they constituted only 2% and 3%, respectively. When the time comes to balance the federal budget and reduce the national deficit, the American public faces difficult choices as to which programs can be reduced. Public health programs, largely discretionary spending, may not fare well in this scenario.

As these stakeholders search for methods to reduce costs and as competition intensifies, efforts to preserve the quality of health care have become increasingly important. An Institute of Medicine study concluded that medical errors account for as many deaths each year as motor vehicle crashes and breast cancer.[13] Despite the difficulty in measuring quality of medical care, it is likely that quality measurement systems will increase substantially.

Almost certainly, health policy issues will become increasingly politicized. The debate on healthcare issues will continue to expand beyond the healthcare community. Many health policy issues may no longer be determined by sound science and practice considerations, but rather by political factors. Changes in the health sector may lead to unexpected divisions and alliances on health policy issues.

The intensity of economic competition in the health sector is likely to continue to increase because of the increasing supply of healthcare personnel and because of the changes in the financing of care. Increased competition is likely to cause realignments among key participants in the healthcare sector, often depending on the particular issue involved. Dialogue and debate among the major stakeholders in the health system will be influenced by the tension between cost containment and regulation; the interdependence of access, quality, and costs; the call for greater accountability; and the slow but steady acceptance of the need for health reform.

The failure of health reform at the national policy level in 1994 did not avert the implementation of significant improvements in both the public or the private components of the health sector. With or without major changes in national health policies, the health system in the United States has been reforming itself incrementally for decades. With the persistence of cost and access as the system's twin critical problems, new approaches and models were both needed and expected. The federal, as well as state, governments have moved to control the costs of Medicaid services, primarily through attempts to enroll nondisabled Medicaid populations into capitated managed care programs. The rapid conversion of Medicaid services to managed care operations and the growth of private managed care organizations pose new issues for the delivery of clinical preventive and public health services.[11] These changes will likely result in fewer clinical preventive and treatment services being provided through public health agencies, but the extent and impact of these shifts is uncertain.

In any event, the underlying investment strategy of the U.S. health system appears to have changed little over recent decades, with more than 95% of the available resources allocated for treatment services, approximately 4% for essential public health services, and a scant 1% for population-based public health services. Without additional investment in prevention and public health approaches, the long-term prospects for controlling costs within the U.S. health system are bleak. The health reform package enacted in 2010 was a significant step toward universal coverage and meaningful health reform, especially in terms of reducing barriers to access for the 45 million Americans on the fringes of the system and who otherwise would continue to incur excessive costs when they inappropriately accessed needed services. Universal access remains a prerequisite for eventual control of costs. Although the Affordable Care Act addressed a variety of health insurance gaps and abuses, it did relatively little to shift the balance in the U.S. health system from treatment to prevention. **Table 3-3** offers a scorecard on the implementation of key Affordable Care Act (also known as Obamacare) components through 2014.

Although progress along the road to reform has been painfully slow, there is evidence that a paradigm shift is already under way. The Pew Health Professions Commission, among other authorities, argues that the American healthcare system of the 21st century will be quite different from its 1990s counterpart. The 21st century health system will be

- More managed, with better integration of services and financing
- More accountable to those who purchase and use health services
- More aware of and responsive to the needs of enrolled populations
- More able to use fewer resources more effectively
- More innovative and diverse in how it provides for health
- More inclusive in how it defines health
- Less focused on treatment and more concerned with education, prevention, and care management
- More oriented to improving the health of the entire population
- More reliant on outcomes data and evidence[14]

These gains, however, will likely be accompanied by pain. The number of hospitals may decline by as much as 50% and the number of hospital beds by even more than that. There will be continued expansion of primary care in community and other ambulatory settings; this will foster replication of services in different settings, a development likely to confuse consumers. These forces also suggest major traumas for the health professions, with projected deficits of some professions, such as nurses and dentists, and surpluses of others, such as physicians and pharmacists.[14] An estimated 100,000–150,000 excess physicians, mainly specialists, could be joined by several hundred thousand excess

nurses as the hospital sector consolidates and by as many as 40,000 excess pharmacists as drug dispensing is automated and centralized. The massive fragmentation among 200 or more allied health fields will likely cause consolidation into multiskilled professions to meet the changing needs of hospitals and other care settings. One of the few professions likely to flourish in this environment will be public health, with its focus on populations, information-driven planning, collaborative responses, and broad definition of health and health interventions.

Where these forces will move the health system is not yet known. To blend better the contributions of preventive and treatment-based approaches, several important changes are needed. There must be a new and more rational understanding of what is meant by "health services." This understanding must include a broad view of health promotion and health protection strategies and must afford these equal standing with treatment-based strategies. Once and for all, health services must be seen to include services that focus on health, as well as those that focus on ill health. The health status of a population is determined by a complex set of considerations which include social determinants that reflect the fundamental causes of many societal ills operating within a social-ecological model of health and illness. Those considerations are very much the focus of the population-focused public health and prevention interventions. A second and companion change needed is to finance this enhanced basic benefit package from the same source, rather than funding public health and most prevention from one source (government resources) and treatment and the remaining prevention activities from private sources (business, individuals, insurance). With these changes, a gradual reallocation of resources can move the system toward a more rational and effective investment strategy.

OUTSIDE-THE-BOOK THINKING 3-5

Which problems and issues of the health system are improved by the Affordable Care Act? Which are not? What forces are most likely to fuel further movement toward major health system reform in America?

TABLE 3-3 Timeline and Implementation Status of Selected Affordable Care Act Health Reform Provisions

Year	Affordable Care Act Provision ✓ = in effect * = delayed or not yet implemented
2010	
✓	Requires the federal government to create a process, in conjunction with states, where insurers have to justify unreasonable premium increases. Provides grants to states for reviewing premium increases.
✓	Appropriates $5 billion for fiscal years 2010 through 2014 and $2 billion for each subsequent fiscal year to support prevention and public health programs.
✓	Provides a $250 rebate to Medicare beneficiaries who reach the Part D coverage gap in 2010. Further subsidies and discounts that ultimately close the coverage gap begin in 2011.
✓	Provides tax credits to small employers with no more than 25 employees and average annual wages of less than $50,000 that provide health insurance for employees. Phase I (2010–2013): tax credit up to 35% (25% for nonprofits) of employer cost; Phase II (2014 and later): tax credit up to 50% (35% for nonprofits) of employer cost if purchased through an insurance Exchange for two years.
✓	Imposes additional requirements on nonprofits hospitals to conduct community needs assessments and develop a financial assistance policy and impose a tax of $50,000 per year for failure to meet these requirements.
✓	Creates a state option to provide Medicaid coverage to childless adults with incomes up to 133% of the federal poverty level. (States will be required to provide this coverage in 2014.)
✓	Creates a temporary program to provide health coverage to individuals with preexisting medical conditions who have been uninsured for at least six months. The plan will be operated by the states or the federal government.
✓	Creates the National Prevention, Health Promotion, and Public Health Council to develop a national prevention, health promotion, and public health strategy.
✓	Extends dependent coverage for adult children up to age 26 for all individual and group policies.
✓	Prohibits individual and group health plans from placing lifetime limits on the dollar value of coverage, rescinding coverage except in cases of fraud, and from denying children coverage based on preexisting medical conditions or from including preexisting condition exclusions for children. Restricts annual limits on the dollar value of coverage (and eliminates annual limits in 2014).
✓	Requires new health plans to provide at a minimum coverage without cost-sharing for preventive services rated A or B by the U.S. Preventive Services Task Force, recommended immunizations, preventive care for infants, children, and adolescents, and additional preventive care and screenings for women.
✓	Permanently authorizes the federally qualified health centers and NHSC programs and increases funding for FQHCs and for the NHSC for fiscal years 2010–2015.
2011	
✓	Requires health plans to report the proportion of premium dollars spent on clinical services, quality, and other costs and provide rebates to consumers if the share of the premium spent on clinical services and quality is less than 85% for plans in the large group market and 80% for plans in the individual and small group markets.
✓	Provides a 10% Medicare bonus payment for primary care services; also, provides a 10% Medicare bonus payment to general surgeons practicing in health professional shortage areas.
✓	Eliminates cost-sharing for Medicare-covered preventive services that are recommended (rated A or B) by the U.S. Preventive Services Task Force and waives the Medicare deductible for colorectal cancer screening tests; authorizes Medicare coverage for a personalized prevention plan, including a comprehensive health risk assessment.
✓	Creates a new Medicaid state option to permit certain Medicaid enrollees to designate a provider as a health home and provides states taking up the option with 90% federal matching payments for two years for health home-related services.

TABLE 3-3 Timeline and Implementation Status of Selected Affordable Care Act Health Reform Provisions (*continued*)

Year	Affordable Care Act Provision ✓ = in effect * = delayed or not yet implemented
2011	
✓	Provides 3-year grants to states to develop programs to provide Medicaid enrollees with incentives to participate in comprehensive health lifestyle programs and meet certain health behavior targets.
*	Provides grants for up to five years to small employers that establish wellness programs. • Funds have yet to be awarded due to budget debates related to the Prevention and Public Health Fund
✓	Requires disclosure of the nutritional content of standard menu items at chain restaurants and food sold from vending machines.
2012	
✓	Allows providers organized as accountable care organizations (ACOs) that voluntarily meet quality thresholds to share in the cost savings they achieve for the Medicare program.
✓	Requires private individual and group health plans to provide a uniform summary of benefits and coverage (SBC) to all applicants and enrollees. The intent is to help consumers compare health insurance coverage options before they enroll and understand their coverage once they enroll.
✓	Requires enhanced collection and reporting of data on race, ethnicity, sex, primary language, disability status, and for underserved rural and frontier populations.
2013	
✓	Provides a one percentage point increase in federal matching payments for preventive services in Medicaid for states that offer Medicaid coverage with no patient cost sharing for services recommended (rated A or B) by the U.S. Preventive Services Task Force and recommended immunizations.
✓	Increases Medicaid payments for primary care services provided by primary care doctors to 100% of the Medicare payment rate for 2013 and 2014 (financed with 100% federal funding).
✓	Creates the Consumer Operated and Oriented Plan (CO-OP) to foster the creation of nonprofit, member-run health insurance companies.
✓	Extends authorization and funding for the Children's Health Insurance Program (CHIP) through 2015 (current authorization is through 2013).
2014	
✓	Expands Medicaid to all individuals not eligible for Medicare under age 65 (children, pregnant women, parents, and adults without dependent children) with incomes up to 138% FPL and provides enhanced federal matching payments for new eligibles.
✓	Allows all hospitals participating in Medicaid to make presumptive eligibility determinations for all Medicaid-eligible populations.
✓	Requires U.S. citizens and legal residents to have qualifying health coverage (there is a phased-in tax penalty for those without coverage, with certain exemptions). • States were given latitude to let people renew insurance policies that fail to meet the law's benefits standards, so that consumers may buy such policies until October 2016 and keep them for one year after that.

(continues)

TABLE 3-3 Timeline and Implementation Status of Selected Affordable Care Act Health Reform Provisions (*continued*)

Year	Affordable Care Act Provision ✓ = in effect * = delayed or not yet implemented
2014	
✓	Creates state-based American Health Benefit Exchanges and Small Business Health Options Program (SHOP) Exchanges, administered by a governmental agency or nonprofit organization, through which individuals and small businesses with up to 100 employees can purchase qualified coverage. Exchanges will have a single form for applying for health programs, including coverage through the Exchanges and Medicaid and CHIP programs. • Online enrollment via SHOPs delayed until November 2014 although small businesses could get coverage directly from an insurer or an insurance agent or broker before online enrollment becomes available. • Implementation of requirement that SHOPs offer two plans delayed until 2015.
✓	Provides refundable and advanceable tax credits and cost sharing subsidies to eligible individuals. Premium subsidies are available to families with incomes between 133–400% of the federal poverty level to purchase insurance through the Exchanges, while cost sharing subsidies are available to those with incomes up to 250% of the poverty level.
✓	Requires guarantee issue and renewability of health insurance regardless of health status and allows rating variation based only on age (limited to a 3 to 1 ratio), geographic area, family composition, and tobacco use (limited to 1.5. to 1 ratio) in the individual and the small group market and the Exchanges.
✓	Prohibits annual limits on the dollar value of coverage.
✓	Creates an essential health benefits package that provides a comprehensive set of services, limiting annual cost-sharing to the Health Savings Account limits ($5,950/individual and $11,900/family in 2010). Creates four categories of plans to be offered through the Exchanges, and in the individual and small group markets, varying based on the proportion of plan benefits they cover.
*	Permits states the option to create a Basic Health Plan for uninsured individuals with incomes between 133-200% FPL who would otherwise be eligible to receive premium subsidies in the Exchange. • Implementation delayed until 2015.
*	Assesses a fee of $2,000 per full-time employee, excluding the first 30 employees, on employers with more than 50 employees that do not offer coverage and have at least one full-time employee who receives a premium tax credit. Employers with more than 50 employees that offer coverage but have at least one full-time employee receiving a premium tax credit, will pay the lesser of $3,000 for each employee receiving a premium credit or $2,000 for each full-time employee, excluding the first 30 employees. • Implementation date moved to: January 1, 2015 for employers with 50—99 employees. • Implementation date moved to January 1, 2016 for employers with 100 or more employees.
✓	Permits employers to offer employees rewards of up to 30%, potentially increasing to 50%, of the cost of coverage for participating in a wellness program and meeting certain health-related standards; establishes 10-state pilot programs to permit participating states to apply similar rewards for participating in wellness programs in the individual market.
2016	
*	Permits states to form healthcare choice compacts and allows insurers to sell policies in any state participating in the compact. • Scheduled implementation date: January 1, 2016
2018	
*	Imposes an excise tax on insurers of employer-sponsored health plans with aggregate expenses that exceed $10,200 for individual coverage and $27,500 for family coverage. • Scheduled implementation date: January 1, 2018

Modified from Kaiser Family Foundation, Kaiser Commission on Medicaid and the Uninsured and Health Care Marketplace Project. Available at http://kff.org/interactive/implementation-timeline/. Accessed March 10, 2014.

Organizations and systems that are unable to achieve their primary objectives and outcomes often justify their existence in terms of how well they do the things they are doing. Our health system is a prime example of this phenomenon. In such cases, the original outcome (here, improved health status) is displaced by a focus on how well the means to that end (the availability of complex and sophisticated services) are being executed. Processes displace outcomes as the prime purpose or mission for that entity. Instead of "doing the right things" to affect health status, the system focuses on "doing things right" (regardless of whether they actually affect population health status). This outcome displacement allows the United States to boast having the best medical care services in the world while having an inadequate health system.

CONCLUSION

Every day in America, decisions are made that influence the health status of individuals and populations. The aggregate of these decisions and the activities necessary to carry them out constitute our health system. It is important to view interventions as linked with health and illness states, as well as with the dynamic processes and multiple factors that move an individual from one state to another. Preventive interventions act at various points and through various means to prevent the development of a disease state or, if it occurs, to minimize its effects to the extent possible. These interventions differ in their linkages with public health practice, medical practice, and long-term care, as well as in their focus on individuals or groups. The framework represents a rational one, reflecting known facts concerning each of its aspects and their relationships with each other.

As this chapter has described, the U.S. health system focuses mainly on disease states and strategies for restoring, as opposed to promoting or protecting, health. It directs the vast majority of human, physical, and financial resources to tertiary prevention, particularly to acute treatment. It focuses disproportionately on individually oriented secondary and tertiary medical care. In so doing, it raises questions as to whether these policies are effective and ethical.

Characterized in the past largely by federalism, pluralism, and incrementalism, the health sector in the United States is finally undergoing fundamental change due in large part to the massive resources it consumes. We are now realizing that this investment strategy is not producing results commensurate with its costs. Health indicators, including those characterizing large disparities in outcomes and access among important minority groups, are not responding to more resources being deployed in the usual ways. How to control costs while moving toward universal access, consistent quality, and improved outcomes will challenge the U.S. healthcare system through the first quarter of the 21st century.

REFERENCES

1. National Center for Health Statistics. *Health, United States, 2013*. Hyattsville, MD: NCHS; 2014.
2. Rust G, Satcher D, Fryer GE, PhD, Robert S. Levine RS, Blumenthal DS. Triangulating on success: innovation, public health, medical care, and cause-specific US mortality rates over a half century (1950–2000). *Am J Public Health*. 2010 April; *100*(Suppl 1): S95–S104. doi: 10.2105/AJPH.2009.164350
3. Leavell HR, Clark EG. *Preventive Medicine for the Doctor in His Community*. 3rd ed. New York: McGraw-Hill; 1965.
4. U.S. Preventive Services Task Force. Guide to Clinical Preventive Services. Accessible at http://www.uspreventiveservicestaskforce.org/index.html. Retrieved June 13, 2014.
5. Lasker RD. *Medicine & Public Health: The Power of Collaboration*. New York: New York Academy of Medicine; 1997.
6. Weil PA, Bogue RJ. Motivating community health improvement: leading practices you can use. *Healthc Exec*. 1999; *14*: 18–24.
7. Brown RE, Elixhauser A, Corea J, Luce BR, Sheingold S. *National Expenditures for Health Promotion and Disease Prevention Activities in the United States*. Washington, DC: Medical Technology Assessment and Policy Research Center; 1991.
8. Core Functions Project, Public Health Service, Office of Disease Prevention and Health Promotion. Health Care Reform and Public Health: A Paper Based on Population-Based Core Functions. Washington, DC: PHS; 1993.
9. Frist B. Public health and national security: the critical role of increased federal support. *Health Aff* (Millwood). 2002; *21*: 117–130.
10. McGlynn EA, Asch SM, Adams J, et al. The quality of health care delivered to adults in the United States. *N Engl J Med*. 2003; *348*: 2635–2645.
11. Halvorson PK, Kaluzny AD, McLaughlin CP. *Managed Care & Public Health*. Gaithersburg, MD: Aspen Publishers; 1998.
12. Blendon RJ. Kaiser/Harvard/KRC National Election Night Survey. Menlo Park, CA: Henry J. Kaiser Family Foundation; 1994.
13. Institute of Medicine. *To Err Is Human*. Washington, DC: National Academy of Sciences; 1999.
14. Pew Health Professions Commission. *Critical Challenges: Revitalizing the Health Professions for the Twenty-First Century*. San Francisco: University of California Center for Health Professions; 1995.

CHAPTER **4**

Law, Government, and Public Health

Public health is not limited to what governmental public health agencies do, although this is a widely held misperception. Still, particular aspects of public health rely on government. For example, the enforcement of laws remains one of those governmental responsibilities important to the public's health and public health practice. Yet, law and the legal system are important for public health purposes above and beyond the enforcement of laws and regulations. Laws at all levels of government bestow the basic powers of government and distribute these powers among various agencies, including public health agencies. Law represents governmental decisions and their underlying collective social values, providing the basis for actions that influence the health of the public.

Decisions and actions that take place outside the sphere of government also influence the health of the public, sometimes even more than those made by our elected officials and administrative agencies. Private sector and voluntary organizations play key roles in identifying factors important for health and advancing actions to promote and protect health for individuals and groups. Public health involves collective decisions and actions; it is often governmental forums that raise issues, make decisions, and establish priorities for action. Many governmental actions reflect the dual roles of government often portrayed on official governmental seals and vehicles of local public safety agencies—to protect and to serve. As they relate to health, the genesis of these two roles lies in separate, often conflicting, philosophies and duties of government. This chapter will examine how these roles are organized in the United States. This examination particularly emphasizes the relationships among law, government, and public health, seeking answers to the following questions:

- What are the various roles for government in serving the public's health?
- What is the legal basis for public health in the United States?
- How are public health responsibilities and roles structured at the federal, state, and local levels?

To review the organization and structure of governmental public health, this chapter will begin with federal public health roles and activities, to be followed, in turn, by those at the state and local levels. The focus is primarily on form and structure, rather than function. In most circumstances, it is logical for form to follow function. Here, however, it is necessary to understand the legal and organizational framework of governmental public health as part of the context for public health practice. The framework established through law and governmental agencies is a key element of public health's infrastructure and one of the basic building blocks of the public health system. This structure is a product of our uniquely American approach to government.

AMERICAN GOVERNMENT AND PUBLIC HEALTH

Former Speaker of the U.S. House of Representatives, Tip O'Neill, frequently observed, "all politics is local." If this is so, public health must be considered primarily a local phenomenon, as well, because politics are embedded in public health processes. After all, public health represents collective decisions as to which health outcomes are unacceptable, which factors contribute to those outcomes, which unacceptable problems will be addressed in view of resource limitations, and which participants need to be involved in addressing the problems. These are political processes, with different viewpoints and values being brought together to determine which collective decisions will be made. All too often, the term politics carries a very different connotation, one frequently associated with overtones of partisan ideologies. However, political processes are necessary and productive, and perhaps the best means devised by humans to meet our collective needs.

The public health system in the United States is a product of many forces that have shaped governmental roles in health. The framers of the U.S. Constitution did not plan for the federal government to deal directly with health or, for that matter, many other important issues. The word *health* does not even appear in that famous document, relegating health to the group of powers reserved to the states and the people. The Constitution explicitly authorized the federal government to promote and provide for the general welfare (in the Preamble and Article I, Section 8) and to regulate commerce (also in Article I, Section 8). Federal powers evolved slowly in the area of health on the basis of these explicit powers and subsequent U.S. Supreme Court decisions that broadened federal authority by determining that additional powers are implied in the explicit language of the Constitution.

The initial duties to regulate international affairs and interstate commerce led the federal government to concentrate its efforts on preventing the importation of epidemics and assisting states and localities, upon request, with their episodic needs for communicable disease control. The earliest federal health unit, the Marine Hospital Service, was established in 1798, partly to serve merchant seamen and partly to prevent importation of epidemic diseases; it evolved over time into the U.S. Public Health Service (PHS).

The power to promote health and welfare, however, did not always translate into the ability to act. The federal government acquired the ability to raise substantial financial resources through the authority to levy a federal tax on income, which was provided by the 16th Amendment in the early 20th century. The ability to raise vast sums generated the capacity to address health problems and needs through transferring resources to state and local governments in various forms of grants-in-aid. Despite its powers to provide for the general welfare and regulate commerce, the federal government could not act directly in most health matters; it could act only through states as its primary delivery system. After 1935, the power and influence of the federal government grew rapidly through its financial influence over state and local programs, such as the Hospital Services and Construction (Hill-Burton) Act of 1946 and, after 1965, through its emergence as a major purchaser of health care through Medicare and Medicaid. As for a public health presence at the federal level, the best-known and most widely respected federal public health agency, now known as the Centers for Disease Control and Prevention (CDC), was not established until 1946.[1]

The emergence of the federal government as a major influence in the health system displaced states from a position they had held since before the birth of the American republic. States were sovereign powers before agreeing to share their powers with the newly established federal government; their sovereignty included powers over matters related to health emanating from two general sources. First, they derived from the police powers of states, which provide the basis for government to limit the actions of individuals in order to control and abate hazards and nuisances. A second source for state health powers lay in the expectation for government to serve those individuals unable to provide for themselves. This expectation had its roots in the Elizabethan Poor Laws and carried over to states in the new American form of government. Despite this common heritage, states assumed these roles quite differently and at different points in time because the evolution of states themselves during the 19th century took place unevenly.

States developed structures and organizations needed to use their police powers to protect citizens from communicable diseases and environmental hazards, primarily from wastes, water, and food. State health agencies developed first in Massachusetts, then across the country, during the latter half of the 19th century. When federal grants became available, especially after 1935, states eagerly sought out federal funding for maternal and child health services, public health laboratories, and other basic public health programs. In so doing, states surrendered some of their autonomy over health issues. Priorities were increasingly dictated by federal grants tied to specific programs and services.

Each state has the ultimate authority to create the political subunits that serve the residents of a particular jurisdiction. In this manner, counties, cities, and other forms of municipalities, townships, boroughs, parishes, and the like are established. Special-purpose districts for every conceivable purpose—from library services and mosquito control to emergency medical services and education—have also abounded. The powers delegated to or authorized for all of these local jurisdictions are established by state legislatures for health and other purposes. Although many big-city health departments were established prior to the establishment of their respective state health agencies, states are free to use a variety of approaches to structuring public health roles at the local level. Because most states use the county form of subdividing the state, counties became the primary local governmental jurisdictions with health roles after 1900.

State constitutions and statutes impart the authority for local governments to influence health. This authority comes in two forms: those responsibilities of the state specifically delegated to local governments and additional authorities allowed through home rule powers. Home rule options permit local jurisdictions to enact a local constitution or charter and to take on additional authority and powers, such as the ability to levy taxes for local public health services and activities.

Counties generally carry out duties delegated by the state. More than two-thirds of U.S. counties have a county commission form of government, with anywhere from 2 to 50 elected county commissioners (supervisors, judges, and other titles are also used).[2] These commissions carry out both legislative and executive branch functions, although they share administrative authority with other local elected officials, such as county clerks, assessors, treasurers, prosecuting attorneys, sheriffs, and coroners. Some counties—generally, the more populous ones—have a county administrator accountable to elected commissioners, and a small number of counties (less than 5%) have an elected county executive.

Local governments in U.S. cities were first on the scene in terms of public health responses, as noted in our discussion of the history of public health. Big-city health agencies remain an important force in the public health system in the United States. However, after about 1875 when states became more extensively involved, the relative role of municipal governments began to erode. Both local and state governments were enticed by the availability of federal funding, finding it preferable to take what they could get from a higher level of government rather than generating their own revenue to finance needed services.

Many forces have been at work to alter the initial relationships among the three levels of government for health roles, including

- Gradual expansion and maturation of the federal government
- Staggered addition of new states and variability in the maturation of state governments
- Population growth and shifts over time
- Ability of the various levels of government to raise revenues commensurate with their expanding needs
- Growth of science and technology as tools for addressing public health and medical care needs
- Rapid growth of the U.S. economy
- Expectations and needs of American society for various services from their government[3,4]

The last of these factors is perhaps the most important. For the first 150 years of U.S. history, there was little expectation that the federal government should intervene in the health and welfare needs of its citizenry. The massive need and economic turmoil of the Great Depression years drastically altered this longstanding value as Americans began to turn to government to help deal with current needs and future uncertainties.

The complex public health network that exists today evolved slowly, with several shifts in relative roles and influence. Economic considerations and societal expectations, both reaching a critical point in the 1930s, set the tone for the rest of the 20th century. In general, power and influence were initially greatest at the local level, residing there until states began to develop their own machinery to carry out their police power and general welfare roles. States then served as the primary locus for these health roles until the federal government began to use its vast resource potential to meet changing public expectations in the 1930s. Federal grant programs for public health and, eventually, personal healthcare service programs soon drove state actions, especially after the 1960s. It was then that several new federal health and social service programs were targeted directly to local governments, bypassing states. At the same time, a new federal-state partnership for the medically indigent (Medicaid) was established to address the national policy concern over the plight of the medically indigent.

Political and philosophical shifts since about 1980 altered roles once again.[3] Debates over federal versus state roles continued throughout the decades that followed, initially resulting in some diminution of federal influence and enhancement of states' rights. However, the Affordable Care Act in 2010 opened the door to further expansion of the federal role in the health arena. In the end, the federal government has acquired the ability to influence the health system through its fiscal muscle power, as well as its research, regulatory, technical assistance, and training roles.

PUBLIC HEALTH LAW

One of the chief organizing forces for public health lies in the system of law. Law has many purposes in the modern world, and many of these are evident in public health laws. Unfortunately, there is no one repository where the entire body of law, even the body of public health law, can be found. This has occurred because laws are products of the legal system, which, in the United States, includes a federal system and 50 separate state-based legal systems. These developed at different times in response to somewhat different circumstances and issues. Common to each is some form of a state constitution, a considerable amount of legislation, and a substantial body of judicial decisions. If there is any road map through this maze, it lies in the federal and state constitutions, which establish the basic framework dividing governmental powers among the various branches of government in ways that allow each to create its own legal structures.

As a result, four different types of law can be distinguished by virtue of their form or authority:

- Constitutionally based law
- Legislatively based law
- Administratively based law
- Judicially based law

A brief description of each of these forms of law follows.

Types of Law

Constitutional law is ultimately derived from the U.S. Constitution, the legal foundation of the nation, in which the powers, duties, and limits of the federal government are established. States basically gave up certain powers (e.g., defense, foreign diplomacy, printing money), ceding these to the federal government while retaining all other powers and duties. Health is not one of those powers explicitly bestowed upon the federal government. States, in turn, have developed their own state constitutions, often patterned after the federal framework, although state constitutions tend to be more clear and specific in their language, leaving less room and need for judicial interpretation. State constitutions provide the broad framework from which states determine which activities will be undertaken and how those activities will be organized and funded. These decisions and actions come in the form of state statutes.

Statutory (legislatively based) law includes all of the acts and statutes enacted by Congress and the various state and local legislative bodies. This collection of law represents a wide range of governmental policy choices, including

- Simple expressions of preferences in favor of a particular policy or service (such as the value of home visits by public health nurses)
- Authorizations for specific programs (such as the authority for local governments to license restaurants)
- Mandates or requirements for an activity to occur or, alternatively, to be prohibited (such as requiring all newborns to be screened for specific metabolic diseases or prohibiting smoking in public places)
- Providing resources for specific purposes (such as the distribution of medications to patients with acquired immune deficiency syndrome)

If the legislative intent is for something to occur, the most effective approaches are generally to require or prohibit an activity.

The basic requirement for statutory-based laws is that they must be consistent with the U.S. Constitution and, for state and local statutes, with state constitutions as well. State laws also establish the various subunits of the state and delineate their responsibilities for carrying out state mandates, as well as the limits of what they can do. At the local level, the legislative bodies of these subunits (e.g., city councils and county commissions) enact ordinances and statutes setting forth the duties and authorizations of local government and its agencies. Laws affecting public health are created at all levels in this hierarchy, but especially at the state and local levels. Among other purposes, these laws establish state and local boards of health and health departments, delineate the responsibilities of these agencies, including their programs and budgets, and establish health-related laws and requirements. Many of these laws are enforced by governmental health agencies.

Administrative law is law promulgated by administrative agencies within the executive branch of government. Rather than enact statutes that include extensive details of a professional or technical nature and to allow greater flexibility in their design and subsequent revision, administrative agencies are provided with the authority to establish law through rule-making processes. These rules, administrative law, carry the force of law and represent a unique situation in which legislative, judicial, and executive powers are carried out by one agency. Administrative agencies include cabinet-level departments, as well as other boards, commissions, and other entities that are granted this power through an enactment of the legislative body.

The fourth type of law is judicial law, also known as common law. This includes a wide range of tradition, legal custom, and previous decisions of federal and state courts. To ensure fairness and consistency, previous decisions are used to guide judgments on similar disputes. This form of law becomes especially important in areas in which laws have not been codified by legislative bodies. In public health, nuisances (unsanitary, noxious, or otherwise potentially dangerous circumstances) are one such area in which few legislative bodies have specified exactly what does and what does not constitute a public health nuisance. In this situation, the common law for nuisances is derived from previous judicial decisions. These determine under what circumstances and for what specific conditions a public health official can take action, as well as the actions that can be taken.

OUTSIDE-THE-BOOK THINKING 4-1

© Alfred Bondarenko/Shutterstock.

What is the legal basis for public health activities in the United States? What differences are there in the public health powers of federal, state, and local governments?

Purposes of Public Health Law

Two broad purposes for public health law can be described: protecting and promoting health and ensuring the protection of rights of individuals in the processes used to protect and promote health. Public health powers ultimately derive from the U.S. Constitution, which bestows the authority to regulate commerce and provide for the general welfare, and from the various state constitutions, which often provide clear but broad authorities, based largely on the police power of the state. States often have reasonably well-defined public health codes. However, there is considerable diversity in their content and scope, despite similarities in their basic sources of power and authority.

Many public health laws are enacted and enforced under what is known as the state's "police power." This is a broad concept that encompasses the functions historically undertaken by governments in protecting the health, safety, welfare, and general well-being of their citizens. A wide variety of laws derive from the police power of the state, a power that is considered one of the least limitable of all governmental powers. The police power of the state can be vested in an administrative agency, such as a state health agency, which becomes accountable for the manner in which these responsibilities are executed. In these circumstances, its use is a duty, rather than a matter of choice, although its form is left to the discretion of the user.

The courts have upheld laws that appear to limit severely or restrict the rights of individuals where these were found to be reasonable, rather than arbitrary and capricious attempts to accomplish government's ends. The state's police power is not unlimited, however. Interference with individual liberties and the taking of personal property are considerations that must be balanced on a case-by-case basis. At issue is whether the public interest in achieving a public health goal outweighs the public interest in protecting civil liberties. Public health laws requiring vaccinations or immunizations to protect the community have generally withstood legal challenges claiming that they infringed upon the rights of individuals to make their own health decisions. A precedent-setting judicial opinion upheld a Massachusetts ordinance authorizing local boards of health to require vaccinations for smallpox to be administered to residents if deemed necessary by the local boards.[5] Such decisions argue that laws that place the common good ahead of the competing rights of individuals should govern society. Similarly, courts have weighed the power of the state to appropriate an individual's property or limit the individual's use of it if the best interests of the community make such an action desirable. In some circumstances, equitable compensation must be provided. Issues of community interest and fair compensation are commonly encountered in dealing with public health nuisances in which an individual's private property can be found to be harmful to others.

OUTSIDE-THE-BOOK THINKING 4-2

© Alfred Bondarenko/Shutterstock.

What is meant by a state's police power, and how is that used in public health?

The various forms of law and the changing nature of the relationships among the three levels of government have created a patchwork of public health laws. Despite its relatively limited constitutionally based powers, the federal government can preempt state and local government action in key areas of public health regulation involving commerce and aspects of communicable disease control. States also have authority to preempt local government actions in virtually all areas of public health activity. Although this legal framework allows for a clear and rational delineation of authorities and responsibilities, a quite variable set of arrangements has arisen. Often, the higher level of government chooses not to exercise its full authority and shifts that authority to a lower level of government. This can be accomplished in some instances by delegating or requiring, and in other instances by authorizing (with incentives), the lower level of government to exercise authorities of the higher level. This has made for a complex set of relationships among the three levels of government and for 50 variations of the theme to be played in the 50 states. These relationships and their impact on the form and structure of governmental public health agencies will be evident in subsequent sections of this chapter.

There have been many critiques of the statutory basis of public health in the United States. A common one is that public health law, not unlike law affecting other areas of society, simply has not kept pace with the rapid and extensive changes in science and technology. Laws have been enacted at different points in time in response to different conditions and circumstances. These laws have often been enacted with little consideration as to their consistency with previous statutes and their overall impact on the body of public health law. For example, many states have different statutes and legal frameworks for similar risks, such as general communicable diseases, sexually transmitted diseases (STDs), and human immunodeficiency virus infections. Confidentiality and privacy provisions, which trace their origins to the vow in the Hippocratic oath not to reveal patient's secrets, are often inconsistent from law to law, and enforcement provisions vary as well. Beyond these concerns, public health laws often lack clear statements of purpose or mission and are not clearly linked to modern public health core function and essential public health services frameworks.

In view of these criticisms, recommendations have been advanced calling for a complete overhaul and recodification of public health law. Recommendations for improvement of the public health codes often call for

- Stronger links with the overall mission and core functions of public health

- Uniform structures for similar programs and services
- Confidentiality provisions to be reviewed and made more consistent
- Clarification of police power responsibilities to deal with unusual health risks and threats
- Greater emphasis on the least restrictive means necessary to achieve the law's intent through use of intermediate sanctions and compulsive measures, based on proven effectiveness
- Fairer and more consistent enforcement and administrative practices

Although these recommendations have been advanced for several decades, little progress has been made at either the federal or state level. At times, states have sought to recodify public health statutes by relocating their placement in the statute books, rather than dealing with the more basic issues of reviewing the scope and allocation of their public health responsibilities so that these are clearly presented and assigned among the various levels of government. The intricacies of public health law often help drive the inner workings of federal, state, and local public health agencies. We will now turn to the form and structure of these agencies.

GOVERNMENTAL PUBLIC HEALTH
Federal Health Agencies

The U.S. Public Health Service (PHS) serves as the focal point for health concerns at the federal level. Although there have been frequent reorganizations affecting the structure of PHS and its placement within the massive Department of Health and Human Services (DHHS), the restructuring completed in 1996 was the most significant in recent decades. The changes were undertaken as part of the federal Reinvention of Government Initiative to bring expertise in public health and science closer to the Secretary of DHHS. In the restructuring, the line authority of the Assistant Secretary for Health over the various agencies within PHS was abolished, with those agencies now reporting directly to the Secretary of DHHS, as illustrated in **Figure 4-1**. The Assistant Secretary for Health became the head of the Office of Public Health and Science (OPHS), a new division reporting to the Secretary that also includes the Office of the Surgeon General. Each of the former PHS agencies became a full DHHS operating division. These eight operating agencies, the OPHS, and the regional health administrators for the 10 federal regions of the country now constitute the PHS. In effect, PHS has become a functional rather than an organizational unit of DHHS. In 2003, several activities related to emergency preparedness and response were moved into the newly

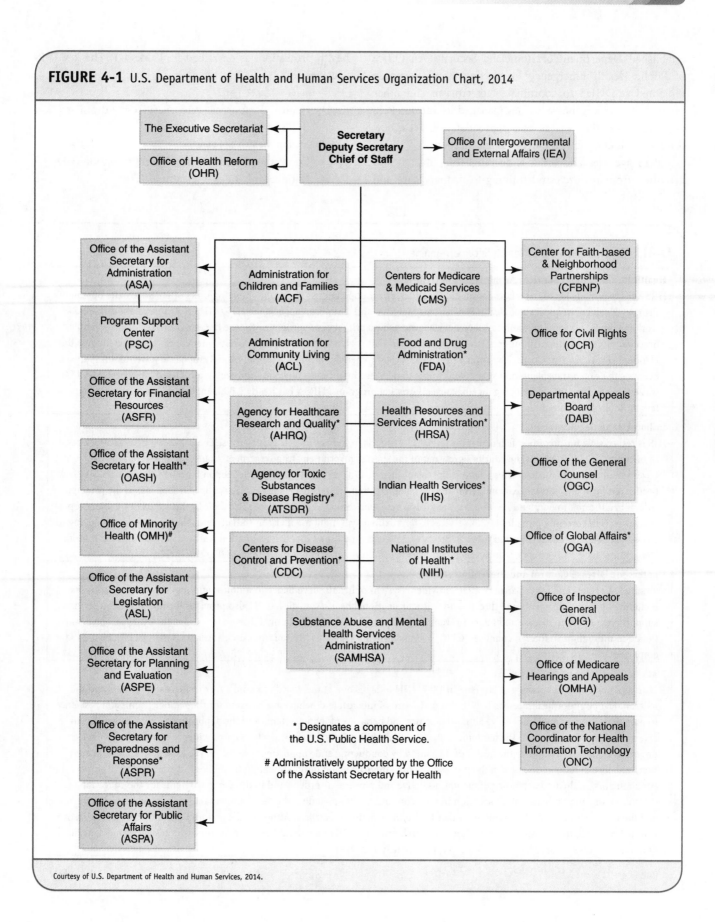

FIGURE 4-1 U.S. Department of Health and Human Services Organization Chart, 2014

established Department of Homeland Security. An Office of Public Health Emergency Preparedness and Response remained at DHHS to coordinate bioterrorism and other public health emergency activities managed by various PHS agencies. These duties were later consolidated under a new Assistant Secretary for Preparedness and Response.

PHS agencies address a wide range of public health activities, from research and training to primary care and health protection, as described in **Table 4-1**. The key PHS agencies are

- Health Resources and Services Administration (HRSA)
- Indian Health Service
- Centers for Disease Control and Prevention (CDC)
- National Institutes of Health (NIH)

TABLE 4-1   U.S. Public Health Service Agencies

Health Resources and Services Administration (HRSA)

HRSA helps provide health resources for medically underserved populations. The main operating units of HRSA are the Bureau of Primary Health Care, Bureau of Health Professions, Maternal and Child Bureau, and the HIV/AIDS Bureau. A nationwide network of community and migrant health centers, augmented by primary care programs for the homeless and residents of public housing, serve more than 10 million Americans each year. HRSA also works to build the healthcare workforce and maintains the National Health Service Corps. The agency provides services to people with AIDS through the Ryan White Care Act programs. It oversees the organ transplantation system and works to decrease infant mortality and improve maternal and child health. HRSA was established in 1982 by bringing together several existing programs. HRSA has nearly 2,000 employees, most at its headquarters in Rockville, Maryland.

Indian Health Service (IHS)

IHS is responsible for providing federal health services to American Indians and Alaska Natives. The provision of health services to members of federally recognized tribes grew out of the special government-to-government relationship between the federal government and Indian tribes. This relationship, established in 1787, is based on Article I, Section 8 of the Constitution, and has been given form and substance by numerous treaties, laws, Supreme Court decisions, and Executive Orders. IHS is the principal federal healthcare provider and health advocate for Native Americans, and its goal is to raise their health status to the highest possible level. IHS currently provides health services to approximately 3 million American Indians and Alaska Natives who belong to more than 564 federally recognized tribes in 35 states. IHS was established in 1924; its mission was transferred from the Interior Department in 1955. Agency headquarters are in Rockville, Maryland. IHS has more than 15,000 employees.

Centers for Disease Control and Prevention (CDC)

Working with states and other partners, CDC provides a system of health surveillance to monitor and prevent disease outbreaks, including bioterrorism events and threats, and maintains national health statistics. CDC also provides for immunization services, supports research into disease and injury prevention, and guards against international disease transmission, with personnel stationed in more than 54 foreign countries. CDC was established in 1946; its headquarters are in Atlanta, Georgia. CDC has 11,000 employees.

National Institutes of Health (NIH)

Begun as a one-room Laboratory of Hygiene in 1887, NIH today is one of the world's foremost medical research centers and the federal focal point for health research. NIH is the steward of medical and behavioral research for the nation. Its mission is science in pursuit of fundamental knowledge about the nature and behavior of living systems and the application of that knowledge to extend healthy life and reduce the burdens of illness and disability. In realizing its goals, NIH provides leadership and direction to programs designed to improve the health of the nation by conducting and supporting research in the causes, diagnosis, prevention, and cure of human diseases; in the processes of human growth and development; in the biological effects of environmental contaminants; in the understanding of mental, addictive and physical disorders; and in directing programs for the collection, dissemination, and exchange of information in medicine and health, including the development and support of medical libraries and the training of medical librarians and other health information specialists. Although the majority of NIH resources sponsor external research, there is also a large in-house research program. NIH includes 27 separate health institutes and centers; its headquarters are in Bethesda, Maryland. NIH has approximately 19,000 employees.

(continues)

TABLE 4-1 U.S. Public Health Service Agencies (*continued*)

Food and Drug Administration (FDA)

FDA ensures that the food we eat is safe and wholesome, that the cosmetics we use won't harm us, and that medicines, medical devices, and radiation-transmitting products such as microwave ovens are safe and effective. FDA also oversees feed and drugs for pets and farm animals. Authorized by Congress to enforce the Federal Food, Drug, and Cosmetic Act and several other public health laws, the agency monitors the manufacture, import, transport, storage, and sale of more than $1 trillion worth of goods annually. FDA has over 15,000 employees. Among its staff, FDA has chemists, microbiologists, and other scientists, as well as investigators and inspectors who visit more than 16,000 facilities a year as part of their oversight of the businesses that FDA regulates. FDA, established in 1906, has its headquarters in Silver Spring, Maryland.

Substance Abuse and Mental Health Services Administration (SAMHSA)

SAMHSA was established by Congress under Public Law 102-321 on October 1, 1992, to strengthen the nation's healthcare capacity to provide prevention, diagnosis, and treatment services for substance abuse and mental illnesses. SAMHSA works in partnership with states, communities, and private organizations to address the needs of people with substance abuse and mental illnesses as well as the community risk factors that contribute to these illnesses. SAMHSA serves as the umbrella under which substance abuse and mental health service centers are housed, including the Center for Mental Health Services (CMHS), the Center for Substance Abuse Prevention (CSAP), and the Center for Substance Abuse Treatment (CSAT). SAMHSA also houses the Office of the Administrator, the Office of Applied Studies, and the Office of Program Services. SAMHSA headquarters are in Rockville, Maryland; the agency has about 600 employees.

Agency for Toxic Substances and Disease Registry (ATSDR)

Working with states and other federal agencies, ATSDR seeks to prevent exposure to hazardous substances from waste sites. The agency conducts public health assessments, health studies, surveillance activities, and health education training in communities around waste sites on the U.S. Environmental Protection Agency's National Priorities List. ATSDR also has developed toxicity profiles of hazardous chemicals found at these sites. The agency is closely associated administratively with CDC; its headquarters are also in Atlanta, Georgia. ATSDR has more than 400 employees.

Agency for Health Care Research and Quality (AHRQ)

AHRQ supports cross-cutting research on healthcare systems, healthcare quality and cost issues, and effectiveness of medical treatments. Formerly known as the Agency for Health Care Policy and Research, AHRQ was established in 1989, assuming broadened responsibilities of its predecessor agency, the National Center for Health Services Research and Health Care Technology Assessment. The agency has about 300 employees; its headquarters are in Rockville, Maryland.

- Food and Drug Administration
- Substance Abuse and Mental Health Services Admini-stration
- Agency for Toxic Substances and Disease Registry
- Agency for Healthcare Research and Quality (AHRQ)

PHS agencies comprise only a small part of DHHS. Other important operating divisions within DHHS include the Administration for Children and Families, the Administration for Community Living, and the massive Centers for Medicare and Medicaid Services (CMS). In addition, there are several administrative and support units for management and the budget.

Beyond DHHS, health responsibilities have been assigned to several other federal agencies, including the federal Environmental Protection Agency (EPA) and the Departments of Homeland Security, Education, Agriculture, Defense, Transportation, and Veterans Affairs, just to name a few. The importance of some of these other federal agencies should not be underestimated in terms of their roles and resources devoted to health purposes. Health-specific agencies at the federal level are a relatively new phenomenon. The first cabinet-level federal human services agency of any kind was the Federal Security Agency in 1939, and PHS itself remained a unit of the Treasury Department until 1944. This historical trivia demonstrates that federal engagement in public health is a relatively recent phenomenon.

The federal government is now the largest purchaser of health-related services, with spending on health representing

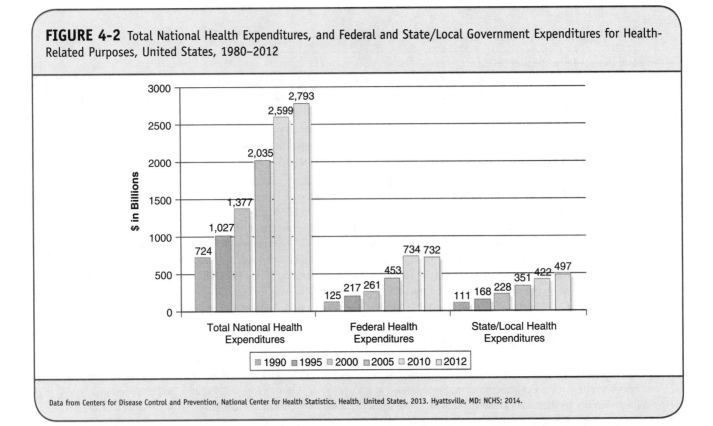

FIGURE 4-2 Total National Health Expenditures, and Federal and State/Local Government Expenditures for Health-Related Purposes, United States, 1980–2012

Data from Centers for Disease Control and Prevention, National Center for Health Statistics. Health, United States, 2013. Hyattsville, MD: NCHS; 2014.

more than one-fourth of the total federal budget. **Figure 4-2** compares total national health expenditures with health expenditures attributed to the federal government and to state and local governments. Escalating costs for healthcare services seriously constrain efforts to reduce the federal budget deficit, and there is little public or political support for additional taxes for health purposes.

It is no simple task to describe the federal budget development and approval process that determines funding levels for federal health programs. Although one-fourth of the federal budget supports health activities, the major share is spent on Medicare and Medicaid. These and other entitlement programs, such as Social Security, comprise two-thirds of the federal budget; this spending is mandatory and cannot be easily controlled. The remaining one-third represents discretionary spending; half of this is related to national defense purposes. Spending for discretionary programs is more readily controlled. Nondefense discretionary spending for health purposes competes with a wide array of programs, including education, training, science, technology, housing, transportation, and foreign aid and is declining as a proportion of all federal spending.

Decisions authorizing and funding health programs are made in an annual budget approval process. The current process is a complex one that establishes ceilings for broad categories of expenditures and then reconciles individual programs and funding levels within those ceilings in omnibus budget reconciliation acts. For discretionary programs, Congress must act each year to provide spending authority. For mandatory programs, Congress may act to change the spending that current laws require. The result is a mixture of substantive decisions as to which programs will be authorized and what they will be authorized to do, together with budget decisions as to the level of resources to be made available through 13 annual appropriations bills. In recent years federal law has imposed a cap on total annual discretionary spending and requires that spending cuts must offset increased mandatory spending or new discretionary programs. This budgetary environment presents major challenges for new public health initiatives and, not infrequently, threatens continued funding for programs that have been operating for decades.

The organization of federal health responsibilities within DHHS is quite complex fiscally and operationally. In federal fiscal year 2015, the overall DHHS budget is about

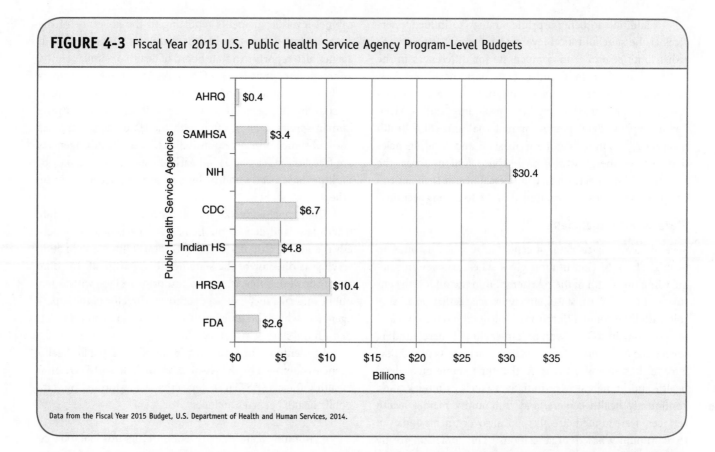

FIGURE 4-3 Fiscal Year 2015 U.S. Public Health Service Agency Program-Level Budgets

Data from the Fiscal Year 2015 Budget, U.S. Department of Health and Human Services, 2014.

$1 trillion.[6] DHHS has nearly 73,000 employees and is the largest grant-making agency in the federal government, with some 60,000 grants each year. DHHS manages more than 300 programs through its 11 operating divisions. The major share of the DHHS budget supports the Medicare and Medicaid programs within HCFA. PHS activities account for less than one-tenth of the DHHS budget.

Budgets for PHS operating divisions in federal fiscal year 2015 range from $30 billion for NIH to $400 million for AHRQ as shown in **Figure 4-3**. Just over 50% of all PHS funds support NIH research activities, and another $32 billion support the remaining PHS agencies with HRSA and CDC together accounting for about $18 billion, which represents only 2% of total DHHS resources and about 0.5% of all federal spending.

As previously described, federal grants-in-aid have long been the prime strategy and mechanism by which the federal government generates state and local action toward health priorities. A variety of approaches to grant making have been used over recent decades. These can be categorized by the extent of restrictions or flexibility imparted to grantees. The greatest flexibility and lack of requirements are associated with revenue-sharing grants. Block grants, including

OUTSIDE-THE-BOX THINKING 4-3

© Alfred Bondarenko/Shutterstock.

What are the primary federal roles and responsibilities for public health in the United States? How do those roles and responsibilities comport with Public Health Service (PHS) agency budget requests for federal fiscal year 2015?

those initiated in the early 1980s, consolidate previously categorical grant programs into a block that generally comes with fewer restrictions than the previous collection of categorical grants. Formula grants are awarded on the basis of some predetermined formula, often based at least partly on need, which determines the level of funding for each grantee. Project grants are more limited in availability and are generally intended for a specific demonstration program or project.

In addition to being a prime strategy to influence services at the state and local level, federal grants also serve to redistribute resources to compensate for differences in the ability of states to fund and operate basic health services. They have also served as a useful approach to promoting minimum standards for specific programs and services. For example, federal grants for maternal and child health promoted personnel standards in state and local agencies that fostered the growth of civil service systems across the country. Other effects on state and local health agencies will be apparent as these are examined in the following sections.

State Health Agencies

Several factors place states at center stage when it comes to health. The U.S. Constitution gives states primacy in safeguarding the health of their citizens. From the mid-19th century until the 1930s, states largely exercised that leadership role with little competition from the federal government and only occasional conflict with the larger cities. Federal funding turned the tables on states after 1935, reaching its peak influence in the 1960s and 1970s. At that time, numerous federal health and human service initiatives (such as model cities, community health centers, and community mental health services) were funded directly to local governments and even to community-based organizations. This practice greatly concerned state officials and served to damage tenuous relationships among the three levels of government. The relative influence of states began to grow once again after 1980, with federal actions restoring some powers and resources to states and their state health agencies. Although states were finding it increasingly difficult to finance public health and medical service programs, they demanded more autonomy and control over the programs they managed, including those operated in partnership with the federal government. Ironically, local governments were making demands on state governments similar to those that states were making on the federal government. States have found themselves uncomfortably in the middle between the two other levels of government as states are one step removed from both the resources needed to address the needs of their citizens and the demands and expectations of the local citizenry.

States carry out their health responsibilities through many different state agencies, although the overall constellation of health programs and services within all of state government is roughly similar across states. In a typical state, there are often two dozen or more state agencies that carry out health responsibilities or activities. Somewhere in the maze of state agencies is an identifiable lead agency for public health. These official health agencies are often freestanding

cabinet-level departments reporting to the governor of the state. In more than one-half of the states, the state health agency also reports to a state board of health or similar entity, although the prevalence of this reporting relationship is declining. Another approach to the organizational placement of state health agencies finds them within a multipurpose human service agency, often with the state's social services and substance abuse responsibilities. State health agencies are freestanding agencies in nearly 30 states and are part of multipurpose health and/or human services agencies in the others.[7]

The official with statutory authority to carry out public health laws and declare public health emergencies is generally the state health officer whose responsibilities also include serving as director of the state health department. In some states, however, this statutory authority resides with other public officials, such as the governor or director of the super-agency in which the state health department is a component, or with the state board of health.

As identified in a recent profile of state public health agencies compiled by the Association of State and Territorial Health Officials (ASTHO), key activities performed by state public health agencies include:

- Running statewide prevention programs like tobacco quit lines, newborn screening programs, and disease surveillance.
- Ensuring a basic level of community public health services across the state, regardless of the level of resources or capacity of local health departments.
- Providing the services of professionals with specialized skills, such as disease outbreak specialists and restaurant and food service inspectors, who bring expertise that is otherwise hard to find, too expensive to employ at a local level, or involves overseeing local public health functions.
- Collecting and analyzing statewide vital statistics, health indicators, and morbidity data to target public health threats and diseases such as cancer.
- Directing statewide investigations of disease outbreaks, environmental hazards such as chemical spills and hurricanes, and other public health emergencies.
- Monitoring the use of funds and other resources to ensure they are used effectively and equitably throughout the state.
- Conducting statewide health planning, improvement, and evaluation.
- Licensing and regulating health care, food service, and other facilities.[7]

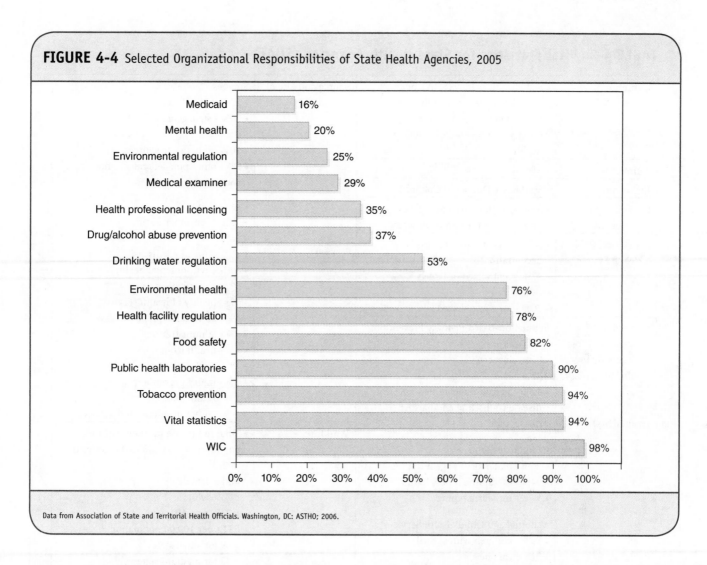

FIGURE 4-4 Selected Organizational Responsibilities of State Health Agencies, 2005

Medicaid	16%
Mental health	20%
Environmental regulation	25%
Medical examiner	29%
Health professional licensing	35%
Drug/alcohol abuse prevention	37%
Drinking water regulation	53%
Environmental health	76%
Health facility regulation	78%
Food safety	82%
Public health laboratories	90%
Tobacco prevention	94%
Vital statistics	94%
WIC	98%

Data from Association of State and Territorial Health Officials. Washington, DC: ASTHO; 2006.

The range of responsibilities for the official state health agency varies considerably in terms of specific programs and services. Staffing levels and patterns also show a wide range, reflecting the diversity in agency responsibilities. The data presented on state health agencies in this chapter are derived from recent surveys of state health officials conducted by ASTHO.[7]

Figure 4-4 illustrates the variability in state health agencies' responsibilities for programs. In 2005, for example, 90% of the official state health agencies administered the Supplemental Food Program for Women, Infants, and Children, vital statistics systems, public health laboratories, and tobacco prevention and control programs. Less than one-half of the state health agencies administered the state Medicaid Program, mental health and substance abuse services, and health professional licensing. Many state health agencies administered programs for environmental health services, most frequently involving food and drinking water safety;

however, only 20% of the state health agencies served as the environmental regulatory agency within their state, which often includes responsibility for clean air, resource conservation, clean water, superfund sites, toxic substance control, and hazardous substances. **Table 4-2** and **Figure 4-5** summarize a wide range of state health agency characteristics and activities. SHAs have made significant progress in completing the three prerequisites for accreditation—state health assessments, state health improvement plans, and agency-wide strategic plans—since 2010 despite budget restrictions and staff reductions.

State health agency responsibilities are anything but fixed in stone. Recent decades witnessed several changes in their public health responsibilities, including more state health agencies taking on preparedness responsibilities and expanding their health planning and development roles. On the other hand, fewer state health agencies are carrying out environmental health and institutional licensing functions

TABLE 4-2   Vital Statistics for State Health Agencies (SHAs)

Definition	• State health agency (SHA), or state department of health, is a department or agency of state government focused on public health.	Source and Use of Funds	Sources • 53%- federal sources • 24% - state general funds • 4% - fees • 10% - other state sources • 9% - other non-federal and non-state sources Use of Funds • 27% - consumer health • 26% - WIC • 10% - infectious diseases • 5% - environmental health • 5% - chronic diseases • 5% - quality of health services • 4% - all-hazards preparedness • 3% - administration • 2% - health laboratory • 1% - vital statistics • 1% - injury prevention • 1% - health data • 10% - other programs and services
Number	• 51		
Jurisdiction Type	• 50 states + District of Columbia		
Organizational Placement	• 58% - freestanding state agency • 42% - unit within umbrella agency		
State-Local Public Health System	• 53% - decentralized or largely decentralized • 27% - centralized or largely centralized • 20% - mixed or shared		

Selected Service Categories Most Frequently Provided by SHAs
 	
(% of SHAs)
	Population-Based Primary Prevention Services
	• 87% - tobacco
	• 85% - HIV
	• 95% - Sexually transmitted disease counseling and partner notification
	
	Laboratory Services
	• 96% - bioterrorism agent testing
	• 94% - foodborne illness testing
	• 94% - influenza typing
	
	Maternal and Child Health Services
	• 59% - children with special healthcare needs
	• 56% - WIC (Supplemental Food Program for Women, Infants and Children)
	• 44% - home visiting services
	
	Access to Healthcare Services
	• 94% - health disparities initiatives
	• 72% - rural health
	• 47% - emergency medical services
		Workforce	• Total full time equivalent (FTE) employees = 101,000 (5,000 fewer than in 2010)
			  ○ 71% female
			  ○ 73% white
			  ○ 93% non-Hispanic
			• FTEs per 100,00 population =
			  ○ 69 for small states
			  ○ 43 for medium states
			  ○ 24 for large states
			• Median FTE employees = 1151

		Governance	• 45% of SHAs relate and/or report to a state board of health • 8% relate and/or report to a similar entity
Expenditures	• Median per capita expenditures = $78 • Mean per capita expenditures = $98	Leadership	• 74% appointed by Governor • 71% with MD degree; 41% with MPH; 10% with DrPH or PhD degree • mean tenure = 3.4 years

Data from Association of State and Territorial Health Officials, Profile of State Health – Volume 3. Washington, DC: ASTHO; 2014.

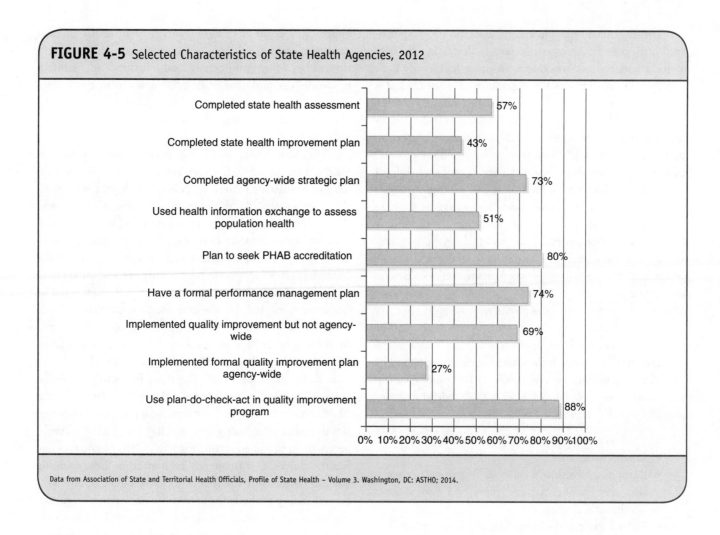

FIGURE 4-5 Selected Characteristics of State Health Agencies, 2012

Completed state health assessment — 57%

Completed state health improvement plan — 43%

Completed agency-wide strategic plan — 73%

Used health information exchange to assess population health — 51%

Plan to seek PHAB accreditation — 80%

Have a formal performance management plan — 74%

Implemented quality improvement but not agency-wide — 69%

Implemented formal quality improvement plan agency-wide — 27%

Use plan-do-check-act in quality improvement program — 88%

0% 10% 20% 30% 40% 50% 60% 70% 80% 90% 100%

Data from Association of State and Territorial Health Officials, Profile of State Health – Volume 3. Washington, DC: ASTHO; 2014.

and some have transferred responsibility for natural disaster preparedness. Notably, all-hazards preparedness and response is now one of the most prevalent of these emerging roles.

In some states regional or district offices carry out state responsibilities and assist local health departments (LHDs). Staff members assigned to district offices often provide consultation and technical assistance to local health agencies especially for purposes of medical oversight, budgetary management, inspectional activities and code enforcement, provision of education and training, and general planning and coordination for activities such as emergency preparedness. More than 50% of the 100,000 full-time equivalent (FTE) employees of state health departments perform their duties from regional, district, or local sites.

With public health responsibilities allocated differently across the various states, data on state public health expenditures are difficult to interpret. These data do not allow for meaningful comparison across states because of the variation

in responsibilities assigned to the official state health agency. Importantly, these data often fail to differentiate between population-based public health activities and personal health services.

OUTSIDE-THE-BOOK THINKING 4-4

© Alfred Bondarenko/Shutterstock.

Access the Web sites of any two U.S. state health departments and compare and contrast the two state-local public health systems in terms of their structure, general functions, specific services, resources, and other important features. Your focus should be on the state-local public health systems in these two states, rather than only the state health agencies!

The organizational placement and specific responsibilities of state health agencies largely determine the size of their budgets and workforce. In order to identify state government expenditures for all public health activities, it is necessary to examine the budgets of multiple state agencies. Data on state health expenditures for fiscal year 2003 indicate that states spent about $10 billion from state sources on population-based public health activities. In addition, states expended another $9 billion of federal funding to support population-based services. Environmental protection, injury prevention, and infrastructure activities were more likely to be funded from state sources. On the other hand, funding for emergency preparedness and chronic disease prevention activity was more likely to come from federal sources. State and federal funds equally supported prevention of epidemics and spread of disease.

In most states, more than a dozen state agencies carry out environmental health roles. This pattern replicates the web of environmental responsibilities among federal agencies, creating a complex system often poorly understood by the private sector and general public. Driving the organization of state responsibilities are several key federal environmental statutes that include

- Clean Air Act
- Clean Water Act
- Comprehensive Environmental Response, Competition, and Liability Act and Superfund Amendments and Reauthorization Act
- Federal Insecticide, Fungicide, and Rodenticide Act
- Resource Conservation and Recovery Act
- Safe Drinking Water Act
- Toxic Substance Control Act
- Food, Drug, and Cosmetic Act
- Federal Mine Safety and Health Act
- Occupational Safety and Health Act

The focus of federal statutes on specific environmental media (water, air, waste) has fostered the assignment of environmental responsibilities to a variety of state agencies other than official state health agencies. The implications of this diversification are important for public health agencies. State health agencies are becoming less involved in environmental health programs; only a handful of states utilize their state health agency as the state's lead agency for environmental concerns. This role has largely shifted to state environmental agencies, although other state agencies are also involved, resulting in state-level environmental strategies shifting from a health-oriented approach to a regulatory approach. Despite their diminished role in environmental concerns, state health agencies continue to address a very diverse set of environmental health issues and maintain epidemiologic and quantitative risk assessment capabilities not available in other state agencies. Linking this important expertise to the workings of other state agencies is a particularly challenging task.[8]

The wide variation in organization and structure of state health responsibilities suggests that there is no standard or consistent pattern to public health practice among the various states. An examination of enabling statutes and state public agency mission statements provides further support for this conclusion. One study found that only 11 of 43 state agency mission statements address the majority of the concepts related to public health purpose and mission in the Public Health in America document.[9] When state public health enabling statutes are examined for consistency with the essential public health services framework (also found in the Public Health in America document), the majority of essential public health services could be identified in only one-fifth of the states. The most frequently identified essential public health services reflected traditional public health activities, such as enforcement of laws, monitoring of health status, diagnosing and investigating health hazards, and informing and educating the public. The essential public health services least frequently referenced in these enabling statutes reflect more modern concepts of public health practice, including mobilizing community partnerships, evaluating the effects of health services, and research for innovative solutions. Only a few states were found to have both enabling statutes and state health agency mission statements highly congruent with the concepts advanced in core functions/essential public health services framework.

State-based public health systems blend the roles of the state health agency and the LHDs in that state. In more than 40 states, all areas of the state are served by an LHD. Where there is no LHD to provide public health services, the state health agency usually provides basic public health coverage. Increasingly, states are using regional or district structures to provide oversight and support for LHDs. In more than two thirds of states, local boards of health also provide direction and oversight of local public health activities.

In sum, states face many challenges related to the fragmentation of public health roles and responsibilities among various state agencies. Central to these are two related challenges: how to coordinate public health's core functions and essential services effectively and how to leverage changes within the health system to instill greater emphasis on population-based preventive services. These are related aims.

Local Health Departments

In the overall structuring of governmental public health responsibilities, LHDs are where the "rubber meets the road." These agencies are established to carry out the critical public health responsibilities embodied in state laws and local ordinances and to meet other needs and expectations of their communities. Although some cities had local public health boards and agencies prior to 1900, the first county health department was not established until 1911. At that time, Yakima County, Washington, created a permanent county health unit, based on the success of a county sanitation campaign to control a serious typhoid epidemic. The number of LHDs grew rapidly during the 20th century, although in recent decades, expansion has been tempered by consolidations.

LHDs should not be considered separately from the state network in which they operate. It is important to remember that states, through their state constitutions and legislatures, establish the types and powers of local governmental units that can exist in that state. In this arrangement, the state and its local subunits, however defined, share responsibilities for health and other state functions. How health duties are shared in any given state depends on a complex set of factors that include state and local statutes, history, need, and expectations.

Local health agencies relate to their state public health systems in one of three general patterns. In most states, LHDs are formed and managed by local government, reporting directly to some office of local government, such as a local Board of Health, county commission, or city or county executive officer. In this decentralized arrangement, LHDs often have considerable autonomy although they may be required to carry out specific state public health statutes.

In some states, oversight of LHDs is shared between the state health agency and local government through the power to appoint local health officers or to approve an annual budget. In other states with decentralized LHDs, some areas of the state lack coverage because the local government chooses not to form a local health agency and the state must provide services in those uncovered areas. This mixed arrangement occurs occasionally in about 20% of the states.

Another 30% of the states use a more centralized approach, in which local health agencies are directly operated by the state or there are no LHDs and the state provides all local health services. Classifying these arrangements as decentralized, centralized, or mixed is useful from the perspective of the state-local public health system. From the perspective of the LHD and the population it serves, however, the LHD is either a unit of local government or a unit of state government or both.

LHDs are established by governmental units, including counties, cities, towns, townships, and special districts, by one of two general methods. The legislative body may create an LHD through enactment of a local ordinance or a resolution, or the citizens of the jurisdiction may create a local board and agency through a referendum. Both patterns are common. Resolution health agencies are often funded from the general funds of the jurisdiction, whereas referendum health agencies often have a specific tax levy available to them. There are advantages and disadvantages to either approach. Resolution health agencies are simpler to establish and may develop close working relationships with the local legislative bodies that create them. Referendum agencies reflect the support of the local electorate and may have access to specific tax levies that preclude the need to compete with other local government funding sources.

Counties represent the most common form of subdividing states. In general, counties are geopolitical subunits of states that carry out various state responsibilities, such as law enforcement (sheriffs and state's attorneys) and public health. Counties largely function as agents of the state and carry out responsibilities delegated or assigned to them. In contrast, cities are generally not established as agents of the state. Instead, they have considerable discretion through home rule powers to take on functions that are not prohibited by state law. Cities can choose to have a health department or to rely on the state or their county for public health services. City health departments often have a wider array of programs and services because of this autonomy. As described previously, the earliest public health agencies developed in large urban centers, prior to the development of either state health agencies or county-based LHDs. This status also contributes to their sense of independence and autonomy. These considerations, as well as the increased demands and expectations to meet the needs of those who lack adequate health insurance, have made many city-based, especially big city-based, LHDs more complex than other LHDs.

Both cities and counties have resource and political bases. Both rely heavily on property and sales taxes to finance health and other services, and both struggle under the limitations of these funding sources. Political resistance to increasing taxes is the major limitation for both. Relatively few counties and cities have imposed income taxes, the form of taxation relied upon by federal and state governments.

Counties play a critical role in the public sector, the extent and importance of which is often overlooked. The overwhelming majority of LHDs are organized at the county level, serving a single county, a city-county, or several counties. As a result, counties provide a substantial portion of the community prevention and clinical preventive services offered in the United States. Counties provide care for tens of millions at a cost of tens of billions from their tax revenues through thousands of sites that include hospitals, nursing homes, clinics, health departments, and mental health facilities. Counties play an explicit role in treatment, are legally responsible for indigent health care in over 30 states, and pay a portion of the nonfederal share of Medicaid in about 20 states. In addition, counties purchase health care for several million county employees.[10]

The National Association of County and City Health Officials (NACCHO) tracks public health activities of LHDs; the most recent survey of LHDs took place in 2013.[10] Data provided in this chapter are derived from this 2013 survey, as well as from several earlier surveys.

One limitation of information on LHDs is that there is neither a clear nor a functional definition of what constitutes a LHD. The most widely used definition calls for an administrative and service unit of local government, concerned with health, employing at least one full-time person, and carrying responsibility for health of a jurisdiction smaller than the state. By this definition, more than 3,000 local health agencies operate in 3,042 U.S. counties. The number of LHDs varies widely from state to state; Rhode Island has none, whereas neighboring Connecticut and Massachusetts each report more than 100 LHDs.

More than two-thirds of LHDs are single-county health agencies, and over 80% operate out of a county base (single county, multicounty, or city-county).[10] Other LHDs function at the city, town, or township levels; some state-operated units also serve local jurisdictions. Although precise numbers are uncertain, it appears that the total number of LHDs has been increasing, from about 1,300 in 1947 to about 2,000 in the mid-1970s to somewhere near 3,000 today.

Authoritative reports going back nearly 70 years have proposed consolidation of small LHDs because of perceived lack of efficiency and coordination of services, inconsistent administration of public health laws, and the inability of small LHDs to raise adequate resources to carry out their prime functions effectively. Consolidations at the county level would appear to be the most rational approach, but only limited progress has been achieved in recent decades.

Most LHDs are relatively small organizations; as illustrated in **Figure 4-6**, 61% serve populations of 50,000 or fewer while 34% of LHDs serve populations of 50,000–499,999. Only 5% of LHDs serve populations of 500,000 or more residents.[10] Fully 90% of the U.S. population is served by an LHD in the medium and large population categories. **Table 4-3** summarizes basic descriptive information on LHDs.

OUTSIDE-THE-BOOK THINKING 4-5

© Alfred Bondarenko/Shutterstock.

Describe the basic structure of a typical local health department (LHD) in the United States in terms of type and size of jurisdiction served, budget, staff, and agency head. (The NACCHO Web site may be useful here!) How does this compare with the LHD serving your community?

Some states set qualifications for local health officers or require medical supervision when the administrator is not a physician. About four-fifths of LHDs employ a full-time health officer. Health officers have a mean tenure of about 9 years. Approximately 15% are physicians. Fewer than one-fourth of LHD directors have graduate degrees in public health.

Local boards of health are associated with most LHDs; in 2013, 70% of LHDs reported working with a local board of health. About 35 states provide for some form of local boards of health. There are an estimated 3,200 local boards of health; about 85% reported an affiliation with an LHD. However, 15% exist independently of any LHD; this pattern is most common in Massachusetts, Pennsylvania, New Hampshire, Iowa, and New Jersey.

Virtually all local boards of health establish local health policies, fees, ordinances, and regulations. **Figure 4-7** indicates that most local boards of health also recommend and/or approve budgets, establish community health priorities, and hire the director of the local health agency. In recent decades, the roles of local boards of health have shifted away from policy making to more advisory duties as local governments have become more directly involved with oversight of their LHDs.

Similar to the situation with state health agencies, data on LHD expenditures lack currency and completeness. Annual LHD expenditures in 2013 ranged from less than

FIGURE 4-6 Small, Medium, and Large LHDs; Percentage of all LHDs and Percentage of Population Served, United States, 2013

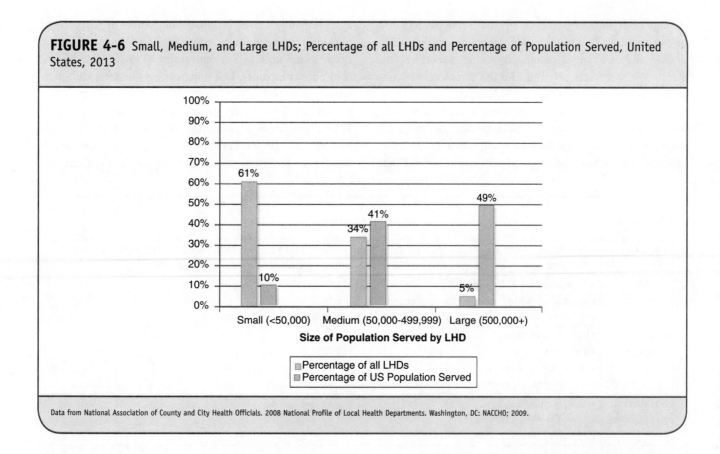

Size of Population Served by LHD

■ Percentage of all LHDs
■ Percentage of US Population Served

Data from National Association of County and City Health Officials. 2008 National Profile of Local Health Departments. Washington, DC: NACCHO; 2009.

$10,000 to over $1 billion. One-half of LHDs had budgets of $1 million or less, and 22% had budgets over $5 million. Total expenditures increase with size of population. LHDs located in metropolitan areas had substantially higher expenditures than their nonmetropolitan area counterparts. The median per capita LHD expenditure level in 2013 was $34 excluding clinical services.

LHDs derived their funding from several sources: local funds (26%), the state (37%, including 17% that were federal funds passing through the state), direct federal funds (2%), Medicaid and Medicare reimbursements (15%), fees (12%), and other sources (8%). Metropolitan LHDs and those serving smaller populations are more dependent on local sources of funding, while LHDs in nonmetropolitan areas and those serving larger populations rely more on state sources.

Revenue from virtually all sources for LHDs had been increasing until the economic recession that began in 2008. The number of FTE workers shows the same pattern. The economic downturn didn't reverse course until 2012 and 2013—well after the official end of recession.

The number of FTE employees also increases with the size of the population served. Only 11% of LHDs employ 125 or more persons, and 68% have 24 or fewer employees. The

number of employees and the number of different occupations and professions are related to LHD population size. Clerical staff, nurses, sanitarians, managers, health educators, and nutritionists are the most common occupational categories.

There is considerable variability in the services provided by LHDs. Top priority areas for LHDs overall are communicable disease control, environmental health, and child health. LHDs serving both large and small populations report similar priorities, although community outreach replaces environmental health as a top priority for the largest local health jurisdictions (those over 500,000 population). Slight differences in priorities are also apparent between metropolitan and nonmetropolitan area LHDs. LHDs in metropolitan areas often include inspections as a high priority, while nonmetropolitan LHDs are more likely to include family planning and home healthcare services as priorities.

Many LHDs provide a common core battery of services that generally includes adult and childhood immunizations, communicable disease control, community assessment, community outreach and education, environmental health services, epidemiology and surveillance programs, food safety and restaurant inspections, health education, and tuberculosis testing. Less commonly, LHDs provide services related to primary care and chronic disease, including cardiovascular disease, diabetes, and glaucoma screening; behavioral and mental health services; programs for the homeless; substance abuse services; and veterinary public health.[12]

LHDs do not always provide these services themselves; increasingly, they contract for these services or contribute resources to other agencies or organizations in the community. Community partners for LHDs include state health agencies, other LHDs, hospitals, other units of government, nonprofit and voluntary organizations, academic institutions, community health centers, the faith community, and insurance companies. LHDs increasingly interact with managed care organizations, although most do not have either formal or informal agreements governing these interactions. Where agreements existed, they were more likely to be formal, to cover clinical and case management services, and to involve the provision (rather than the purchase) of services.

TABLE 4-3 Vital Statistics for Local Health Departments (LHDs)

Definition	• An administrative and service unit of state or local government, concerned with health, employing at least one full-time person, and carrying responsibility for health of a jurisdiction smaller than the state
Number	• Approximately 3200 using the above definition; 2532 in NACCHO sampling frame • Functional definition would reduce number considerably • Ranges from zero in Rhode Island and Hawaii to more than 100 in seven states
Jurisdiction Type	• 68% - single county • 8% - multicounty • 20% - city or town • 4% - other (mostly multiple cities and towns)
Jurisdiction Population	• 61% - <50,000 • 34% - 50,000—499,999 • 5% - 500,000 and greater
Services Most Frequently Provided by LHDs	• 91% - communicable disease surveillance • 90% - adult immunizations • 90% - childhood immunizations • 83% - tuberculosis screening • 78% - environmental health surveillance • 78% - food service establishment inspection • 76% - tuberculosis testament • 72% - food safety education • 69% - population-based nutrition services • 69% - schools and daycare centers inspection
Expenditures	• Mean - $7,220,000 • 25% - < $500,000 • 22% - > $5,000,000 • Median per capita expenditures: $34 (excluding clinical revenue); $39 (all sources)
Source of Funds (from 2008 survey)	• 25% - local • 20% - state • 17% - federal funds passed through state • 2% - federal direct to local agency • 10% - Medicaid reimbursement • 5% - Medicare reimbursement • 11% - fees • 7% - other • 2% - not specified

TABLE 4-3 Vital Statistics for Local Health Departments (LHDs) *(continued)*

Workforce	• Total full-time equivalent (FTE) employees = 146,000 (20,000 fewer than in 2008)
	• Median number of employees = 20
	• Median FTE employees = 17
	  ○ 61% of LHDs with < 25 FTE
	  ○ 13% of LHDs with >100 FTE
	• Median FTEs in selected occupational categories employed by LHDs

Population Served

	<10,000	10,000—24,999	25,000—49,999	50,000—99,999	100,000—249,999	250,000—499,999	500,000—999,999	1,000,000+
All LHD Staff	4	9	15	28	64	130	251	453
Manager	0.7	1	1	2	2	4	14	17
Nurse	1	2.8	4	6	12	19	34.5	44.5
Physician	0	0	0	0	0.3	1	1.7	3
Environmental Health Worker	0.1	1	1.8	3	7	14	25	34
Licensed Practical or Vocational Nurse (LPN/LVN)	0	0	0	0	0	0	2	3
Epidemiologist	0	0	0	0	0	1	2	6
Community Health Worker	0	0	0	0	0.5	2	6	20
Health Educator	0	0	0.6	1	1.7	3	5	9.9
Nutritionist	0	0	0.6	1	3	5	8.5	20.9
Information Systems Specialist	0	0	0	0	0	1	2	4.5
Public Information Specialist	0	0	0	0	0	0	1	1
Emergency Preparedness Staff	0	0.2	0.5	1	1	2	4	5
Behavioral Health Professional	0	0	0	0	0	0	1	0
Laboratory Worker	0	0	0	0	0	0	2	10
Oral Health Care Professional	0	0	0	0	0	0	0	1
Administrative/ Clerical	1	2.5	4	6.8	14	28.3	48.5	101.5

Governance	• 80% of LHDs relate and/or report to a local board of health • for 66% of local boards of health, members of the board are appointed to their positions
Leadership	• more than one-half of local health officers are women • one-fifth of all local health officers have doctoral-level degrees • mean tenure = 8.7 years

Data from National Association of County and City Health Officials, 2013 National Profile of Local Health Departments. Washington, DC: NACCHO; 2014.

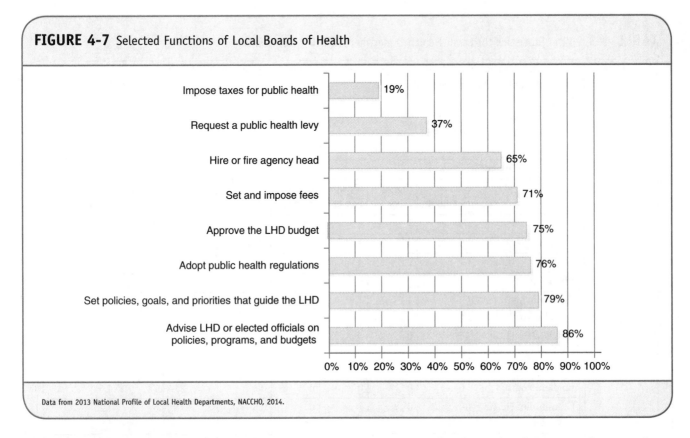

FIGURE 4-7 Selected Functions of Local Boards of Health

Function	Percentage
Impose taxes for public health	19%
Request a public health levy	37%
Hire or fire agency head	65%
Set and impose fees	71%
Approve the LHD budget	75%
Adopt public health regulations	76%
Set policies, goals, and priorities that guide the LHD	79%
Advise LHD or elected officials on policies, programs, and budgets	86%

Data from 2013 National Profile of Local Health Departments, NACCHO, 2014.

INTERGOVERNMENTAL RELATIONSHIPS

In terms of public health roles, no level of government predominates. The relationships between and among the three levels of government have changed considerably over time in terms of their relative importance and influence. This is especially true for the federal and local roles. The federal government had little authority and little ability to influence health priorities and interventions until after 1930. Since that time, it has exercised its influence primarily through financial leverage on both state and local governments, as well as on the private medical care system. The massive financing role of the federal government has moved it to a position of preeminence among the various levels of government in actual ability to influence health affairs. This is evident in the federal share of total national health expenditures and the federal government's role in implementing the Affordable Care Act. However federal public health spending represents only about 1% of total federal health spending, one-fourth less than in 2005 (**Figure 4-8**). This suggests that the relative federal commitment to public health has declined somewhat over recent decades. The federal proportion of total public health activity spending shows a similar pattern (**Figure 4-9**), declining from 20% in 2010 to 15% in 2012. **Figure 4-10** traces public health activity spending from 1980 to 2012.

In recent decades, political initiatives have sought to diminish the powerful federal role and return some of its authority back to the states. However, little in the form of meaningful transfer of authority or resource control has

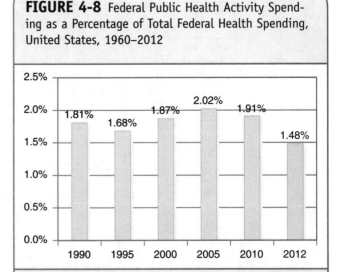

FIGURE 4-8 Federal Public Health Activity Spending as a Percentage of Total Federal Health Spending, United States, 1960–2012

Year	Percentage
1990	1.81%
1995	1.68%
2000	1.87%
2005	2.02%
2010	1.91%
2012	1.48%

Data from Centers for Medicare and Medicaid Services, National Health Accounts (NHA), selected years, 1960–2012.

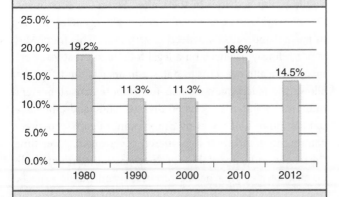

FIGURE 4-9 Federal Public Health Activity Spending as a Percentage of Total Public Health Activity Spending, United States, 1960–2012

Data from Centers for Medicare and Medicaid Services, National Health Accounts (NHA), selected years, 1960–2012.

taken place through 2014. It is likely that the federal government's fiscal muscle will sustain its current upper hand in its relationships with state and local government.

Local government has experienced the greatest and most disconcerting change in relative influence over the 20th century. Prior to 1900, local government was the primary locus of action, with the development of both population-based

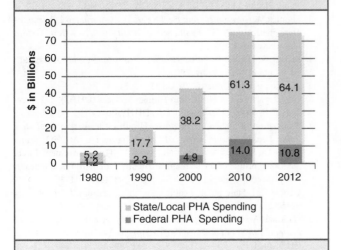

FIGURE 4-10 Federal and State/Local Public Health Activity Spending, United States, 1980–2012

Data from Centers for Medicare and Medicaid Services, National Health Accounts (NHA), selected years, 1980–2012.

interventions for communicable disease control and environmental sanitation and locally provided charity care for the poor. However, the massive problems related to simultaneous urbanization and povertization of the big cities spawned needs that could not be met with local resources alone. States often viewed local governments in general and LHDs in particular as their delivery system for programs and services. In any event, the power of states and the growing influence of financial incentives through grant programs of both federal and state government acted to alter local priorities. Priorities were being established by higher levels of government more often than through local determinations of needs. Although the demands and expectations were being directed at local governments, key decisions were being made in state capitals and in Washington, DC. Unfortunately there are signs that local governments across the country are looking for opportunities to reduce their health roles for both clinical services and population-based interventions where they can. The perception is that the responsibility for clinical services lies with federal and state government or the private sector and that even traditional public health services can be effectively outsourced. How these actions will comport with the widespread belief that services are best provided at the local level raises serious questions regarding new roles of oversight and accountability that are not easily answered. Local governments have lost control over priorities and policies; they bridle under the regulations and grant conditions imposed by state and federal funding sources. As costs increase, grant awards fail to keep pace; however, even with Obamacare wholly or partly uninsured individuals will continue to look to local government for services. These rising expectations and increasing costs are occurring at a time when local governments are unable and unwilling to seek additional tax revenues. The complexities of organizing and coordinating community-wide responses to modern public health problems and risks also push local government to look elsewhere for solutions.

OUTSIDE-THE-BOOK THINKING 4-6

© Alfred Bondarenko/Shutterstock.

What is the basis for the historic and ongoing tension between the powers of the federal government and the powers of states in public health matters?

States were slow to assume their extensive powers in the health arena but have been major players since the latter half of the 19th century. Although the growing influence of the federal government since 1930 displaced states as the most important level of government, their relative role has strengthened since about 1980. Still, states have become secondary players in the health sector. Most states lack the means, political as well as statutory, to intervene effectively in the portion of the health sector located within their jurisdictional boundaries. This is further complicated by their tradition of imitating the federal health bureaucracy whenever possible through the decentralization of health roles and responsibilities throughout dozens of administrative agencies. Coordination of programs, policies, and priorities has become exceedingly difficult within state government. Still, the widely disparate circumstances from state to state make for laboratories of opportunity in which innovative approaches can be developed and evaluated.

The relationship between state and local government in public health has traditionally been tenuous and difficult. Just as the federal government views the states, states themselves have come to view local governments as just another way to get things done. As a result, states have turned to other parties, such as community-based organizations, and have begun to deal directly with them, leaving local government on the sidelines. This undervaluing of LHDs, when coupled with competing priorities, such as education, public safety, and transportation, within local governments, presents major challenges for the future of public health services in the U.S. Instead of becoming stronger allies, these forces are working to pull apart the fabric of the national public health network.

These ever-changing and evolving relationships call into question whether the governmental public health network can be strengthened through a more centralized approach involving greater federal leadership and direction.[11] With a continued emphasis on decentralization, some states may truly be laboratories of innovation and offer creative solutions. There are many examples of creative policies and programs at the state level, but there are also many examples of state creativity being stifled by the federal government. The history of state requests for waivers of Medicaid requirements is a case in point. Many states waited several years or more for federal approval of the waivers necessary to begin innovative programs, and some of the more creative proposals were actually rejected. Still, it can be argued that state political processes are more reflective of the different political values that must be reconciled for progressive policies to develop.

CONCLUSION

Public health activities in the United States are coordinated by a network of state and local public health agencies working in partnership with the federal government. This framework is precariously balanced on a legal foundation that gives primacy for health concerns to states, a financial foundation that allows the federal government to promote consistency and minimum standards across 50 diverse states, and a practical foundation of LHDs serving as the point of contact between communities and their three-tiered government. Over time, the relative influence of these partners has shifted dramatically because of changing needs, resources, and public expectations. The challenges to this dynamic organizational structure are many. There are increasing calls for government to turn over many public programs to private interests and growing distrust of government, in general. These developments make it easy to forget that many of the public health achievements of the past century would not have been possible without a serious commitment of resources and leadership by those in the public sector. In any event, it is clear that the organizational structure of public health—its form—intimately reflects the structure of government in the United States. The extent to which public health's form facilitates or impedes its effective functioning is the focus of an upcoming chapter.

REFERENCES

1. Centers for Disease Control and Prevention. History of CDC. *MMWR.* 1996; *45*: 526–528.
2. Centers for Disease Control and Prevention. *Profile of State and Local Public Health Systems 1990.* Atlanta, GA: CDC; 1991.
3. Shonick W. *Government and Health Services: Government's Role in the Development of the U.S. Health Services 1930–1980.* New York: Oxford University Press; 1995.
4. Pickett G, Hanlon JJ. *Public Health Administration and Practice.* 9th ed. St. Louis, MO: Mosby; 1990.
5. *Jacobson v Massachusetts.* 197 US 11 (1905).
6. U.S. Department of Health and Human Services (DHHS). *The Fiscal Year 2015 Budget.* Washington, DC: DHHS; 2014.
7. Association of State and Territorial Health Officials. *Profile of State Public Health, Volume Three, 2012.* Washington, DC: ASTHO; 2014.
8. Burke TA, Shalauta NM, Tran NL, Stern BS. The environmental web: a national profile of the state infrastructure for environmental health and protection. *J Public Health Manage Pract.* 1997; *3*: 1–12.
9. Gebbie KM. State public health laws: an expression of constituency expectations. *J Public Health Manage Pract.* 2000; *6*: 46–54.
10. National Association of County and City Health Officials. *2013 National Profile of Local Health Departments.* Washington, DC; NACCHO; 2014.
11. Turnock BJ, Atchison C. Governmental public health in the United States: the implications of federalism. *Health Aff.* 2002; *6*: 68–78.

CHAPTER **5**

Twenty-First Century Community Public Health Practice

The Institute of Medicine's (IOM) landmark report in 1988, *The Future of Public Health*, stimulated important changes in the U.S. public health system.[1] The IOM report rearticulated the mission, substance, and core functions of public health and challenged the public health community to think more strategically, plan more collectively, and perform more effectively. Exciting opportunities afforded by broader participation through engaging communities and other stakeholders, heightened public expectations for addressing threats and emergencies, and the potential for better integration of public health and medical care activities have energized these efforts. These developments brought change to the public health system while offering new hope for achieving improved health outcomes through public health practice. This chapter examines the link between public health's functions and public health practice, focusing on the organizing concepts for modern public health practice and how these have advanced new standards for public health practice. Key questions to be addressed in this chapter are as follows:

- What have been public health's main functions over the past century?
- What are the core functions of public health today?
- How are these functions translated into practice?
- What are the current standards for community public health practice?

Improvement science asserts that results reflect the systems that produce them. In other words, every system is perfectly designed to achieve the exact results it gets. This somewhat elliptical wisdom underscores a major challenge confronting efforts to enhance the results of public health practice: Improving health outcomes calls for improving the basic processes of public health practice. However, as some additional reasoning from the improvement scientists warns, to improve something, we must be able to control it; to control it, we must be able to understand it; and to understand it, we must be able to measure it. Measurement relies on operational definitions for the concepts of interest. Improving the performance of public health functions is an agenda that defines, measures, understands, and controls the processes that constitute public health practice.

For nearly 100 years, the public health community has been grappling with this agenda, with only limited success along the way.[2] For much of the 20th century, an adequate conceptual framework for defining the public health system was lacking. As a result, past efforts generally focused on measuring aspects of the public health system that only indirectly or partially characterized the functions carried out in public health practice. This limited opportunities for understanding, controlling, and improving public health practice and health outcomes. Nonetheless, these efforts paved the way for developments that were subsequently jump-started by the 1988 IOM report.

PUBLIC HEALTH FUNCTIONS AND PRACTICE BEFORE 1990

Over much of the past century, the mission and purpose of public health (what it is) and its functions (how it addresses its mission) were viewed as synonymous with the provision of public health services. In fact, public health's services were frequently characterized as its functions. Public health was known more by its deeds than its intent. As a result, early efforts to describe and measure public health practice focused primarily on measuring aspects of important public health services.

The earliest attempts to define and measure public health practice in the United States date back to 1914. Before that time, public health functions were primarily those identified in the broad statutes of state and local governments, centering on the prevention and control of infectious diseases. In 1914, however, a survey catalogued the various services of state health agencies, as well as their role in fostering the development of local health departments (LHDs). This study concluded that even though public health agencies were carrying out a wide variety of programs and services they were missing their mark. Much of what was being done through public health agencies had little effect on community health status, and there was actually much that these agencies could have been doing that would have reduced mortality and morbidity.[3] Public health practice was evaluated using a scoring system that placed greater weight on some public health activities and services than on others, allowing a basis for comparisons across agencies. Key elements of this approach were soon incorporated into local public health assessment initiatives orchestrated by the American Public Health Association (APHA).

In 1921, the first report of APHA's Committee on Municipal Health Department Practice called for the systematic collection and analysis of information on local public health practice to support the development of standards for LHDs serving the nation's largest municipalities. The committee had determined that LHDs and the communities they served would benefit from standards that would ensure a consistent level of public health services from one jurisdiction to another. The committee also sought to identify characteristics of LHD practice that produce the best results. An elaborate survey instrument and process were established; more than 80 big-city health departments were reviewed in the initial effort.

The need to examine public health practice outside the nation's large cities, especially in the growing number of county-based LHDs, was soon apparent. In 1925, the committee was reconstituted as the Committee on Administrative Practice to assess more broadly the status of public health practice in the United States. The new committee developed the first version of an "Appraisal Form" to be used as a self-assessment tool by local health officers. The intent was to measure the immediate results attained from local public health services. Examples of these immediate results follow:

- Birth and death records adequately catalogued and analyzed
- Various vaccinations provided for specific age groups
- Health problems in school-aged children identified and treated
- Tuberculosis cases hospitalized and treated
- Laboratory tests performed[4]

Successive iterations of the Appraisal Form appeared through the 1920s and 1930s; these were well received by the public health community, although there were occasional concerns that quantity was being emphasized over quality. Local health officers were able to compare their ratings with those of other public health agencies. The basis for comparison was a numerical rating score, based on aggregated points awarded across key administrative and service areas. Comparative ratings were used to improve health programs, advocate for resources, summarize health agency activities in annual reports, and engage other health interests in the community. Agency ratings often attracted considerable public interest, resulting in both good and bad publicity for local agencies. Despite the initial intent to emphasize immediate results, however, the major focus of the ratings remained on measuring the more concrete aspects of public health practice, such as staff, clinic sites, patient visits, and the number of services rendered.

In 1943, a new instrument, the "Evaluation Schedule," which was scored centrally by the APHA Committee on Administrative Practice, replaced the self-assessment approach used in the Appraisal Form. The scores for health agencies of varying size and type were widely disseminated so that individual LHDs could directly compare

TABLE 5-1   Public Health Practice Performance Measures from 1947 Evaluation Schedule

1. Hospital beds: percentage in approved hospitals
2. Practicing physicians: population per physician
3. Practicing dentists: population per dentist
4. Water: percentage of population in communities over 2,500 served with approved water
5. Sewerage: percentage of population in communities over 2,500 served with approved sewerage systems
6. Water: percentage of rural schoolchildren served with approved water supplies
7. Excreta disposal: percentage of rural schoolchildren served with approved means of excreta disposal
8. Food: percentage of food handlers reached by group instruction program
9. Food: percentage of restaurants and lunch counters with satisfactory facilities
10. Milk: percentage of bottled milk pasteurized
11. Diphtheria: percentage of children under 2 years given immunizing agent
12. Smallpox: percentage of children under 2 years given immunizing agent
13. Whooping cough: percentage of children under 2 years given immunizing agent
14. Tuberculosis: newly reported cases per death, 5-year period
15. Tuberculosis: deaths per 100,000 population, 5-year period
16. Tuberculosis: percentage of cases reported by death certificate
17. Syphilis: percentage of cases reported in primary, secondary, and early latent stage
18. Syphilis: percentage of reported contacts examined
19. Maternal: puerperal deaths per 1,000 total births, 5-year rate
20. Maternal: percentage of antepartum cases under medical supervision seen before the sixth month
21. Maternal: percentage of women delivered at home under postpartum nursing supervision
22. Maternal: percentage of births in hospital
23. Infant: deaths under 1 year of age per 1,000 live births, 5-year rate
24. Infant: deaths from diarrhea and enteritis under 1 year per 1,000 live births, 2-year rate
25. Infant: percentage of infants under nursing supervision before 1 month
26. School: percentage of elementary children with dental work neglected
27. Accidents: deaths from motor accidents per 100,000 population, 5-year rate
28. Health department budget: cents per capita spent by health department

Data from American Public Health Association, Committee on Administrative Practice. *Evaluation Schedule for Use in Study and Appraisal of Community Health Programs.* New York, NY: APHA; 1947.

their performance in meeting community needs with that of their peers. **Table 5-1** lists some of the key performance measures included in the 1947 version of the Evaluation Schedule.

To develop a blueprint for a national network of LHDs that would provide every American with public health coverage, the Committee on Administrative Practice established a Subcommittee on Local Health Units. The subcommittee's major report (widely known as the Emerson Report) in 1945 was a landmark for recommendations regarding local public health practice. The Emerson Report became the postwar plan for public health in the United States. The report's far-reaching recommendations called

for a minimum population base of 50,000 people for each LHD and included state-by-state proposals for networks of LHDs that would cover all Americans while reducing the number of LHDs by about 50% through consolidation of smaller units.[5]

The Emerson Report gave increased prominence to six basic services believed to represent local government's public health responsibilities to its citizens: vital statistics, environmental sanitation, communicable disease control, maternal and child health services, public health education, and public health laboratory services.[5,6] This was not a new formulation for local public health services. Rather, it was essentially the same package of services that had been considered the

TABLE 5-2   Basic Six Services of Local Public Health

1. Vital statistics—collection and interpretation.
2. Sanitation.
3. Communicable disease control, including immunization, quarantine, and other measures such as identifying communicable disease carriers and distributing vaccines to physicians as well as doing immunizations directly.
4. Maternal and child health (MCH), consisting of prenatal and postpartum care for mothers and babies and supervision of the health of schoolchildren. In some places, immunization of children was handled by the MCH program.
5. Health education, including instruction in personal and family hygiene, sanitation and nutrition, given in schools, at neighborhood health center classes, and in home visits.
6. Laboratory services to physicians, sanitarians, and other interested parties.

Data from Shonick W. *Government and Health Services: Government's Role in the Development of U.S. Health Services 1930–1980.* New York: Oxford University Press; 1995.

standard of practice among LHDs for several decades. Over time, these services had become widely known as the six basic functions of public health ("Basic Six"); **Table 5-2** describes the Basic Six. With the added impetus of the Emerson Report, these six activities became the cornerstone for structuring local public health practice. Although the report's extensive recommendations never became national public policy, they promoted positive changes in many states.

The Committee on Administrative Practice stimulated considerable interest in local public health practice. After about 1950 and continuing into the 1980s, there were repeated efforts to reexamine and redefine the boundaries of local public health practice. This search for mission redefinition is evident in a series of APHA policy statements from 1950 to 1970.[6] In a 1950 APHA statement on LHD services and responsibilities, the Basic Six were presented as desirable minimal services, and several new "optimal" responsibilities were identified: recording and analysis of health data, health education and information, supervision and regulation, provision of direct environmental health services, administration of personal health services, and coordination of activities and services within the community. Another APHA policy statement in 1963 added seventh and eighth services to the Basic Six: operation of health facilities and area-wide planning and coordination. Then, in 1970, APHA adopted another policy statement, expanding on these concepts and calling for increased involvement of state and LHDs in coordinating, monitoring, and assessing the adequacy of health services in their jurisdictions. The evolution of these various characterizations of public health practice is traced in **Table 5-3**.

In the closing decades of the 20th century, important new expectations for local public health practice emerged. Inadequate access to medical care was increasingly identified as a significant impediment to promoting and improving community health. This resulted in local health departments increasingly serving a safety net function. This expanded direct service provision role moved LHDs into new territory, beyond the boundaries of the expanded six functions that characterized public health practice throughout the first half of the 20th century. There was considerable debate as to whether this new role was appropriate, as well as whether LHDs should play leadership roles within their communities in integrating medical and community health services. The movement into medical care was controversial from its inception. Hanlon, in examining the future of LHDs in 1973, urged official public health agencies to withdraw from the business of providing personal health services (whether preventive or therapeutic) and instead to "concentrate upon [their] important and unique potential as community health conscience and leader"[7(p901)] in promoting the establishment of sound social policy. Despite these admonitions, direct medical care services increased among LHDs throughout the 1960s, 1970s, and 1980s, largely as a result of new federal and state grant programs. LHDs were becoming significant providers of safety-net medical services, joining public hospitals and community health centers in this important role.

Quietly emerging through these developments was a unique concept that began to shift the emphasis from the services of public health to its mission and functions. This concept, often characterized as *a governmental presence at the local level* (AGPALL), emerged in the 1970s in the process of fashioning model standards for communities to participate in establishment of the 1990 national health objectives.[8] As described in **Table 5-4**, AGPALL asserts that local government, acting through various means, is ultimately responsible and accountable for ensuring that minimum standards are met in the community. Every locality is served by a unit of government that has responsibility for the health of that locality and population. This responsibility can be executed through an organization other than the official public health agency, but government, through its presence and interest in health, is responsible to see that necessary, agreed-on services are available, accessible, acceptable, and of good quality.

TABLE 5-3 Expansion of the Basic Six Public Health Services, 1920–1980

Initial "Basic Six"
- Vital statistics
- Sanitation
- Communicable disease control
- Maternal and child health
- Health education
- Laboratory services

"Optimal" Services in 1950s
- Basic Six as minimal level
- Analysis and recording of health data
- Health education and information
- Supervision and regulation
- Provision of direct environmental health services
- Administration of personal health services
- Coordination of activities and services within the community

Added in 1960s
- Operation of health facilities
- Area-wide planning and coordination

Added in the 1970s
- Coordinating, monitoring, and assessing the adequacy of health services

Data from Shonick W. *Government and Health Services: Government's Role in the Development of U.S. Health Services 1930–1980*. New York: Oxford University Press; 1995.

TABLE 5-4 Governmental Presence at the Local Level

The concept of governmental presence at the local level is based upon a multifaceted, multitiered governmental responsibility for ensuring that standards are met—a responsibility that often involves agencies in addition to the public health agency at any particular level. Regardless of the structure, every community must be served by a governmental entity charged with that responsibility, and general-purpose government must assign and coordinate responsibility for providing and ensuring public health and safety services. Where services in any area covered by standards are readily available, government may also (but need not also) be involved in delivery of such services. Conversely, where there is a gap in service availability, it is the responsibility of government to have, or to develop, the capacity to deliver such services. Where county and municipal responsibilities overlap, agreements on division of responsibility are necessary.

In summary, government at the local level has the responsibility for ensuring that a health problem is monitored and that services to correct that problem are available. The state government must monitor the effectiveness of local efforts to control health problems and act as a residual guarantor of services where community resources are inadequate, recognizing of course that state resources are also limited.

Reproduced from the U.S. Conference of City Health Officials, National Association of County Health Officials, Association of State and Territorial Health Officials, American Public Health Association, and U.S. Department of Health, Education and Welfare, Public Health Service, Centers for Disease Control. Model Standards for Community Preventive Health Services [Preamble to original model standards]. Public Health Service: Atlanta, GA; 1978.

The AGPALL concept emphasizes the leadership and change agent dimensions of community public health practice; however, exercising leadership to serve the community's health is neither simple nor straightforward. The complexities of 20th century health problems and their contributing factors often called for collaborative, rather than command-and-control solutions. Key to identifying and solving important community health problems is the ability to engage diverse interests and build constituencies. The AGPALL concept suggests that modern public health practice involves more than the provision of services. This broader view of public health's functions was powerfully reinforced by the IOM report.

PUBLIC HEALTH FUNCTIONS AND PRACTICE AFTER 1990

The forecast for the public health system provided in the 1988 IOM report (appropriately titled *The Future of Public Health*) was more dismal than many had expected. After all, the infrastructure of the national public health system had grown substantially throughout the century, especially in terms of LHD coverage of the population. There was widespread acceptance that appropriate community services should include chronic disease prevention and medical care, in addition to the basic six services. Also, importantly, health status had never been better. Nevertheless, the HIV/AIDS epidemic had emerged, and there was no shortage of intractable health and social issues being placed on the public health agenda. Resources to meet these challenges were greatly limited, in part because of the insatiable appetite of the medical care delivery system for every available health dollar. These forces acted together to dissipate public appreciation and support for public health, and the IOM feared that public health would not be able to overcome these challenges without a new vision that would engender the support of the public, policy makers, the media, the medical establishment, and other key stakeholders.

The vision articulated in the IOM report was grounded in a broader view of public health functions than had existed in the past. Throughout earlier decades, the services provided by public health agencies had come to be viewed by many as public health's functions. In identifying three core functions, the IOM report suggested that the function to serve—whether described in terms of specific services or as the more abstract concept of assurance—incompletely characterizes the unique role of public health in our society. Public health interventions represent the products of carrying out public health's core functions, rather than the functions themselves. The IOM examination explicated three public health core functions: assessment, policy development, and assurance.[1]

Assessment calls for public health to regularly and systematically collect, assemble, analyze, and make available information on the health of the community, including statistics on health status, community health needs, and epidemiologic and other studies of health problems. Not every agency is large enough to conduct these activities directly; intergovernmental and interagency cooperation is essential. Nevertheless, each agency bears the responsibility for seeing that the assessment function is fulfilled. This basic function of public health cannot be delegated.[1(p7)]

Policy development calls for public health to serve the public interest in the development of comprehensive public health policies by promoting the use of the scientific knowledge base in decision making about public health and by leading in developing public health policy. Agencies must take a strategic approach, developed on the basis of a positive appreciation for the democratic political process.[1(p8)]

Assurance calls for public health to ensure their constituents that services necessary to achieve agreed on goals are provided, either by encouraging actions by other entities (private or public), by requiring such action through regulation or by providing services directly. Each public health agency is to involve key policy makers and the general public in determining a set of high-priority personal and community-wide health services that government will guarantee to every member of the community. This guarantee should include subsidization or direct provision of high-priority personal health services for those unable to afford them.[1(p8)]

This new core function framework resonated widely within the public health community; its broader characterization of the important functions of public health led to the definition and measurement of their operational aspects, facilitating assessment of their performance. Several key aspects of the assessment, policy development, and assurance functions are processes that identify and address health problems; others are processes (e.g., services and other interventions) generated to ensure that these problems are addressed. To explicate the core functions and provide a framework for characterizing modern public health practice, a work group representing the national public health organizations developed the essential public health services framework.[9] Since 1995, virtually all national and state public health initiatives have adopted the essential public health services framework as the foundation for efforts to characterize, measure, and improve the performance of public health practice. Unfortunately, the use of the term services in the essential public health services framework can be a source of confusion. Although they are not services in the same sense that most people view clinical services (e.g., immunizations) or community preventive services (e.g., fluoridating water), the essential public health services are important processes that operationalize the core functions— assessment, policy development, and assurance—into actionable elements of public health practice.

Public health strives to identify health problems and their causative factors, develop strategies to address these problems, and see that these strategies are implemented in a way that achieves the desired goals. Whereas a comprehensive description for public health practice is yet to be agreed on, the best depiction of what contemporary public health practice is all about can be found in the mission, vision, and functions outlined in the Public Health in America statement.[10] This one-page document articulates a vision (healthy

OUTSIDE-THE-BOOK THINKING 5-1

© Alfred Bondarenko/Shutterstock.

Review the organization of health responsibilities in the state of your choice and describe how public health's core functions and essential services are distributed among various offices and agencies of state government beyond the state health department.

people in healthy communities), a mission (promoting physical and mental health and preventing disease, injury, and disability), and statements of what public health practice does and how it accomplishes these ends. As presented in **Table 5-5**, these statements offer a framework for establishing and measuring practice standards for public health systems, organizations, and workers. The processes embodied in the essential public health services and their links to the

TABLE 5-5   Relationship of Public Health in America Statement to Public Health Practice

Public Health in America Elements	Relationship to Public Health Practice
Vision: Healthy people in healthy communities **Mission:** Promote physical and mental health and prevent disease, injury, and disability	Vision and mission statements for public health practice
Public Health	
• Prevents epidemics and the spread of disease • Protects against environmental hazards • Prevents injuries • Promotes and encourages healthy behaviors • Responds to disasters and assists communities in recovery • Ensures the quality and accessibility of health services	Statements of the broad categories of outcomes affected by public health practice; sometimes viewed as what public health does
Essential Public Health Services	
1. Monitor health status to identify community health problems 2. Diagnose and investigate health problems and health hazards in the community 3. Inform, educate, and empower people about health issues 4. Mobilize community partnerships to identify and solve health problems 5. Develop policies and plans that support individual and community health efforts 6. Enforce laws and regulations that protect health and ensure safety 7. Link people with needed personal health services and ensure the provision of health care when otherwise unavailable 8. Ensure a competent public health and personal healthcare workforce 9. Evaluate effectiveness, accessibility, and quality of personal and population-based health services 10. Research for new insights and innovative solutions to health problems	Statements of the processes of public health practice that affect public health outcomes; sometimes viewed as how public health does what it does

Data from Public Health Functions Steering Committee. *Public Health in America.* Washington, DC: PHS; 1994.

three core functions are critical to an understanding of modern public health practice.

Assessment in Public Health

Two important processes (or essential public health services) characterize the assessment function of public health: (1) monitoring health status to identify community health problems and (2) diagnosing and investigating health problems and health hazards in the community.

Monitoring health status to identify community health problems encompasses:

- Accurate, ongoing assessment of the community's health status
- Identification of threats to health
- Determination of health service needs
- Attention to the health needs of groups that are at higher risk than the total population
- Identification of community assets and resources that support the public health system in promoting health and improving quality of life
- Use of appropriate methods and technology to interpret and communicate data to diverse audiences
- Collaboration with other stakeholders, including private providers and health benefit plans, to manage multisectoral integrated information systems

Diagnosing and investigating health problems and health hazards in the community encompass:

- Access to a public health laboratory capable of conducting rapid screening and high-volume testing
- Active infectious disease epidemiology programs
- Technical capacity for epidemiologic investigation of disease outbreaks and patterns of infectious and chronic diseases and injuries and other adverse health behaviors and conditions

Policy Development for Public Health

The assessment function and its related processes provide a foundation for policy development and its key processes, including (1) informing, educating, and empowering people about health issues; (2) mobilizing community partnerships to identify and solve health problems; and (3) developing policies and plans that support individual and community health efforts.

Informing, educating, and empowering people about health issues encompass:

- Community development activities

- Social marketing and targeted media public communication
- Provision of accessible health information resources at community levels
- Active collaboration with personal healthcare providers to reinforce health promotion messages and programs
- Joint health education programs with schools, churches, work sites, and others

Mobilizing community partnerships to identify and solve health problems encompasses:

- Convening and facilitating partnerships among groups and associations (including those not typically considered to be health related)
- Undertaking defined health improvement planning process and health projects, including preventive, screening, rehabilitation, and support programs
- Building a coalition to draw on the full range of potential human and material resources to improve community health

Developing policies and plans that support individual and community health efforts encompasses:

- Leadership development at all levels of public health
- Systematic community-level and state-level planning for health improvement in all jurisdictions
- Development and tracking of measurable health objectives from the community health plan as a part of a continuous quality improvement strategy
- Joint evaluation with the medical healthcare system to define consistent policy regarding prevention and treatment services
- Development of policy and legislation to guide the practice of public health

OUTSIDE-THE-BOOK THINKING 5-2

© Alfred Bondarenko/Shutterstock.

How are the essential public health services related to public health's three core functions? How are these operationalized in public health practice?

Assurance of the Public's Health

Whereas assessment and policy development set interventions into motion, the assurance function keeps them on track through five important processes: (1) enforcing laws and regulations that protect health and ensure safety; (2) linking people to needed personal health services and ensuring the provision of health care when otherwise unavailable; (3) ensuring a competent public health and personal healthcare workforce; (4) evaluating effectiveness, accessibility, and quality of personal and population-based health services; and (5) researching for new insights and innovative solutions to health problems.

Enforcing laws and regulations that protect health and ensure safety encompasses:

- Enforcement of sanitary codes, especially in the food industry
- Protection of drinking water supplies
- Enforcement of clean air standards
- Animal control activities
- Follow-up of hazards, preventable injuries, and exposure-related diseases identified in occupational and community settings
- Monitoring quality of medical services (e.g., laboratories, nursing homes, and home healthcare providers)
- Review of new drug, biologic, and medical device applications

Linking people to needed personal health services and ensuring the provision of health care when otherwise unavailable (sometimes referred to as outreach or enabling services) encompass:

- Assurance of effective entry for socially disadvantaged people into a coordinated system of clinical care
- Culturally and linguistically appropriate materials and staff to ensure linkage to services for special population groups
- Ongoing care management
- Transportation services
- Targeted health education/promotion/disease prevention to high-risk population groups

Ensuring a competent public and personal healthcare workforce encompasses:

- Education, training, and assessment of personnel (including volunteers and other lay community health workers) to meet community needs for public and personal health services

- Efficient processes for licensure of professionals
- Adoption of continuous quality improvement and lifelong learning programs
- Active partnerships with professional training programs to ensure community-relevant learning experiences for all students
- Continuing education in management and leadership development programs for those charged with administrative/executive roles

Evaluating effectiveness, accessibility, and quality of personal and population-based health services encompasses:

- Assessing program effectiveness
- Providing information necessary for allocating resources and reshaping programs

Researching for new insights and innovative solutions to health problems encompasses:

- Full continuum of innovation, ranging from practical, field-based efforts to fostering change in public health practice to more academic efforts to encourage new directions in scientific research
- Continuous linkage with institutions of higher learning and research
- Internal capacity to mount timely epidemiologic and economic analyses and conduct health services research

The important processes embodied in the essential public health services framework underscore the complexities of public health practice. The essential public health services framework is relevant to both programs and organizations and is evident in virtually any public health intervention (although to different degrees), constituting what might be considered generic public health practice. The core functions and essential services framework demonstrate that public health practice is more than a collection of programs and services; it embodies the AGPALL concept and the tools to carry out that role.

COMMUNITY HEALTH ASSESSMENT AND IMPROVEMENT TOOLS

The delineation of core functions and essential public health services fortified the foundation for public health practice.[11] Over the two decades after the appearance of the IOM report, several important new tools for public health practice came onto the scene to build on this foundation.

Mobilizing for Action through Planning and Partnerships

Among the early post-IOM report initiatives, the Assessment Protocol for Excellence in Public Health (APEXPH), developed by the National Association of County and City Health Officials (NACCHO), in collaboration with other national public health organizations, had an extensive and positive influence on public health practice.[12] Even greater reach and impact are expected from the second generation of this tool, *Mobilizing for Action through Planning and Partnerships* (MAPP).[13]

OUTSIDE-THE-BOOK THINKING 5-3

© Alfred Bondarenko/Shutterstock.

Determine whether your LHD has completed a community health assessment and/or improvement process. If it has, what approaches and tools were used? What were the products and results? If it has not, why?

The original APEXPH was a tool for organizational self-assessment and improvement for LHDs, as well as a simple and effective community needs assessment process. APEXPH provided a means for LHDs to enhance their organizational capacity and strengthen their leadership role in their communities. APEXPH guided health department officials in two principal areas of activity: (1) assessing and improving the organizational capacity of the agency, and (2) working with the local community to improve the health status of its citizens. There were three principal parts to this process:[12]

1. An organizational capacity assessment—self-assessed key aspects of operations, including authority to operate, community relations, community health assessment, public policy development, assurance of public health services, financial management, personnel management, and program management, resulting in an organizational action plan that set priorities for correcting perceived weaknesses.
2. A community health assessment process—guided formation of a community advisory committee that identified health problems requiring priority attention and then set health status goals and programmatic

objectives. The aim was to mobilize community resources in pursuit of locally relevant public health objectives consistent with the Healthy People objectives.
3. Completing the cycle—ensured that the activities from the organizational and community processes were effectively carried out and that they accomplished the desired results through policy development, assurance, monitoring, and evaluation activities.

After its appearance in 1991, APEXPH steadily gained acceptance with the majority of all LHDs using all or part of APEXPH during the 1990s. Although the decade's experience with APEXPH was highly positive, opportunities for strengthening the tool became apparent. Heightened interest in community health improvement efforts, widespread acceptance of the essential public health services as the framework for public health practice, the need to strategically engage a wider range of community interests, and the opportunity to formalize and activate local public health systems converged to suggest that an even more strategic approach to community health improvement was needed.

The development of MAPP addressed these needs in the form of a robust tool of public health practice that could be used by communities with effective LHD leadership to create a local system that ensures the delivery of health services essential to protecting the health of the public.[13] Distinguishing features of MAPP include:

- Incorporation of strategic planning concepts—to assist LHDs in more effectively engaging their communities, securing resources, and managing the process of change. Visioning, contextual environment assessment, strategic issue identification, and strategy formulation principles are among the strategic planning concepts embedded in MAPP.
- Grounding in local public health practice—to ensure that the process is practical, flexible, and user friendly. The instruments rely heavily on the previous experiences and successes of typical communities through vignettes, case studies, and other examples.
- A focus on the local public health system—to broaden community health improvement efforts by recognizing and including all public and private organizations contributing to public health at the local level.

Because public health involves more than what public health agencies do, MAPP provides a framework for actualizing this assertion through:

- A common approach for assessing local public health systems—to promote consistent quality of public health practice from community to community and state to state. The essential public health services framework provides the measures used to assess local public health systems consistent with other national and state efforts to promote a basic set of public health performance standards.

- Expansion of the basic indicators for health status—to reflect better the demographic and socioeconomic determinants of health, community assets, environmental and behavioral risks, and quality of life. MAPP includes a core set of measures for all communities and an extended menu of additional measures for use, where appropriate.
- Recognition that community themes and strengths play an important role in community health improvement efforts—to balance overreliance on data and expert opinion, provide new insights into factors affecting community health, and increase buy-in and active participation as stakeholders feel their concerns and opinions are important to the process.

The model developed for MAPP incorporates interrelated and interactive components. To be practical for use in widely diverse communities and to meld basic strategic planning concepts with public health and community health improvement concepts, MAPP is both simple and complex, as illustrated in **Figure 5-1**. There is no fixed or even preferred sequencing of its components. The boundaries of the model identify the four assessments that comprise the MAPP process; these are usually completed after visioning has taken place but before strategic issues are identified in the steps indicated in the center of the model. Each element of the model is briefly described here:

- Organizing for success/partnership development—involves establishing values and outcomes for the process and determining the scope, form, and timing for planning process, as well as its participants.
- Visioning—involves developing a shared vision of the ideal future for the community, which serves to provide the process with focus, purpose, direction, and buy-in.
- Four MAPP assessments—these inform the planning process and drive the identification of strategic issues. All are critical to the success of the process, although there is no prescribed order in which they need to be undertaken. The four strategic assessments are described below:
  1. Community themes and strengths assessment—involves the collection of inputs and insights from

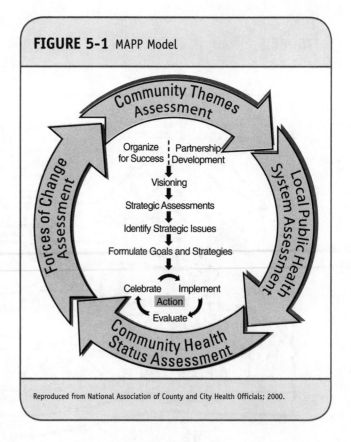

FIGURE 5-1 MAPP Model

Reproduced from National Association of County and City Health Officials; 2000.

throughout the community in order to understand issues that residents feel are important.
  2. Local public health assessment—involves an analysis of mission, vision, and goals through the use of performance measures for the essential public health services. Both strengths and areas for improvement are identified.
  3. Community health status assessment—involves an extensive assessment of indicators in 11 domains, including asset mapping and quality of life; environmental health; socioeconomic, demographic, and behavioral risk factors; infectious diseases; sentinel events; social and mental health; maternal and child health; health resource availability; and health status indicators.
  4. Forces of change assessment—identifies broader forces affecting the community, such as technology and legislation.
- Identify strategic issues—involves fundamental policy questions for achieving the shared vision, arising from the information developed in the previous phases. Some are more important than others and require action.

FIGURE 5-2 MAPP as a Road Map for Community Public Health Systems

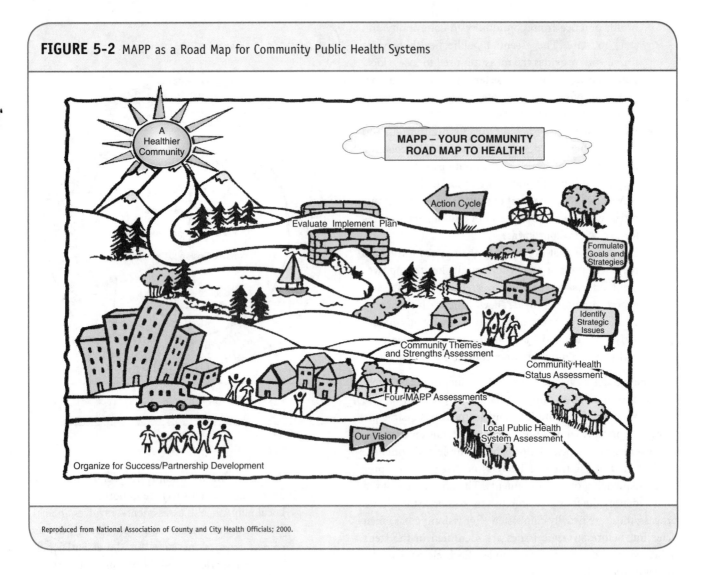

- Formulate goals and strategies—involves developing and examining options for addressing strategic issues, including questions of feasibility and barriers to implementation. Preferred strategies are selected.
- The action cycle—involves implementation, evaluation, and celebration of achievements after LHD leaders have selected and agreed-upon strategies.

As depicted in **Figure 5-2**, MAPP offers a virtual road map for community public health systems. Widespread use of MAPP began in 2001, and after only a few years, its impact was apparent in an evaluation of early adopters.[14] LHDs, other local government agencies, hospitals, and social service providers were the most frequent community participants in the MAPP process, as shown in **Figure 5-3**. Educational institutions, nonprofit organizations, community residents,

local businesses and employers, and civic interest groups were the most frequently identified new partners. Managed care organizations, health professional organizations, environmental agencies, and neighborhood organizations were substantially less likely to be engaged in the MAPP process. LHDs reported that the most frequent results from MAPP were the strengthened existing partnerships, an increased understanding of community health problems, and greater community engagement.

Other Community Health Assessment and Improvement Tools

In addition to the essential public health services framework and the APEXPH/MAPP processes, the IOM report stimulated several other important initiatives to promote core

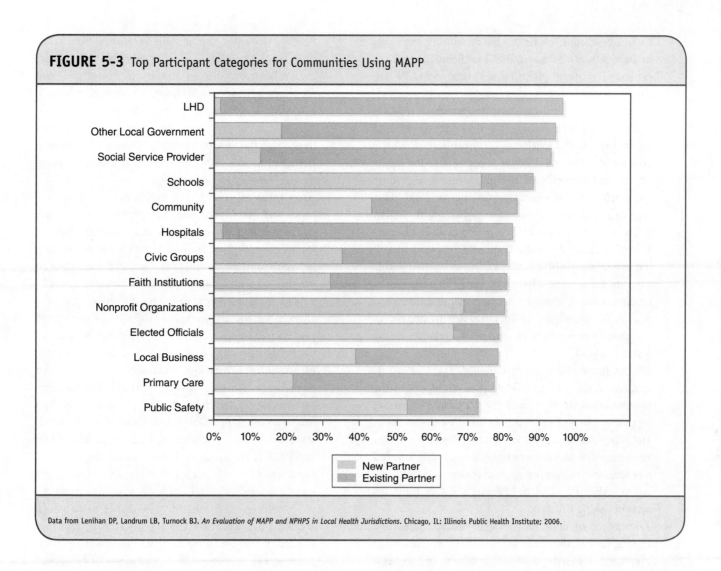

FIGURE 5-3 Top Participant Categories for Communities Using MAPP

New Partner
Existing Partner

Data from Lenihan DP, Landrum LB, Turnock BJ. *An Evaluation of MAPP and NPHPS in Local Health Jurisdictions*. Chicago, IL: Illinois Public Health Institute; 2006.

function-related performance, especially for the assessment and policy development functions. One of the first community health planning tools to be widely used was the Planned Approach to Community Health (PATCH), a process for community organization and community needs assessment that emphasizes community mobilization and constituency building. PATCH focuses on orienting and training community leaders and other community participants in all aspects of the community needs assessment process and includes excellent documentation and resource materials. Although originally developed by the Centers for Disease Control and Prevention (CDC) to focus on chronic health conditions and stimulate health promotion and disease prevention interventions, PATCH is flexible enough to be used in a wide variety of community health needs assessment applications.

Yet another important tool for addressing public health core functions and their associated processes is the Model

Standards framework.[8] The steps outlined for community implementation of the Model Standards process link many of the various core function-related tools; these steps represent, in effect, a pathway for organizations to participate in community health improvement activities. The steps include:

1. Assessment of organizational role. Communities are organized and structured differently. As a result, the specific roles of local public health organizations will vary from community to community. This essential first step is to reexamine organizational purpose and mission and develop a long-range vision through strategic planning involving its internal and external constituencies. The resulting mission statement and long-range vision serve to guide the organization (leadership and board, as well as employees) and to define it for its community partners. This critical step

should be completed before the remaining steps can be successfully addressed. Part 1 of APEXPH and the expanded strategic planning elements of MAPP are useful in accomplishing this task.

2. Assessment of organizational capacity. After a mission and role have been defined, it is necessary to examine an organization's capacity to carry out its role in the community. This calls for an assessment of the major operational elements of the organization, including its structure and performance for specific tasks. This type of organizational and local public health system self-assessment is best carried out through broad participation from all levels. Both APEXPH and MAPP include hundreds of indicators that can be used in this capacity assessment. These indicators can be modified or eliminated if they are deemed inappropriate, and additional indicators can also be used. This step serves to identify strengths and weaknesses relative to the mission and role.

3. Development of a capacity-building plan. The development of a capacity-building plan incorporates the organization's strengths and prioritizes its weaknesses so that the most important are addressed first. As in any plan, specific objectives for addressing these weaknesses are developed, responsibilities are assigned, and a process for tracking progress over time is established. Again, APEXPH and MAPP are valuable tools for accomplishing this task.

4. Assessment of community organizational structure. Having looked internally at its capacity and ability to exercise its leadership role for identifying and addressing priority health needs in the community, the public health organization must assess the key stakeholders and necessary participants for a community-wide needs assessment and intervention initiative. This is often a long-term and continuous process in which the relationship of all important community stakeholders and partners (e.g., the health agency, community providers of health-related services, community organizations, community leaders, interest groups, the media, and the general public) is assessed. This step determines how and under whose auspices community health planning will take place within the community. Both APEXPH/MAPP and PATCH processes support the successful completion of this step.

5. Organization of community. This step calls for organizing the community so that it represents a strong constituency for public health and will participate collaboratively in partnership with the health agency.

Specific strategies and activities will vary from community to community but will generally include hearings, dialogues, discussion forums, meetings, and collaborative planning sessions. The specific roles and authority of community participants should be clarified so that the process is not perceived as one driven largely by the health agency and so-called experts. Both APEXPH/MAPP and PATCH are useful for completing this step.

6. Assessment of community health needs. The actual process of identifying health problems of importance to the community is one that must carefully balance information derived from data sets with information derived from the community's perceptions of which problems are most important. Often, community readiness to mitigate specific problems greatly increases the chances for success, as well as support for the overall process within the community. In addition to generating information on possible health problems, this step gathers information on resources available within the community. This step serves to provide the information necessary for the community's most important health problems to be identified. The community needs assessment tools provided in both APEXPH/MAPP and PATCH are useful in accomplishing this step.

7. Determination of local priorities and community health resources. After important health problems are identified, decisions must be made as to which are most important for community action. This step requires broad participation from community participants in the process so that priorities will be viewed as community rather than agency-specific priorities. Debate and negotiation are essential for this step, and there are many approaches to coming to consensus around specific priorities. Both APEXPH/MAPP and PATCH support this step.

8. Selection of outcome objectives. After priorities are determined, the process must establish a target level to be achieved for each priority problem. For this step, the Model Standards process is especially useful in linking community priorities to national health objectives and establishing targets that are appropriate for the current status and improvement possible from a community intervention. This step also calls for negotiation within the community because deployment and reallocation of resources may be needed to achieve the agreed-upon target outcomes. In addition to Model Standards, both APEXPH/MAPP and PATCH can be useful in accomplishing this step.

9. Development of intervention strategies. This step is one of determining strategies and methods of achieving the outcome objectives established for each priority health problem. This can be quite difficult and, at times, contentious. For some problems, there may be few or even no effective interventions. For others, there may be widely divergent strategies available, some of which may be deemed unacceptable or not feasible. After agreement is reached as to strategies and methods, responsibilities for implementing and evaluating interventions will be assigned. With community-wide interventions, overall coordination of efforts may also need to be addressed as part of the intervention strategy.

10. Implementation of intervention strategies. After the establishment of goals, objectives, strategies, and methods, specific plans of action for the intervention are developed, and specific tasks and work plans are developed. Clear delineation of responsibilities and time lines is essential for this step.

11. Continuous monitoring and evaluation of effort. The evaluation strategy for the intervention will track performance related to outcome objectives, as well as process objectives and activity measures over time. If activity measures and process objectives are being accomplished, there should be progress toward achieving the desired outcome objectives. If this does not occur, the selected intervention strategy needs to be reconsidered and revised.

OUTSIDE-THE-BOOK THINKING 5-4

© Alfred Bondarenko/Shutterstock.

What features are similar among MAPP, PATCH, CHIP, and Model Standards? What features differ? What role do these tools play in carrying out public health's core functions at the local level?

In 1996, and again in 2002, the IOM revisited issues addressed in its 1988 report, concluding that different organizations, leadership, and political and economic realities were transforming how public health carried out its core functions and essential services.[15,16] On one hand, market-driven health care was forcing public health to clarify and strengthen its public role in a predominantly private health system. On the other, public health was increasingly identifying and working with a variety of entities within the community that shape community health and well-being. Another important IOM report in 1997 advanced an expanded community health improvement planning (CHIP) model that extended the tools developed earlier in the decade and the steps described previously here.[17] Its main features are its expanded perspective on the wide variety of factors that influence health, its support for broad participation by community stakeholders, and its emphasis on the use of performance measures to ensure accountability of partners and track progress over time.

Community health assessments leading toward community health improvement plans increased in quantity as well as quality during the 25 years between 1988 and 2013. A survey conducted by NACCHO in 2013 found that more than two-thirds of local health jurisdictions (LHJs) nationwide had conducted a community health assessment in the past 5 years (58% within the past 3 years) and only 11% either had not completed one or were not planning one in the near future. Similar results were reported for community health improvement plans and organizational strategic plans, although at somewhat lower levels.[18] Those LHDs not planning to conduct assessments, CHIPs, and strategic plans were primarily the smallest local health jurisdictions with few full-time employees. State health agencies have also been active in completing state health assessments, statewide health improvement plans, and agency-wide strategic plans, as demonstrated in **Figure 5-4**. State agency commitment to these planning activities provides an additional impetus for LHDs.

In most communities, LHDs serve as the primary instigators of community health assessments or serve as the lead agency or full partner in a community-wide coalition that assumes responsibility for the assessment. A provision of the Affordable Care Act health reform legislation requires nonprofit hospitals to engage in community health assessments at least every 3 years and encourages hospitals to collaborate with public health agencies where possible. **Figure 5-5** documents that two-thirds of LHDs either had already been collaborating with their local hospitals by 2013 or were in discussions to incorporate hospitals into their existing community health assessment efforts.

Community Engagement

Communities remain the battlefields on which public health threats are met and public health challenges are addressed in the 21st century. There was steady growth in the armamentarium of community public health practice during the

FIGURE 5-4 State Health Agency (SHA) and Local Health Department (LHD) Participation in Health Assessment, Health Improvement Planning, and Strategic Planning Activities, United States, 2012 and 2013

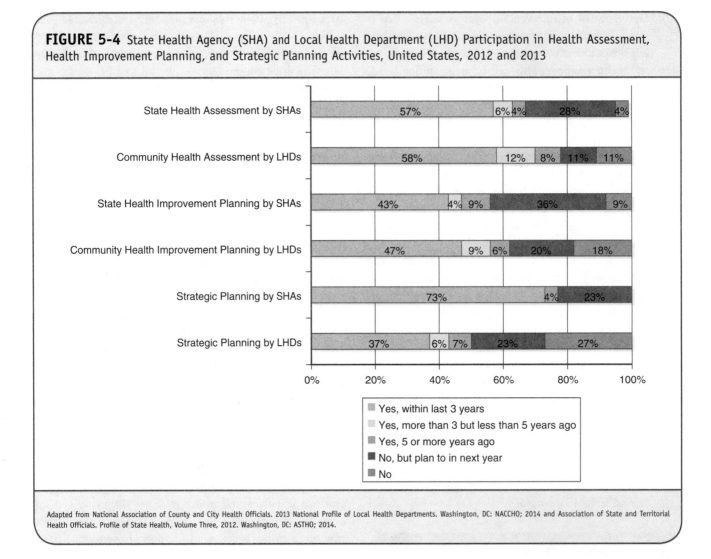

Adapted from National Association of County and City Health Officials. 2013 National Profile of Local Health Departments. Washington, DC: NACCHO; 2014 and Association of State and Territorial Health Officials. Profile of State Health, Volume Three, 2012. Washington, DC: ASTHO; 2014.

late 20th century in the form of community health assessment and improvement tools based on the core functions and essential public health services framework. Community health improvement is grounded in the realization that more doctors, more clinics, and more sophisticated diagnostic and treatment advances will not alleviate the major health problems facing Americans. Instead, the greatest gains will come from what people do or do not do for themselves, individually and collectively. Acting collectively can take place at many levels; at the community level, it often works best.

The notion of community is an elusive concept. Generally, communities are aggregates of individuals who share common characteristics or other bonds. One person can be part of many different communities. One definition views community as the associative, self-generated gathering of common people who have sufficient resources in their lives to cope with life's demands and not suffer ill health. This definition of community focuses on the capacity of communities to achieve their health goals through the effective use of their own assets. It differs considerably from the view of communities as locations in which health problems reside and health services are delivered. Rather than focusing on the level of individual actions and behaviors, it recognizes the importance of social determinants of health and of the environmental and policy levels for public health responses. Community public health practice revolves around engaging communities to work collectively on their own behalf. Community engagement is the process of working collaboratively with groups of people who are affiliated by geographic proximity, special interests, or similar situations, with respect to issues affecting their well-being. Although community engagement is a relatively recent phenomenon for many governmental public

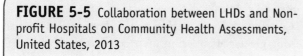

FIGURE 5-5 Collaboration between LHDs and Non-profit Hospitals on Community Health Assessments, United States, 2013

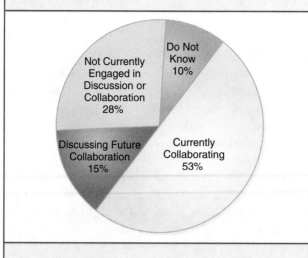

Data from National Association of County and City Health Officials. *2013 National Profile of Local Health Departments*. Washington, DC: NACCHO; 2014.

health organizations, health education specialists have been using these principles for decades, based on the simple guiding principle of starting where the people are.[19]

This positive approach emphasizes that all communities have assets. All too often, communities have been viewed solely in terms of their needs and problems. The implication of these different perspectives is important. If communities are viewed from their needs, the policies and interventions will be based on needs. If they are to be viewed from their assets, the policies and interventions will be based on the community's capacities, skills, and assets. Community health improvement seldom occurs from the actions of outside interests; the most successful community development efforts are driven by the commitment of those investing themselves and their resources in the effort. Identifying community assets is possible through approaches that catalog and actually map the basic building blocks that will be used to address important community health problems.[20] Primary building blocks include those community assets that are most readily available for community health improvement, including both individual and organizational assets. Individual assets include the skills, talents, and experiences of residents, individual businesses, and home-based enterprises, as well as personal income. Organizational assets include associations of businesses, citizen associations, cultural organizations, communications organizations, and religious organizations. Secondary building blocks are private,

public, and physical assets, which can be brought under community control and used for community improvement purposes. These include private and nonprofit organizations (higher educational institutions, hospitals, social service agencies), public institutions and services (public schools, police, libraries, fire departments, parks), and physical resources (vacant land, commercial and industrial structures, housing, energy, and waste resources).

In addition to community engagement and asset-mapping strategies, performance measurement offers another tool for community health improvement activities. Performance measures are also not new to public health practice. The use of performance measures to track progress toward community or national health objectives and to monitor programs has long been standard practice. The CHIP proposed by the IOM in its report on performance monitoring, however, takes performance measurement to a new level. In these processes, performance measures serve to hold communities (acting through stakeholders and partnerships) accountable for actions for which they have accepted responsibility.[17] This supports the development of a shared vision and a collaborative and integrative approach to community problem solving for the purpose of improving health status. It offers a pathway for stakeholders and partners to assume responsibility collectively and to marshal their resources and assets in pursuit of agreed-upon objectives.

The CHIP model incorporates a problem identification and prioritization cycle, followed by an analysis and implementation cycle. This second cycle develops, implements, and evaluates health intervention strategies that address priority community health problems. The distinguishing feature of this approach is the emphasis on measurement to link performance and accountability on a community-wide basis, rather than solely on the LHD or another public entity. Several recommendations were developed to operationalize the community health improvement concept, including:

- Communities should base a health improvement process on a broad definition of health and a comprehensive conceptual model of how health is produced within the community.
- A CHIP should develop its own set of specific, quantitative performance measures, linking accountable entities to the performance of specific activities expected to lead to the production of desired health outcomes in the community.
- A CHIP should seek a balance between strategic opportunities for long-term health improvement and goals that are achievable in the short term.

- Community conditions guiding CHIPs should strive for strategic inclusiveness, incorporating individuals, groups, and organizations that have an interest in health outcomes; can take actions necessary to improve community health; or can contribute data and analytic capabilities needed for performance monitoring.
- A CHIP should be centered in a community health coalition or similar entity.[17]

Numerous useful tools and guides are available via the Internet to support the expanded community health improvement efforts in models such as CHIP, MAPP, and similar initiatives. Prominent among these tools are CDC's Principles of Community Engagement, the Community Tool Box (developed by the University of Kansas), and the *Healthy People 2020* Tool Kit (produced by the Public Health Foundation).[21-23]

The maturation of community-driven models of public health practice was fostered in part by the National Turning Point Initiative.[24] Funded jointly by the Kellogg Foundation and Robert Wood Johnson Foundation, Turning Point sought to transform and strengthen the public health infrastructure at the state and local levels, in effect, reforming public health practice. More than twenty states participated in Turning Point through statewide and local partnerships that brought together a broad spectrum of health interests to develop a shared vision and strategic plans to improve statewide public health systems. The collaborations in the various Turning Point sites varied significantly, nurturing and developing many different models for systems change.

The Healthy Communities framework represents another successful model for community health improvement, using health as a metaphor for a broader approach to building community.[25] Because health cuts across lines of race, ethnicity, class, culture, and sector, the focus on a healthy community enables the entire community to collaborate in community renewal. Healthy Communities is based on the belief that change in public policies and actions will occur only when people act together to participate directly in the public work of our society and problems occur. A key to success involves community institutions using their organizational skills, relationships, in-kind resources, and credibility to engage the rest of the community in mobilizing the creativity and resources of the community to improve health and well-being. Focusing on systems change, Healthy Communities seeks to build broad citizen participation that encourages new players and honors diversity. It looks to build true collaborations between business, government, nonprofit organizations, and citizens stimulating the community and political will to act together.

Community-based health policy development is also receiving greater attention in these collaborations and partnerships. Public policy serves as a guide to influence governmental decisions and action at any jurisdictional level, thereby affecting what would otherwise occur.[26] For the health and well-being of communities, policies indicate broad directions toward important goals, cutting across many different stakeholders and affecting large populations. Policies focus on both goals and the means to achieve those goals, often affecting the decisions and actions of individual organizations. At the community level, health policy has many options, such as more and better health services to address unmet needs in the community or advocacy for broader support to improve the conditions influencing health in the community. Increasingly, community-driven public health initiatives are tackling the broader social and community factors, even as they seek to ensure that gaps in services are somehow met.

Little research is available to elucidate the value of community-driven health policy development initiatives. There is some evidence that widespread initiation of CHIPs increases the frequency with which key policy development components take place. Policy development may be the public health core function most heavily impacted by CHIPs. The increase in performance of specific practices related to the core functions has been greatest for those related to policy development, and generally, the baseline level of measures of policy development lags behind that of assessment and assurance where CHIPs have not been implemented.

Together, these strategies, initiatives, and tools can make substantial contributions to improving public health practice in the United States. In addition, there is reason to believe that improvement is needed in view of assessments of performance that were completed over recent decades.

OUTSIDE-THE-BOOK THINKING 5-5

© Alfred Bondarenko/Shutterstock.

You are the administrator of a typical county-based LHD in a largely rural state. Your newly elected county board chairman has ordered you to come up with new health-related initiatives that will improve the health of the county's residents. How would you approach this charge?

STRATEGIC PLANNING, STANDARDS, AND ACCREDITATION

Community health assessments, and community health improvement plans offer public health organizations an opportunity to reexamine their mission, vision, and goals and to better align their strategic direction with community needs and priorities. Strategic planning has become a third pillar of modern public health practice that is now institutionalized in a process that accredits state and local public health agencies through the Public Health Accreditation Board.

Strategic planning has long been recognized as an effective management practice and tool among private sector organizations. More recently, the practice has become widely established among nonprofit and public sector organizations. Strategic planning encompasses a series of key steps from laying the groundwork through implementing, evaluating, and revising the plan. Preplanning calls for identifying key stakeholders, assessing the availability of necessary information, and developing a plan, process, and timeline for the strategic planning project. These preparatory activities provide a foundation for the critically important step of developing clear statements of mission, vision, and values.

Many strategic planning processes begin with the identification of core values for the organization with the input of key stakeholders and after careful consideration of both formal and informal mandates for the organization. An initial mission statement is then developed as well as a vision statement that articulates where the organization wants to be in the future. The vision statement is critical here, as it characterizes the difference between where an organization is and where it wants to be. This sets the stage for the identification of strategic issues that must be addressed for the vision to be achieved. **Figure 5-6** illustrates the key components of an organizational strategic planning process.

Examination of strategic issues depends in part on the availability of relevant information. Existing reports and data may or may not be useful. Additional data and information are often needed, as are appropriate methods of summarizing data and information for the analysis step that follows.

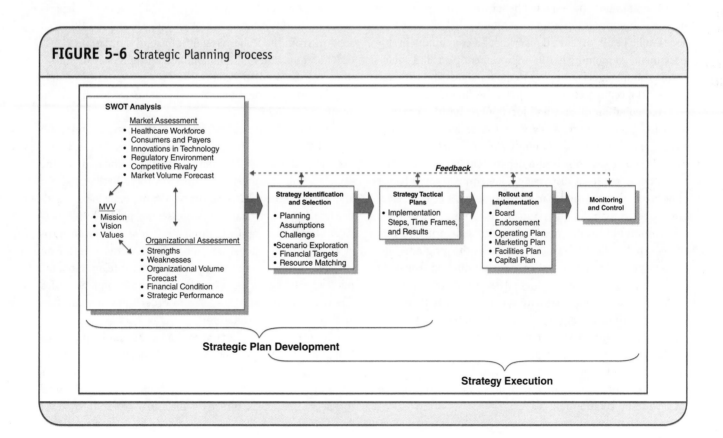

FIGURE 5-6 Strategic Planning Process

Many methods are used to analyze data for strategic planning purposes, although one commonly used approach is the SWOT/SWOC Analysis. In this method, strengths, weaknesses, opportunities, and threats (or challenges) are identified as quadrants of an analysis matrix. Making these dimensions explicit facilitates the identification of emerging trends, cross-cutting themes, and ultimately, key strategic issues and priorities.

It is these key strategic issues and priorities that drive the strategic plan in the form of its strategies, goals and objectives, timelines, accountabilities, and evaluation framework. These are captured in a strategic planning document that is widely communicated to staff and stakeholders.

As the plan is implemented, activities and objectives are monitored closely using quality improvement practices that emphasize outcomes, yet foster flexibility to shift strategies when results dictate the need to do so. Revisions and updates for the original strategic plan should be viewed as the rule, rather than the exception. It is equally important that results be shared widely among staff and stakeholders.

Strategic plans for public health organizations benefit greatly from preexisting community health assessments and community health improvement plans. Together, these three tools define the minimal requirements for an effective public health organization. It should not be surprising that these three elements comprise the basic prerequisites for PHAB accreditation. Public health organizations without a community health assessment, community health improvement plan, and strategic plan simply aren't living up to the standards and expectations of 21st century community public health practice.

Accreditation of state and local public health organizations has been a controversial idea for decades. For many years, the public health community did not view the observation, "If you've seen one health department, you've seen one health department" as disparaging. For some, it was a badge of honor in that health departments should differ from each other due to their unique populations, political structures, and community health needs. As discussed earlier in this chapter, public health was long viewed as the programs and services provided, which understandably differed from one community or state to another. After the IOM report in 1988, however, a view that core functions rather than programs and community services defined a public health organization promoted a view that health departments should in fact be more alike than different. These commonalities offered a template for common standards to be developed and applied through national or state strategies to promote their widespread adoption.

Standards are basically explicit performance expectations. Progress towards the development of public health practice standards came quickly after 1990. At the national level, CDC collaborating with the major national public health practice organizations developed the National Public Health Performance Standards Program.[27] These standards were based on the 10 essential public health services framework and designed so that they could be used in several applications that would synergize their adoption. These national standards could be used by health departments for self-assessment and improvement. The standards or a subset of the standards could also be used for national surveillance purposes to determine how many health departments or what proportion of the population were being served by a health department meeting some level of these standards. The standards framework could also be adopted or adapted by states, which would then require or incentivize their LHDs to meet the standards. Finally, some external entity could apply the standards through a national voluntary accreditation program.

NACCHO extended and focused the content of the national public health performance standards in the development of a panel of standards, again based largely on the essential public health services framework, that constituted an operational definition of a functional local health department.[28] Relatively soon thereafter with substantial financial support from the Robert Wood Johnson Foundation, NACCHO and the other national public health practice organizations collaborated to explore the feasibility and ultimately established a national voluntary program for public health agency accreditation.

The standards and process for the national program were developed by the Public Health Accreditation Board over several years.[29] The PHAB standards focused on the same catalog of concepts captured in the NPHPS program and the operational definition of a functional local health department. Once again the 10 essential public health services served as organizing domains. The accreditation process calls for an extensive self-assessment activity before an on-site verification and review by a site visit team. Notably, public health agencies must demonstrate completion of a CHA, CHIP, and strategic plan in order to even submit an application for accreditation.

In 2013, PHAB announced the initial cohort of accredited public health agencies. Additional approvals steadily followed as many agencies sought to be early adopters. Surveys of local and state health agencies, document that demand for accreditation is already substantial. As indicated in

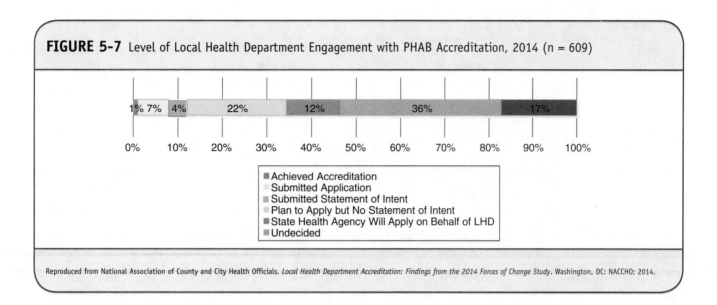

FIGURE 5-7 Level of Local Health Department Engagement with PHAB Accreditation, 2014 (n = 609)

1% 7%   4%   22%   12%   36%   17%

0%   10%   20%   30%   40%   50%   60%   70%   80%   90%   100%

- Achieved Accreditation
- Submitted Application
- Submitted Statement of Intent
- Plan to Apply but No Statement of Intent
- State Health Agency Will Apply on Behalf of LHD
- Undecided

Reproduced from National Association of County and City Health Officials. *Local Health Department Accreditation: Findings from the 2014 Forces of Change Study.* Washington, DC: NACCHO; 2014.

Figure 5-7, by early 2014, nearly one-half of LHDs had either been accredited or entered the pipeline for accreditation by submitting an application or letter of intent, or by indicating that they planned to submit a letter of intent or apply through their state health agency.[30] Only 17% of LHDs indicated that they did not intend to seek accreditation, virtually guaranteeing that PHAB will be busy reviewing applicants for years to come. Interest among state health agencies was even higher with 80% either already applying or planning to apply as of later 2012.[31]

CONCLUSION

For more than a century, public health has sought to measure its efforts through standards that reflected its mission to promote and protect population health and well-being. The 1988 IOM report emphasized the need for stronger assessment and policy development functions to complement the long-standing view that public health's role is one of assurance. The essential public health services framework operationalizes the core functions and serves as the organizing construct for modern public health practice standards. For public health organizations, those standards are achieved in part through community health assessments, community health improvement plans, and organizational strategic plans. These activities are now recognized by the Public Health Accreditation Board as prerequisites for recognition by that body, further establishing the core functions and essential public health services framework as the bedrock of modern public health practice.

REFERENCES

1. Institute of Medicine, Committee on the Future of Public Health. *The Future of Public Health.* Washington, DC: National Academy Press; 1988.
2. Turnock BJ, Handler AS. From measuring to improving public health practice. *Annu Rev Public Health.* 1997; *18:* 261–282.
3. Vaughan HF. Local health services in the United States: the story of CAP. *Am J Public Health.* 1972; *62:* 95–108.
4. American Public Health Association, Committee on Administrative Practice. Appraisal form for city health work. *Am J Public Health.* 1926; *16*(Suppl): 1–65.
5. Emerson H, Luginbuhl M. *Local Health Units for the Nation.* New York, NY: Commonwealth Fund; 1945.
6. Shonick W. *Government and Health Services: Government's Role in the Development of U.S. Health Services 1930-1980.* New York, NY: Oxford University Press; 1995.
7. Hanlon JJ. Is there a future for local health departments? *Health Serv Rep.* 1973; *88:* 898–901.
8. American Public Health Association. *Healthy Communities 2000: Model Standards.* Washington, DC: American Public Health Association; 1991.
9. Harrell JA, Baker EL. The essential services of public health. *Leadership Public Health.* 1994; *3:* 27–31.
10. Public Health Functions Steering Committee. *Public Health in America.* Washington, DC: U.S. Public Health Service; 1994.
11. Corso LC, Wiesner PJ, Halverson PK, Brown CK. Using the essential services as a foundation for performance measurement and assessment of local public health systems. *J Public Health Manage Pract.* 2000; *6:* 1–18.
12. National Association of County and City Health Officials. *Assessment Protocol for Excellence in Public Health.* Washington, DC: National Association of County and City Health Officials; 1991.
13. National Association of County and City Health Officials. *Mobilizing for Action through Planning and Partnerships.* Washington, DC: National Association of County and City Health Officials; 2000.
14. Lenihan DP, Landrum LB, Turnock BJ. *An Evaluation of MAPP and NPHPS in Local Public Health Jurisdictions.* Chicago, IL: Illinois Public Health Institute; 2006.

15. Institute of Medicine. *Healthy Communities: New Partnerships for the Future of Public Health*. Washington, DC: National Academy Press; 1996.

16. Committee on the Future of the Public's Health in the 21st Century, Institute of Medicine. *The Future of the Public's Health in the 21st Century*. Washington, DC: National Academy Press; 2003.

17. Institute of Medicine. *Improving Health in the Community: A Role for Performance Monitoring*. Washington, DC: National Academy Press; 1997.

18. National Association of County and City Health Officials. *2013 National Profile of Local Health Departments*. Washington, DC: National Association of County and City Health Officials; 2014.

19. Minkler M. Ten commitments for community health education. *Health Educ Res Theory Pract*. 1994; 9: 527–534.

20. McKnight JL, Kretzmann J. Mapping community capacity. *New Designs*. 1992; Winter: 9–15.

21. Centers for Disease Control/ATSDR Committee on Community Engagement. *Principles of Community Engagement*. Atlanta, GA: Centers for Disease Control; 1997.

22. University of Kansas. Community Tool Box. http://ctb.ku.edu/en. Accessed September 27, 2014.

23. Public Health Foundation. *Healthy People 2010 Tool Kit*. Washington, DC: American Public Health Foundation; 1999.

24. Berkowitz B. Collaboration for health improvement: models for state, community, and academic partnerships. *J Public Health Manage Pract*. 2000; 6: 67–72.

25. Norris T. Healthy communities. *Natl Civic Rev*. 1997; *86*: 3–10.

26. Milio N. Priorities and strategies for promoting community-based prevention policies. *J Public Health Manage Pract*. 1998; 4: 14–28.

27. Centers for Disease Control and Prevention, Public Health Practice Program Office. Available at www.cdc.gov/nphpsp/.

28. National Association of County and City Health Officials. *Operational Definition of a Functional Local Health Department*. Washington, DC: NACCHO; 2005.

29. Public Health Accreditation Board. Available at www.phaboard.org. Accessed June 14, 2014.

30. National Association of County and City Health Officials. *Local Health Department Accreditation: Findings from the 2014 Forces of Change Study*. Washington, DC: NACCHO; 2014.

31. Association of State and Territorial Health Officials. *Profile of State Health, Volume Three, 2012*. Washington, DC: ASTHO; 2014.

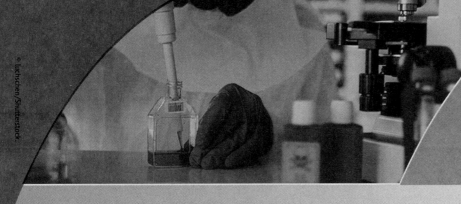

CHAPTER 6

Public Health Emergency Preparedness and Response

Given an emergency situation with public health implications (such as H1N1 influenza, massive flooding, or bioterrorism threats), identify the critical components necessary for an effective response. Key aspects of this competency expectation include being able to

- Differentiate among the various types of public health emergencies and disasters, including their definitions and related terminology
- Describe why emergencies and disasters are problems in which the public health system must be an integral participant across a range of activities
- Describe the roles, responsibilities and competencies expected of public health workers in emergency preparedness and response
- Define terrorism and bioterrorism and identify category A, B, and C biologic agents and their unique characteristics and relevance to bioterrorism events and threats, and
- Describe recent governmental public health initiatives for public health emergency preparedness and response

PUBLIC HEALTH ROLES IN EMERGENCY PREPAREDNESS AND RESPONSE

Public health crossed the threshold of the new century as an admittedly important but poorly understood contributor to American society. Despite its contributions to population health status and quality of life throughout the 20th century, the visibility and economic valuation of public health activities remained low. This situation changed rapidly after the terrorist attacks on the World Trade Center and Pentagon on September 11, 2001, and the bioterrorism events spreading anthrax through the United States postal system the following month. The nation responded quickly in the aftermath of these events, elevating terrorism, bioterrorism preparedness,

and emergency response to the top of the national agenda. Within months, several billion dollars were made available to federal, state, and local public health agencies for public health preparedness and response activities, with additional funding allocated annually thereafter. This explosion of attention, resources, and expectations typifies the history of public health in America—a dramatic health-related event spotlights a largely neglected public health infrastructure resulting in a rapid infusion of resources to resuscitate the system.

This chapter describes the decisions made and actions taken to enhance public health emergency preparedness and response, as well as some of the successes, failures, and lessons learned along the way. The intent is to chronicle why and how public health emergency preparedness and response is emerging as one of the hallmarks of public health practice in 21st century America. Toward that end, this chapter focuses on several key questions:

- What is public health preparedness?
- What are the key components of preparedness?
- Is the public health system adequately prepared?
- What is needed to become fully prepared?

The core functions and essential public health services framework for modern public health responses is organized around six major functions:

- Preventing epidemics and the spread of disease
- Protecting against environmental hazards
- Preventing injuries
- Promoting and encouraging healthy behaviors

- Responding to disasters and assisting communities in recovery
- Ensuring the quality and accessibility of health services[1]

Although only one of these functions explicitly refers to public health's role in responding to emergencies, all six drive the public health approach to emergency preparedness and response. Public health emergency preparedness and response efforts seek to prevent epidemics and the spread of disease, protect against environmental hazards, prevent injuries, promote healthy behaviors, and ensure the quality and accessibility of health services. Each of these is expected by the public and each is evident in effective preparedness and response related to public health emergencies. Together they make preparedness and response a special and particularly critical component of modern public health practice.

For public health emergencies, preparedness and response are inextricably linked.[2] Preparedness is based on lessons learned from both actual and simulated response situations. Effective response is all but impossible without extensive planning and thoughtful preparation. Public health roles in health-related emergencies illustrate both facets.

Public Health Surveillance

Many public health emergencies are readily apparent, but others may not manifest themselves immediately. Effective preparedness and response rely on monitoring disease patterns, investigating individual case reports, and using epidemiologic and laboratory analyses to target public health intervention strategies. For example, foodborne illness outbreaks may involve individuals who remain in the same location after being exposed, making it easier to identify a common exposure pattern when these individuals seek medical care. Alternatively, an exposure at a convention or family reunion is more difficult to detect because individuals may present for medical care far from the location of exposure. Whether within the same community or in distant locations, it is often difficult for individual medical practitioners to recognize that an outbreak or widespread epidemic is occurring. Prompt recognition and reporting of cases to health authorities is a critical link in the public health chain of protection. New approaches to public health surveillance include biosurveillance and syndromic surveillance, the early detection of abnormal disease patterns and nontraditional early disease indicators, such as pharmaceutical sales, school and work absenteeism, and animal disease events. Multiple large data sets can be mined and analyzed for nontraditional markers of disease, which can lead to more rapid detection and response efforts.

OUTSIDE-THE-BOOK THINKING 6-1

© Alfred Bondarenko/Shutterstock.

What constitutes vulnerability in populations living in disaster-prone areas? Provide a concrete example from a disaster that has drawn media attention in recent years.

Epidemiologic Investigation and Analysis

Once a disease event is reported, public health agencies can uncover unusual patterns that help identify outbreaks and continuing risks. Public health professionals may use sophisticated analytic tools, such as pattern recognition software and geographic information systems, to determine patterns in disease cases. These surveillance activities help to ensure that disease outbreaks are identified quickly and that appropriate response actions, such as the issuance of health alerts for area providers and communication with response partners, are initiated. Many current disease surveillance systems act in a passive manner (i.e., they rely on providers to initiate disease reports); however, public health agencies are increasingly using active surveillance activities, such as when public health workers proactively seek information from providers and other sources to monitor disease trends. In the event of an actual or threatened public health emergency, active surveillance activities are deployed and/or expanded.

Surveillance activities trigger more extensive and focused epidemiologic investigations in order to determine the identity, source, and modes of transmission of disease agents. Epidemiologic investigations seek to determine what is causing the disease, how the disease is spreading, and who is at risk. Answers to these questions inform efforts to mount rapid and effective interventions. Methods of obtaining epidemiologic information, often characterized as disease detective activities, include contacting patients, obtaining detailed information on location and types of possible exposures, and examining both clinical specimens (such as blood and urine) and environmental samplings (such as food, water, air, and soil). Epidemiologic investigations require trained personnel and, in many cases, are quite intensive in terms of the quantity and quality of human resources needed. Laboratory capacity to support these investigations is critical.

Laboratory Investigation and Analysis

In many situations, laboratories provide the definitive identification of causative agents, both biological and chemical, and through various fingerprinting activities link cases to a common source. Capabilities to identify rare or unusual diseases are often not present in every community, necessitating linkages with higher level laboratories. Specimens may be sent for analysis and confirmation to a regional or state public health laboratory or possibly even to a CDC reference laboratory (laboratories are rated in terms of the level of safety they provide). Some specialized capabilities found at these higher level laboratories include serotyping to determine the antigenic profile of a microorganism and DNA fingerprinting to not only identify the type of microorganism causing an infectious disease but to also pinpoint the particular strain of bacterium or virus involved. In this way, public health authorities can determine if reported disease cases are part of the same outbreak, and therefore linked to a common source. Public health laboratories must rely on specialized protective laboratory equipment and facilities because of the dangerous agents with which they work. Some agents, such as smallpox, require special biocontainment equipment and procedures.

Intervention through Effective Countermeasures

The primary reason for collecting, analyzing, and sharing information on disease is to control that disease. Expending resources for surveillance and analysis makes little sense if actions do not follow. Interventions that protect individuals from risks associated with environmental hazards are many, including setting standards for health and safety, inspecting food production and importation facilities, monitoring environmental conditions, abating conditions that foster infectious disease (e.g., insect and animal control), and enforcing private-sector compliance with established standards. Disease and injury risks associated with these biologic and chemical hazards, whether naturally occurring or initiated by man, are reduced through rigorous monitoring and enforcement activities. Public health agencies also play a substantial role in remediation of environmental hazards by decontaminating sites and facilities after they are identified. The extent of remediation necessary can vary greatly, just as the nature and extent of the contamination varies with different disease agents and their ability to remain viable outside a human host or animal/insect vector.

Risk Communication

Epidemiologic and laboratory investigations drive the initiation of actions intended to limit the spread of disease and to prevent additional cases in the community. The range of possible actions can be quite broad, including restraining the activities of individuals through isolation and quarantine and imposing temporary or permanent barriers around sources of contamination (e.g., sealing buildings, closing restaurants, and cutting off water supplies). In severe and unusual circumstances, special emergency powers may be put into effect limiting human and animal travel and/or restricting certain types of business activity. In these situations, the importance of effective public education and information activities to communicate risk to the public cannot be overstated. Commonly encountered examples include notices to boil drinking water when contaminated water supplies are suspected and product recalls and food safety advisories for potentially contaminated food products. The dissemination of information on mail handling practices during the anthrax attacks in late 2001 served both public education and risk communication purposes.

Promoting and encouraging healthy behaviors during public health emergencies represents another public health intervention strategy. It is not uncommon in the event of a natural disaster or terrorist attack for the most devastating effects to take the form of social disruption and infrastructure damage. The psychological effects of fear and terror, together with disruption of infrastructure components such as electricity, water, and safe housing, may create more casualties than any initial terrorist's biologic or chemical assault. Such conditions can also foster toxicity and infectious disease threats, such as occurred with the mass evacuation of the area around the World Trade Center leading to the abandonment of food supplies in surrounding homes and restaurants. Public health officials in New York City took steps to secure these premises to avoid the proliferation of rodents and other pests that otherwise could have resulted in secondary health threats.

Preparedness Planning

Organizing responses to emergencies is an important public health role that ensures the availability and accessibility of medical and mental health services. Preparedness and planning cannot eliminate all biologic, chemical, radiation, and mass casualty threats. But coordinated, community-wide planning for emergency medical and public health responses ensures that emergency medical services and medical treatment services are deployed in a rapid and effective manner. Such planning foresees the need for public health measures to be activated in order to ensure the safety of responders and to prevent secondary effects caused by further disease transmission and injury risk. Planning for these coordinated responses includes monitoring available response resources, establishing action protocols, simulating emergency events to improve readiness, training public and private sector personnel, assessing communication capabilities, supplies, and resources, and maintaining relationships with partner organizations to improve coordination. Hazard vulnerability analyses are an especially important planning tool that rate and rank the risk of specific emergencies for communities.

OUTSIDE-THE-BOOK THINKING 6-2

© Alfred Bondarenko/Shutterstock.

What are the basic functions that public health organizations perform in response to emergencies and disasters? When and how should the organization identify these functions?

Community-Wide Response

Public sector agencies play an important, but not exclusive, role in community-wide responses to emergencies. In many response situations, private sector medical care providers deliver the bulk of the triage and treatment services needed when a mass casualty emergency occurs. Although less involved with direct care, public sector agencies play key roles in coordinating and overseeing the delivery of services as well as communicating with providers, the media, and the public. Supervision of decontamination and triage often falls to public health authorities. Countermeasures such as antibiotics, antitoxins, and chemical antidotes as well as prophylactic medications and vaccines must be obtained, deployed, and delivered. Public health plays an active role in situations necessitating deployment of Strategic National Stockpile (SNS) pharmaceuticals, supplies, and equipment. In some situations, public health professionals also provide direct medical care. Public health also contributes through mobilization of regional and national assets and resources when local resources are overwhelmed. Some emergency situations, such as the anthrax attacks of 2001, prompted public fear and overreactions resulting in mountains of unknown powdery substances being tested and thousands of individuals unnecessarily initiating prophylactic antibiotic treatments. That situation and others over recent years argue that the worried well can stress response systems even more than those actually affected.

Unique Aspects of Bioterrorism Emergencies

Across the spectrum of possible public health emergency scenarios, bioterrorism threats represent a particularly challenging form of public health emergency. Bioterrorism is the threatened or intentional release of biologic agents (viruses, bacteria, or their toxins) for the purpose of influencing the conduct of government or intimidating or coercing a civilian population to further political or social objectives. These agents can be released by way of the air (as aerosols), food, water, or insects. Biologic agents with significant bioterrorism potential are listed in **Table 6-1**. Category A includes organisms that pose a risk to national security because of several factors. These organisms can be easily disseminated or transmitted from person to person, and they result in high mortality rates and have the potential for major public health impact. In addition, these organisms are likely to cause public panic and social disruption, thereby requiring special action for public health preparedness. Category B agents are the second highest priority organisms. These are moderately easy to disseminate, result in moderate morbidity rates and low mortality rates, and require specific enhancements of the CDC's diagnostic capacity and enhanced disease surveillance. The third highest priority agents fall into Category C and include emerging pathogens that could be engineered for mass dissemination in the future because of availability, ease of production and dissemination, and potential for high morbidity and mortality rates with major public health impact.

Biologic, chemical, radiation, and mass casualty threats that are intentionally inflicted differ from naturally occurring disease and injury threats in a number of important aspects. Central to these differences, bioterrorism is a criminal act requiring its prevention and response to include criminal justice, military, and intelligence agencies that are not likely to be familiar with naturally occurring disease outbreaks. Law enforcement agencies, including the Federal Bureau of Investigation, have lead responsibility for responding to a bioterrorism attack. In addition, bioterrorism attacks may involve disease agents that occur infrequently in nature and with which neither public health officials nor clinicians have had much experience. It is increasingly possible to genetically engineer chimeras to create, for example, microorganisms that blend the pathogenic qualities of multiple disease

TABLE 6-1 Biologic Agents with Bioterrorism Potential

Category A
- Anthrax (Bacillus anthracis)
- Botulism (Clostridium botulinum toxin)
- Plague (Yersinia pestis)
- Smallpox (variola major)
- Tularemia (Francisella tularensis)
- Viral hemorrhagic fevers (filoviruses [e.g., Ebola, Marburg] and arenaviruses [e.g., Lassa, Machupo])

Category B
- Brucellosis (Brucella species)
- Epsilon toxin of Clostridium perfringens
- Food safety threats (e.g., Salmonella species, Escherichia coli O157:H7, Shigella)
- Glanders (Burkholderia mallei)
- Meloidosis (Burkholderia pseudomallei)
- Psittacosis (Chlamydia psittaci)
- Q fever (Coxiella burnetii)
- Ricin toxin from Ricinus communis (castor beans)
- Staphylococcal enterotoxin B
- Typhus fever (Rickettsia prowazekii)
- Viral encephalitis (alphaviruses [e.g., Venezuelan equine encephalitis, eastern equine encephalitis, western equine encephalitis])
- Water safety threats (e.g., Vibrio cholerae, Cryptosporidium parvum)

Category C
- Emerging infectious diseases such as Nipah virus and hantavirus

Reproduced from Centers for Disease Control and Prevention; 2010.

agents. Because such organisms do not exist in nature, they would be completely unknown to public health and medical experts. Attacks related to biologic or chemical threats initiated by a bioterrorist would not likely follow known epidemiologic patterns, diminishing the value of using past experience with disease transmission and manifestation to identify the source or cause.

It is likely that bioterrorists would seek to be covert, expending great energy and attention to ensure the delayed discovery of the disease to maximize the population's exposure. Intentional outbreaks may develop in multiple locations simultaneously, thereby straining local, state, and federal response efforts. With many emerging and reemerging infectious disease threats (e.g., Ebola Virus, Sudden Acute Respiratory Syndrome, West Nile Virus, hantavirus), it is increasingly difficult to predict the precise nature of the next public health emergency. It could result from a chance mutation of a microorganism or it could result from the intentional act of terrorists. Multiple threats are possible, necessitating preparedness and response systems that can address a wide variety of unknown and unanticipated hazards. This concept of multiple threats and unknown hazards has led many terrorism experts to advocate for a robust public health infrastructure capable of responding to many different forms of emergencies.

Protecting the public from infectious diseases and other threats is one of the major roles of public health in modern society. This role took on a new meaning after the national security was threatened by the events of September 11, 2001, and the anthrax attacks that were initiated less than a month later. **Figure 6-1 and Figure 6-2** summarize the time lines and pathways for the most infamous bioterrorism attack in U.S. history. Initially focused on bioterrorism threats and events, this new role of public health emergency preparedness and response for all types of emergencies and disasters has emerged as central to what public health professionals and organizations are expected to perform in 21st century America.

Workplace Preparedness

Public health emergencies, including those related to terrorism, have many different visages and many different venues. Yet most of the direct victims of terrorism in the United States in recent years have been people at work, including the victims of the bombing of the federal building in Oklahoma City, those who died in the World Trade Center and the Pentagon on September 11, 2001, and the victims who contracted anthrax transmitted through the mail later in that same year.

Acts of terrorism intend to make people feel powerless and believe that they cannot take steps to prevent such incidents or mitigate their consequences. But experience to date in battling other workplace safety risks suggests that there are steps that can be taken by employers and employees. The workplace is, in effect, a key line of defense for homeland security. This is recognized formally in the formation and scope of responsibilities for the new federal Department of Homeland Security (DHS) as well as in the response of the business community after 2001 in taking tangible steps to enhance security.

FIGURE 6-1 Epidemic Curve for 22 Cases of Bioterrorism-Related Anthrax, United States, 2001

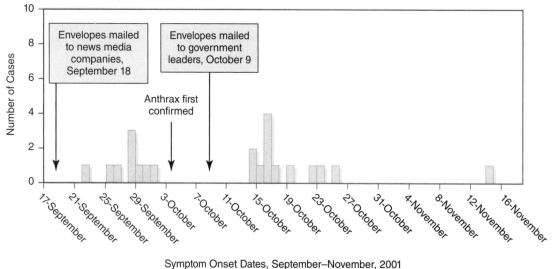

Reprodcued from Jernigan DB, Raghunathan PL, Bell BP, et al. Investigation of bioterrorism-related anthrax, United States, 2002: epidemiologic findings. *Emerging Infectious Diseases*. 2002; 8(10): 1019–1028.

FIGURE 6-2 Cases of Anthrax Associated with Mailed Paths of Implicated Envelopes and Intended Target Sites, United States, 2001

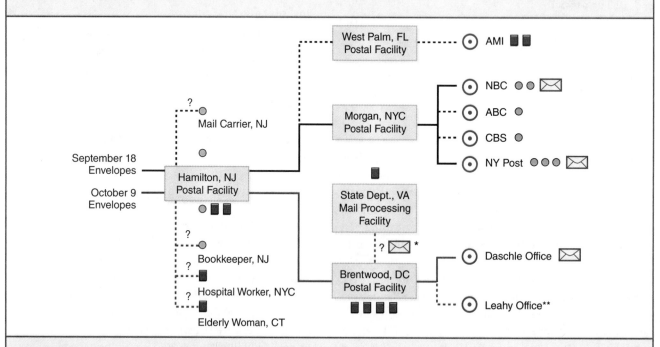

Reprodcued from Jernigan DB, Raghunathan PL, Bell BP, et al. Investigation of bioterrorism-related anthrax, United States, 2002: epidemiologic findings. *Emerging Infectious Diseases*. 2002; 8(10): 1019–1028.

NATIONAL PUBLIC HEALTH PREPAREDNESS AND RESPONSE COORDINATION

The terrorist events of 2001 resulted in a series of new national policies and priorities to safeguard American citizens at home. One major development was the creation of the Department of Homeland Security (DHS) with extensive authority and powers related to domestic terrorism and security. In accord with the Homeland Security Act of 2002, several important public health functions were transferred into the new DHS in 2003, including the SNS of emergency pharmaceutical supplies and medical equipment. Responsibilities for SNS were subsequently transferred from DHS to CDC. The new federal agency immediately became part of the American everyday experience through activities providing timely and detailed information about threat levels to the public, government agencies, first responders, transportation hubs, and the private sector.

The establishment of a new federal agency, however, did not substantially alter the configuration of public health responsibilities within the system of operational federalism described in our earlier examination of law, government, and public health. Federal agencies are significant contributors, but public health remains largely a state responsibility, with the bulk of this activity taking place at the local level. For public health emergencies, including national disasters such as Hurricane Katrina in 2005 and bioterrorism events or threats, preparedness and coordinated response across all levels of government are critical. Nonetheless, there are significant issues related to intergovernmental relationships, resource deployment, and financing that make public health emergencies especially difficult challenges for the public health system. The following sections examine key aspects of the structure, operations, and issues in public health emergency preparedness and response at the national, state, and local levels.

Federal Agencies and Assets

Several dozen separate federal departments and agencies have roles in preparing for or responding to public health emergencies, including bioterrorist attacks. Within this constellation of agencies, the Department of Health and Human Services (DHHS) and DHS play the most important public health roles.

Prior to 2003, DHHS was the primary federal agency responsible for the medical and public health response to emergencies (including major disasters and terrorist events). Beginning in 2003, DHHS now shares center stage with the new DHS. DHHS discharges its responsibilities through several operating agencies, including the following:

- CDC: CDC works with state public health agencies to detect, investigate, and prevent the spread of disease in communities. CDC provides support to state public health agencies in a variety of ways, including financial assistance, training programs, technical assistance and expert consultation, sophisticated laboratory services, research activities, and standards development. The Office of Public Health Preparedness and Response coordinates efforts across the various CDC centers, institutes, and offices. CDC now has operational responsibility for deployment of SNS resources during emergencies.

- Health Resources and Services Administration (HRSA): HRSA was the agency originally responsible for a state grant program to facilitate regional hospital preparedness planning and to upgrade the capacity of hospitals and other healthcare facilities to respond to public health emergencies until this program was transferred to the Office of the Assistant Secretary for Preparedness and Response. HRSA is also generally responsible for healthcare workforce development, including grant programs for curriculum development and continuing education for health professionals on bioterrorism preparedness and response.

- Food and Drug Administration (FDA): FDA has responsibilities both for ensuring the safety of the food supply and for ensuring the safety and efficacy of pharmaceuticals, biologics, and medical devices. FDA fulfills its food safety responsibilities in partnership with the Department of Agriculture, which is responsible for the safety of meat, poultry, and processed egg products.

- National Institutes of Health (NIH): NIH conducts and supports biomedical research, including research targeted at the development of rapid diagnostics and new and more effective vaccines and antimicrobial therapies.

- Office of the Assistant Secretary for Preparedness and Response (ASPR) within DHHS sets overall policy direction and coordinates public health emergency preparedness and response activities across the various DHHS agencies. This office now administers the hospital preparedness program, formerly managed by HRSA.

In 2003, 23 federal agencies, programs, and offices were fashioned into the new federal DHS. The new agency sought to bring a coordinated approach to national security from emergencies and disasters, both natural and man-made.

DHS actively promotes an "all-hazards" approach to disasters and homeland security issues. The Federal Emergency Management Agency (FEMA), formerly an independent agency, became one of the major branches of the new DHS responsible for emergency preparedness and response, tasked with responding to, planning for, recovering from, and mitigating against disasters under authority provided by the federal Stafford Act (**Table 6-2**).

Within DHS, the Emergency Preparedness and Response Directorate coordinates emergency medical response in the event of a public health emergency, including the National Disaster Medical System and the Metropolitan Medical

Response Systems (these are described later in this chapter). Other major directorates (divisions) of the new DHS include Border and Transportation Security, Science and Technology, Information Analysis and Infrastructure Protection, and Management.

Within DHS, the chief medical officer has primary responsibility for medical issues related to natural and man-made disasters and terrorism. In the aftermath of Hurricane Katrina, the Pandemic and All-Hazards Preparedness Act (PAHPA) of 2006 clarified the roles and responsibilities of DHS and DHHS. Several programs, including the National Disaster Medical System, were moved from DHS to DHHS.

Other federal agencies also carry important responsibilities related to bioterrorism and public health emergency preparedness. The Environmental Protection Agency responds to emergencies involving chemicals and other hazardous substances. The Department of Defense indirectly supports public health preparedness through various research efforts on biologic and chemical weapons, intelligence gathering related to terrorism threats, and civil support functions in the event of an emergency that results in severe social unrest. The Department of Justice has lead responsibility for assessing and investigating terrorist threats, including those related to bioterrorism, and provides funds and assistance to emergency responders (police, fire, ambulance, and rescue personnel) at state and local levels. The Department of Veterans Affairs purchases drugs and other therapeutics for the SNS and operates one of the nation's largest healthcare systems, which could provide critical surge capacity in the event of a mass casualty event. Several other federal agencies, including the Departments of Transportation, Commerce, and Energy, also have potential roles to play in preparing for and responding to a public health emergency.

National Incident Management System

Prior to the establishment of the new DHS, the management of large-scale health events was complicated by the involvement of many different federal agencies. States have established a similar web of agencies to manage disasters and other emergencies, with each developing its own form of an incident management system. In order to ensure greater consistency across states and for interfaces between the federal government and states, a National Incident Management System (NIMS) was prescribed by a presidential directive in 2003 to cover all incidents (natural and unnatural) for which the federal government deploys emergency response assets. The Secretary of Homeland Security is responsible for the development and implementation of NIMS. Its success depends in large part on the establishment of consistent

---

TABLE 6-2   Robert T. Stafford Disaster Relief and Emergency Assistance Act

The Congress hereby finds and declares that (1) because disasters often cause loss of life, human suffering, loss of income, and property loss and damage; and (2) because disasters often disrupt the normal functioning of governments and communities, and adversely affect individuals and families with great severity; special measures, designed to assist the efforts of the affected States in expediting the rendering of aid, assistance, and emergency services, and the reconstruction and rehabilitation of devastated areas, are necessary.

It is the intent of Congress, by this Act, to provide an orderly and continuing means of assistance by the Federal Government to State and local governments in carrying out their responsibilities to alleviate the suffering and damage which result from such disasters by—

(1) revising and broadening the scope of existing disaster relief programs;

(2) encouraging the development of comprehensive disaster preparedness and assistance plans, programs, capabilities, and organizations by the States and by local government;

(3) achieving greater coordination and responsiveness of disaster preparedness and relief programs;

(4) encouraging individuals, States, and local governments to protect themselves by obtaining insurance coverage to supplement or replace governmental assistance;

(5) encouraging hazard mitigation measures to reduce losses from disasters, including development of land use and construction regulations; and

(6) providing Federal assistance programs for both public and private losses sustained in disasters.

P.L. 93-288, as amended.

approaches within the states as to roles and responsibilities for both public health agencies and the hospital community (including their supporting healthcare systems) in managing emergencies at the state and regional levels and developing and deploying incident management plans at substate levels.

Bioterrorism and other public health incidents fall within the scope of NIMS. To this end, DHHS has the initial lead responsibility for the federal government and deploys assets as needed within the areas of its statutory responsibility (such as the Public Health Service Act and the Federal Food, Drug, and Cosmetic Act) while keeping the Secretary of Homeland Security apprised regarding the course of the incident and nature of the response operations.

While NIMS is used for all events, the National Response Plan (NRP) is implemented for incidents requiring federal coordination. The NRP is another key provision of the Homeland Security Act of 2002 and Homeland Security Presidential Directive 5. The purpose of NRP is to align federal coordinating, structures, capabilities, and resources into a unified, all-discipline, and all-hazards approach to domestic incident management. It is based on the premise that incidents are typically managed at the lowest possible geographic, organizational, and jurisdictional level. NRP does not alter or impede the ability of federal agencies to carry out their specific authorities under applicable laws, executive orders, and directives. It establishes the coordinating structures, processes, and protocols required to integrate the specific statutory and policy authorities of various federal departments and agencies in a collective framework for action to include prevention, preparedness, response, and recovery activities. The NRP distinguishes between events that require the secretary of DHS to manage the federal response for incidents of national significance and the majority of incidents occurring each year that are handled by responsible jurisdictions or avenues through other established authorities and existing plans.

Under the NRP, DHS assumes responsibility for coordinating federal response operations, including those involving public health components, under certain conditions. DHS coordinates the federal government's resources utilized in response to or in recovery from terrorist attacks, major disasters, or other emergencies if and when any of the following four conditions applies:

1. A federal department or agency acting under its own authority has requested the assistance.
2. The resources of state and local authorities are overwhelmed and federal assistance has been formally requested by state and local authorities.

3. More than one federal department or agency has become substantially involved in responding to the incident.
4. DHS has been directed to assume responsibility for managing the domestic incident by the president.[3]

For states and local governments to gain full benefit from the emergency response assets of the federal government, states must develop incident management systems that are interoperable with NIMS. Beginning in 2004, adherence to and compatibility with NIMS became a condition of all grants and other awards from federal agencies for any aspect of state or local emergency preparedness and response. NRP compliance was required as well after 2006.

The Pandemic and All-Hazards Preparedness Act (PAHPA) legislation of 2006 and 2013 reauthorized and restructured key components of public health preparedness and response efforts in DHS and DHHS. PAHPA also addressed lessons learned from the flawed federal response to Hurricane Katrina and growing concerns over a possible global flu pandemic. Central to the restructuring of federal roles and responsibilities was the establishment of a national health security strategy for public health emergency preparedness and response, including a full assessment of federal, state, and local public health and medical capabilities. Key elements of the national health security strategy in PAHPA focused on:

- Public health workforce enhancements including revitalization of the Commissioned Corps and loan repayment programs to increase the number of public health professionals working in shortage areas;
- Vaccine tracking and distribution to improve effective distribution of seasonal flu vaccine supplies;
- Enhanced all-hazards medical surge capacity through use of mobile medical assets and federal facilities during emergencies, expanding the Medical Reserve Corps and establishing a single nationwide network of systems for the purpose of advance registration of volunteer health professionals;
- Biomedical research and development for vaccine and drug development to combat pandemic flu emergencies; and
- Grants to state and local government to improve detection and response capabilities for pandemic flu.

Federal Emergency Medical Assets

Several national emergency response assets are available to state and local governments from the new DHS. These include the National Disaster Medical System (NDMS), the Metropolitan Medical Response System (MMRS), and the Strategic National Stockpile (SNS).

The NDMS now operates within the Office of Emergency Preparedness and Response within DHHS. NDMS brings together medical services from DHHS, DHS, Defense, and Veterans Affairs to augment local emergency medical services during a disaster or other large-scale emergency. The NDMS has several operational components, including Disaster Medical Assistance Teams (DMATs), Disaster Mortuary Teams (DMORTs), Federal Coordinating Centers, and Management Support Units.

DMATs are self-sustaining squads of licensed, actively practicing, volunteer professional and paraprofessional medical personnel who provide emergency medical care at the site of a disaster or other emergency. DMAT teams often triage, stabilize, and prepare patients for evacuation in mass casualty situations. They are sent into these situations to supplement, rather than supplant or replace, local capacity. Once activated, these professionals are federalized, allowing them to practice with their current professional licenses in any jurisdiction. DMORTs include mortuary, dental, and forensic specialists who serve to augment the services of local coroners and medical examiners. Portable temporary mortuaries for mass casualty situations are provided when needed. Management support units provide command, coordination, and communication capabilities for DMATs and DMORTs and other federal assets. Federal Coordinating Centers recruit hospitals to participate in the NDMS and recruit health workers for the DMATs and DMORTs.

The MMRS, involving more than 100 metropolitan communities, integrates existing emergency response systems at the local level, including emergency management, medical and mental health providers, public health agencies, law enforcement, fire departments, emergency medical services, and the National Guard. The MMRS seeks to develop a unified regional response to mass casualty events. MMRS was transferred from DHHS when the new DHS was established in 2003.

The SNS ensures the availability and rapid deployment of life-saving pharmaceuticals, antidotes, other medical supplies, and equipment necessary to counter the effects of nerve agents, biologic pathogens, and chemical agents. The SNS stands ready for immediate deployment to any U.S. location in the event of a terrorist attack using a biologic toxin or chemical agent directed against a civilian population. In the event of possible bioterrorist attack, a 12-hour push package containing 50 tons of stockpile materials can be immediately dispatched to predetermined Receipt, Store, and Storage sites identified in state bioterrorism response plans. There are twelve 12-hour push packages centrally located around the U.S. for immediate deployment. Detailed deployment activities for SNS materials are prescribed in state and local emergency response plans.

Federal Funding for Public Health Preparedness Infrastructure

Although multiple agencies provide federal funding for emergency preparedness, federal support for the public health infrastructure at the state and local levels is provided largely from grants and cooperative agreements with CDC. In 1999, for the first time, CDC awarded more than $40 million for bioterrorism preparedness to states and cities for enhanced laboratory and electronic communication capacity and another $32 million to establish a national pharmaceutical stockpile to ensure availability of vaccines, prophylactic medicines, chemical antidotes, medical supplies, and equipment needed to support a medical response to a biologic or chemical terrorist incident. At the time, these appeared to be large sums. In the wake of September 11, 2001, and the anthrax attacks the following month, increased concerns regarding homeland security led to a $2.1 billion FY 2002 appropriation for CDC's antiterrorism activities, over a 20-fold increase from FY 1999 levels. The FY 2002 supplemental appropriations nearly $1 billion for grants to states and localities to upgrade state and local capacity. Roughly similar levels of funding were provided throughout the first decade of the new century, although steady reductions marked the years of the second decade. The state and local activities impacted by this funding are described in subsequent sections of this chapter.

STATE AND LOCAL PUBLIC HEALTH PREPAREDNESS AND RESPONSE COORDINATION

State Agencies and Assets

Similar to the federal pattern, states rely on a variety of agencies to deliver public health emergency services. Also similar to the federal model, these functions tend to be concentrated within a limited number of agencies at the state level, with the state health department and state emergency management agency playing the most significant roles. Most state health departments are freestanding agencies (i.e., not part of a larger human services agency), and many have responsibility for emergency medical service systems within the state. However, most states have an environmental health agency that is separate from the state health agency. Although these states may have an environmental health section within the health agency, the environmental health agency is charged with monitoring environmental contaminants and remediation of hazardous conditions. Nearly all states have a separate emergency management agency (patterned after FEMA), and some states have established their own Departments of Homeland Security. In responding to a public health emergency, the state public health agency works collaboratively with the state emergency management agency as well as with the state environmental protection, law enforcement, public safety, and transportation agencies and, in some instances, the National Guard.

States execute their powers and authority to act in public health emergencies through various state public health laws. There are concerns that existing public health laws may be inadequate in some states because they are obsolete and fragmented. A Model Public Health Emergency Powers Act was designed to assist states in examining and enhancing their legal framework for public health emergencies. The model act addresses key issues related to preparedness, surveillance, protection of persons, management of property, and public information and communications.[4]

Considerable differences exist among states in the breadth and depth of services provided within their jurisdictions and the degree to which public health service delivery responsibilities are delegated to local governments. In general, however, state governments are ultimately responsible for ensuring adequate response to a public health emergency and tend to play certain key roles in preparedness and response, regardless of how decentralized a particular public health system might be. Except in the largest metropolitan local public health departments, local public health officials rely on state personnel and capacity for a number of key functions, including advanced laboratory capacity, epidemiologic expertise, and serving as a conduit for federal assistance.

OUTSIDE-THE-BOOK THINKING 6-3

© Alfred Bondarenko/Shutterstock.

Describe three or more provisions of public health statutes that are important elements of public health emergency response plans.

States participate in an interstate agreement whereby one or more states can provide resources, equipment, services, and other needed support to another state during an emergency incident. This mutual aid agreement, the Emergency Management Assistance Compact (EMAC), covers licensing, credentialing, workers compensation, and reimbursement, allowing personnel to focus on the emergency at hand. EMAC personnel integrate into the existing structures of the requesting state. Of the more than 65,000 personnel deployed to Louisiana, Mississippi, and Alabama for Hurricanes Katrina and Rita in 2005, nearly 4,000 were health and medical personnel.

Incident Command Systems

In order to manage resources effectively and facilitate decision making during emergencies, incident command systems (ICS) are in wide use by police, fire, and emergency management agencies. Initially adopted for the fire service, ICS eliminates many common problems related to communication, terminology, organizational structure, span of control, and other differences across different disciplines and agencies in response to a critical incident. Critical incidents include any natural or man-made event, civil disturbance, or any other occurrence of unusual or severe nature that threatens to cause or actually causes the loss of life or injury to citizens and/or severe damage to property.

In managing critical incidents, clear goals and objectives are established and communicated to responders, response plans are utilized, communications are effective, and resources are utilized in a timely and effective manner. ICS should not be considered an additional set of procedures; rather the system must become part of routine operations, with personnel fully trained in its use and standard operating procedures reflective of the capabilities actually available.

One important key to effective ICS is the ability to size up the incident scene and make the initial call for resources. This allows responders to get control of the incident rather than playing catch-up for the rest of the incident. Appropriate initial size-up prevents unnecessary injury or loss of life, property or environmental damage, and negative perceptions of the responding agencies.

Key components of ICS include

- Common terminology—Major organizational functions and units are named; in multiple incidents, each incident is named. Common names are used for personnel, equipment, and facilities. Clear terms are used in radio transmissions (e.g., codes, such as "10" codes, are not used).

- Modular organization—ICS develops "top down" from the first unit involved based on the specific incident's management needs. Each ICS is staffed with a designated incident commander (responsible for safety, liaison, and information) with other functions (operations, planning, logistics, finance/administration) staffed as needed.
- Integrated communications—ICS uses a common communications plan and redundant two-way communications.
- A unified command structure—This is necessary when the incident is within a single jurisdiction with multiple agencies involved, or the incident is multijurisdictional, or individuals representing different agencies or jurisdictions share common responsibilities. All agencies involved contribute to the unified command process by determining overall goals and objectives, planning jointly for tactical activities, conducting integrated tactical operations, and maximizing the use of assigned resources.
- Consolidated action plans—Written action plans are necessary when the incident is complex and/or when several agencies and/or jurisdictions are involved. Action plans include specific goals, objectives, and support -activities.
- A manageable span of control—The number of subordinates one supervisor can manage effectively should be between three and seven, with five being optimal.
- Designated incident facilities—These include the command post from which all incident operations, direction, control, coordination, and resource management are directed. Command posts can be fixed or mobile but need adequate communications capabilities.
- Comprehensive resource management—This maximizes resource use, consolidates control, reduces communications load, provides accountability, and reduces freelancing.

The emergency management team functions at the emergency operations center (EOC) where it coordinates strategic decisions through the incident command structure. Ideally, the team should be isolated from the confusion, media, and weather during the incident. EOC participants must have adequate authority and decision-making capability. EOC decisions could include issuing curfews, circumventing normal bidding processes, emergency appointments, permanent or temporary relocation, emergency demolition of unsafe properties, or implementation of prophylaxis to

populations. The EOC is supported operationally by incident command posts in the field, which are responsible for tactical decisions as well as oversight and command of responders at the scene.

Effective emergency operations plans and standard operating procedures simplify decision making during incidents. Training makes implementation of decisions easier for subordinates. When the level of preparation and practice exercises is inadequate, emergency operations plans can become overwhelmed by common incidents and unable to deal with those that are not fully anticipated. In such circumstances, decision making becomes complex and challenging. A comprehensively planned and frequently exercised organizational system is necessary to overcome these pitfalls.

As ICS has become increasingly accepted as an effective framework for responding to incidents, its use has extended to other settings. For example, there has been much progress in development and deployment of hospital emergency ICSs and tabletop exercises for hospitals. Several states have expanded on the ICS concept to develop standardized emergency management systems that formally incorporate ICS, mutual aid agreements, and multijurisdictional and interagency cooperation at the substate level, resulting in coordinated and unified decisions throughout the state.

Local Agencies and Assets

The front line of response to public health emergencies is at the local level, where LHDs work collaboratively with other first responders, such as fire and rescue personnel, emergency medical service providers, law enforcement officers, hazardous materials teams, physicians, and hospitals in preparing for and managing the consequences of health-related emergencies. Although the relationships between state and local public health agencies vary greatly from state to state, and even from local jurisdiction to local jurisdiction within the same state, local government has significant responsibilities for dealing with emergencies in virtually all states. First responders play key roles in:

- Recognizing public health emergencies, including those that result from terrorist attacks
- Identifying unique personal safety implications associated with the emergency situation
- Identifying security issues that are unique to the event or to the emergency medical system response
- Understanding basic principles of patient care based upon the type of emergency event encountered

Focusing on the services most directly related to emergency preparedness and response, the vast majority of LHDs carry out activities related to epidemiology and surveillance, communicable disease control, food safety, and restaurant inspections.[5] Relatively few LHDs operate laboratory services, air quality, animal control, or water inspections.

In those cases in which the LHD is not responsible for these services, they are typically delivered by another local government agency (e.g., a fire department or environmental services agency), a private agency (hospital or ambulance service), or the state. Even when services are offered by an LHD, they may be quite limited in terms of scope or hours of availability. For example, although nearly one-half of LHDs report providing laboratory services, these services may be quite limited in nature (e.g., to support tuberculosis and sexually transmitted disease testing). Many LHDs that report having laboratory services are likely to rely on state public health labs for more specialized diagnostic needs.

The state of readiness among LHDs has increased since 2001, when only about one-fourth of LHDs had completed a comprehensive emergency response plan with another one-fourth indicating that planning was underway. Deployment of LHD staff to assist in emergencies is limited by the size and qualifications of the agency's workforce. More than one-half of all LHDs have 20 or fewer staff members.[5] Larger agencies generally have much higher staffing levels and a more comprehensive range of expertise. **Figure 6-3** illustrates the range of LHD activities related to emergency preparedness and response in 2013. Nearly 60% of LHDs reported responding to an emergency event in the previous year. **Figure 6-4** demonstrates the percentage of LHDs responding to specific events or participating in drills and exercises related to those emergencies. **Table 6-3** catalogs the range and types of drills and exercises.

The configuration of LHDs within a state or in a multistate metropolitan area also varies across the country. Several states organize local public health activities at a regional or district level. Other states have virtually hundreds of LHDs that serve towns or townships, some in counties or districts served by a larger LHD. Some communities have no LHD at all. Organizing preparedness and response efforts in these different circumstances presents special problems in terms of multijurisdictional response, surge capacity, backup, and mutual aid agreements. Several capacity assessment and enhancement tools are available from NACCHO and CDC to assist local assessment of readiness.[6–8]

Medical Reserve Corps are locally based volunteer response teams that can be deployed in emergency situations.

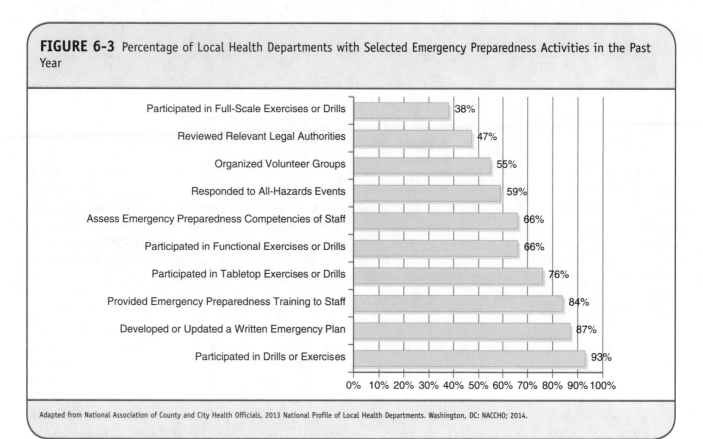

FIGURE 6-3 Percentage of Local Health Departments with Selected Emergency Preparedness Activities in the Past Year

Participated in Full-Scale Exercises or Drills — 38%
Reviewed Relevant Legal Authorities — 47%
Organized Volunteer Groups — 55%
Responded to All-Hazards Events — 59%
Assess Emergency Preparedness Competencies of Staff — 66%
Participated in Functional Exercises or Drills — 66%
Participated in Tabletop Exercises or Drills — 76%
Provided Emergency Preparedness Training to Staff — 84%
Developed or Updated a Written Emergency Plan — 87%
Participated in Drills or Exercises — 93%

Adapted from National Association of County and City Health Officials, 2013 National Profile of Local Health Departments. Washington, DC: NACCHO; 2014.

FIGURE 6-4 Percentage of Local Health Departments Responding to a Specific All-Hazards Event or Participating in a Drill or Exercise for that Event in the Past Year

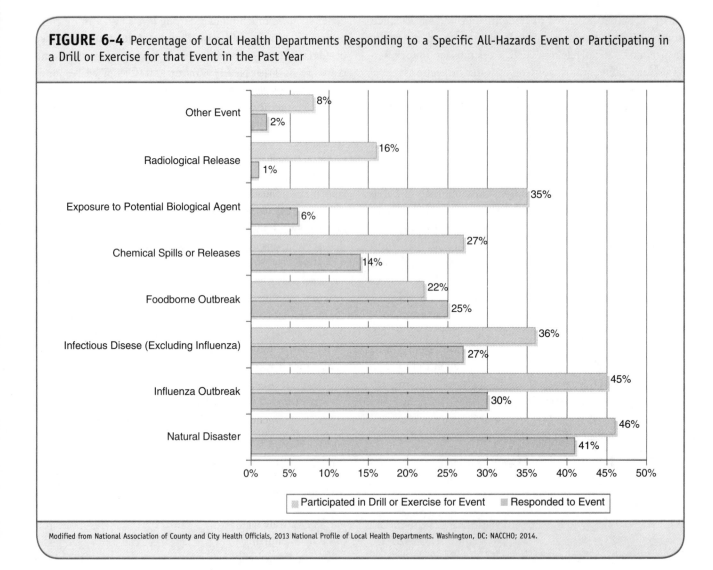

Modified from National Association of County and City Health Officials, 2013 National Profile of Local Health Departments. Washington, DC: NACCHO; 2014.

These multidisciplinary teams often have ongoing relationships with local public health agencies and other community medical care providers that may include volunteer work on health promotion and screening projects or assistance with mosquito control activities in communities where West Nile Virus presents a risk. During emergencies, Medical Reserve Corps teams play predetermined roles such as providing local surge capacity for triage and medical care or assisting with deployment of SNS materials. Several hundred communities already participate in the Medical Reserve Corps program, either through start-up funding from the HRSA or through local resources.

Education and training for frontline workers has been a continuing challenge for local agencies in order for them to assess and address the training needs of key public health professionals, infectious disease specialists, emergency department personnel, and other healthcare (including mental health) providers. Emergency preparedness competencies (**Table 6-4**) for all public health workers serve as the focal point for these assessment, enhancement, and recognition efforts. A more extensive panel of bioterrorism and emergency readiness competencies for various categories of public health workers is also in wide use.[9]

Private Healthcare Providers and Other Partners

In nearly all communities, government agencies play a central role in preparing for and responding to public health emergencies. Often overlooked, however, is the critical contribution made by private sector healthcare providers, pharmaceutical manufacturers, agricultural producers, the food industry, and other private sector interests. An important example is the role played by alert health professionals who

TABLE 6-3 Types of Emergency Exercises

Exercise	Activities that can be undertaken by an agency or group of agencies to test their readiness to respond to emergencies or to evaluate the adequacy of their response plan and success of their training program
Orientation seminar or workshop	An exercise carried out to familiarize new staff with the agency's emergency response activities or current staff to new or changing information or procedures or to bring together response agencies for better understanding and coordination
Drill	An exercise limited to a specific response activity and conducted to instruct thoroughly through repetition and practice
Tabletop	An exercise conducted in a conference room setting with situations presented as verbal or written problems or questions intended to generate discussion of actions to be taken based on the emergency plan and standard operating procedures. Basic tabletop exercises use group process to solve problems. Advanced play uses prescripted messages.
Functional	An exercise usually conducted at the site where the event would normally take place such as the command center and designed to evaluate the capabilities of the disaster response system.
Full scale	An exercise designed to test a major portion of the emergency operations plan, evaluate the operational capability of emergency responders in an interactive manner over an extended period of time, and mobilize field personnel and resources.

Adapted from Center for Health Policy, Columbia University School of Nursing. *Defining Emergency Exercises: A Working Guide to the Terminology Used in Practicing Emergency Responses in Communities and Public Health Agencies.* New York, NY: Columbia University School of Nursing, Center for Health Policy; 2004.

are trained to recognize potential emergency situations and report these suspicions to public health officials. Clinicians in Florida played a major role in first identifying and then linking anthrax cases with bioterrorism in 2001. Hospital emergency rooms and physicians' offices are where most individuals who have contracted an infectious disease or are exposed to dangerous chemicals encounter their community's emergency response system. That encounter should trigger an appropriate response if the condition is one that represents a threat to others. Every state has incorporated requirements in state statute that call for physicians, laboratories, and other health providers to notify public health officials when specific notifiable diseases or conditions are encountered. Some states include a general provision that physicians should report "unusual" infectious diseases. Despite these laws and regulations, compliance with disease reporting physicians remains spotty for a variety of reasons. The requirements and the reporting procedures may not be understood by some physicians. Others believe reporting is not worth the time and effort. Reporting from laboratories is more complete, but concerns exist as to whether laboratories serving multiple jurisdictions are fully aware of differences in requirements among the jurisdictions served.

In addition to playing an important role in identifying potential public health emergencies, healthcare providers play a critical role in responding to the medical consequences

of those emergencies, especially in mass casualty situations. For the relatively rare disease threats associated with bioterrorism, healthcare providers often have only limited experience dealing with these conditions and look to public health authorities for clinical guidance. Through the development of community-wide emergency response plans, public health agencies, private sector delivery systems, hospitals, physicians, pharmacies, nursing homes, and others are mobilized in the event of an emergency to provide needed treatment to those affected by disease and to provide prophylactic care to those at risk for exposure to disease. State and federal laws that confer tax-exempt status on hospitals typically require those institutions to provide significant community benefit, including the provision of emergency medical services and participation in regional emergency medical service planning. Funds for hospital preparedness, including staff training and preparedness planning, are provided by DHHS and channeled through state health departments.

Other private sector interests also contribute to public health emergency preparedness. Although NIH makes significant investments in the development of new vaccines and antimicrobial agents, pharmaceutical manufacturers represent the primary source of funding for research and development. Efforts to encourage industry interest in the development of vaccines and other countermeasures include incentives such as liability protections, antitrust waivers,

TABLE 6-4   Emergency Preparedness Core Competencies for All Public Health Workers

All Public Health Workers must be competent to
- Describe the public health role in emergency response in a range of emergencies that might arise (e.g., "The department provides surveillance, investigation, and public information in disease outbreaks and collaborates with other agencies in geological, environmental, and weather emergencies.").
- Describe the chain of command in emergency response.
- Identify and locate the agency emergency response plan (or the pertinent portion of the plan).
- Describe his/her functional role(s) in emergency response and demonstrate his/her role(s) in regular drills.
- Demonstrate correct use of all communication equipment used for emergency communication (e.g., phone, fax, radio).
- Describe communication role(s) in emergency response—within the agency using established communication systems, with the media, with the general public, and personal (with family, neighbors).
- Identify limits to own knowledge/skill/authority and identify key system resources for referring matters that exceed these limits.
- Recognize unusual events that might indicate an emergency and describe appropriate action (e.g., communicate clearly within chain of command).
- Apply creative problem solving and flexible thinking to unusual challenges within his/her functional responsibilities and evaluate effectiveness of all actions taken.

Public Health Leaders/Administrators must also be competent to
- Describe the chain of command and management system ("incident command system") or similar protocol for emergency response in the jurisdiction.
- Communicate the public health information, roles, capacities, and legal authority to all emergency response partners—such as other public health agencies, other health agencies, and other governmental agencies—during planning, drills, and actual emergencies. (This includes contributing to effective community-wide response through leadership, team building, negotiation, and conflict resolution.)
- Maintain regular communication with emergency response partners. (This includes maintaining a current directory of partners and identifying appropriate methods for contacting them in emergencies.)
- Ensure that the agency (or the agency unit) has a written, regularly updated plan for major categories of emergencies that respects the culture of the community and provides for continuity of agency operations.
- Ensure that the agency (or agency unit) regularly practices all parts of emergency response.
- Evaluate every emergency response drill (or actual response) to identify needed internal and external improvements.
- Ensure that knowledge and skill gaps identified through emergency response planning, drills, and evaluation are addressed.

Public Health Professionals must also be competent to
- Demonstrate readiness to apply professional skills to a range of emergency situations during regular drills (e.g., access, use, and interpret surveillance data; access and use lab resources; access and use science-based investigation and risk assessment protocols; identify and use appropriate personal protective equipment).
- Maintain regular communication with partner professionals in other agencies involved in emergency response. (This includes contributing to effective community-wide response through leadership, team building, negotiation, and conflict resolution.)
- Participate in continuing education to maintain up-to-date knowledge in areas relevant to emergency response (e.g., emerging infectious diseases, hazardous materials, and diagnostic tests).

Public Health Technical and Support Staff must also be competent to
- Demonstrate the use of equipment (including personal protective equipment) and skills associated with his/her functional role in emergency response during regular drills.
- Describe at least one resource for backup support in key areas of responsibility.

Data from Bioterrorism & Emergency Readiness Competencies for All Public Health Workers, Centers for Disease Control and Prevention, 2003.

patent extensions, and long-term contracts. Similarly, activities to improve the safety and security of the food supply will rely on the agricultural and food production industries to make necessary upgrades to their processes and to seek innovative ways to minimize disease threats.

Public Perceptions and Expectations

The flurry of activity to improve public health emergency preparedness and response capabilities is understandable. The public is highly concerned over the possibility of terrorist attacks of all types. Fears of possible anthrax or smallpox attacks are nearly as high as concerns of conventional explosives, airline hijacking or bombings, and attacks using

radioactive, toxic, or hazardous materials as weapons.[10] Among these potential terrorist weapons, concerns persist that smallpox will be used, related in part to the attention placed on smallpox at the national level with the initiation of smallpox preparedness programs that include vaccinations for key medical and first responder personnel. Although the public believes that the country is better prepared for a biologic or chemical attack than it was prior to 2002, the public perceives that the current level of preparedness is not high enough and more needs to be done. Public health leaders have been concerned that the emphasis on bioterrorism would reduce efforts on other public health problems and issues. **Figure 6-5** and **Figure 6-6** suggest that this concern

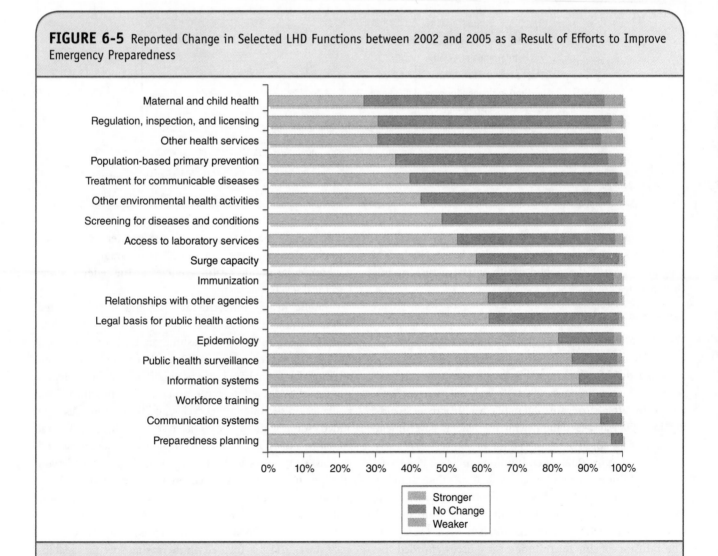

FIGURE 6-5 Reported Change in Selected LHD Functions between 2002 and 2005 as a Result of Efforts to Improve Emergency Preparedness

Data from National Associaiton of County and City Health Officials. 2005 National Profile of Local Health Departments. Washington, DC: NACCHO; 2006.

FIGURE 6-6 Percentage of States Reporting Stronger Infrastructure and Programs Because of Emergency Preparedness Efforts

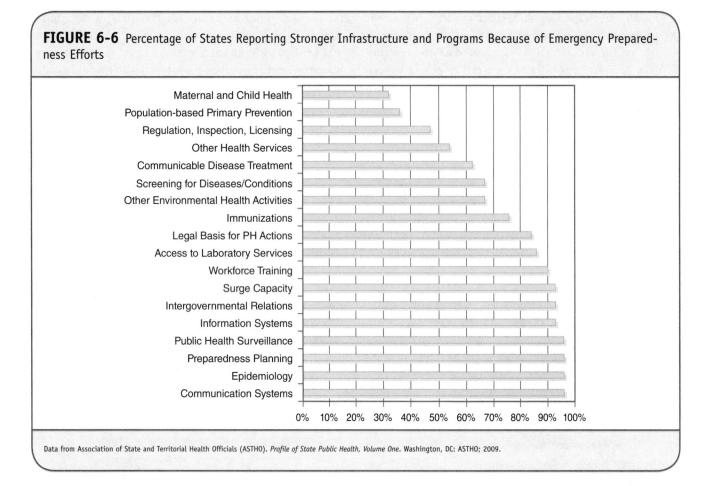

Data from Association of State and Territorial Health Officials (ASTHO). *Profile of State Public Health, Volume One.* Washington, DC: ASTHO; 2009.

may be unfounded as evidence suggests that preparedness funding has actually served to strengthen key public health programs as well the public health infrastructure in the United States.

State and Local Preparedness Grants

With the public health infrastructure increasingly viewed as a frontline defense against terrorism and homeland security priority, federal funding for public health purposes increased dramatically beginning in 2002. To put this increase into perspective, total governmental public health activity spending in 2000 was $43 billion, with the federal government accounting for approximately $5 billion.[11]

Beginning in 2002, federal funding increased by more than $2 billion, with about one-half of that amount directed to state and local governments for public health infrastructure improvements. Similar levels were funded through 2010 with reductions implemented thereafter. The infusion of this magnitude of resources afforded the opportunity to address serious and longstanding gaps in

public health protection and foster greater consistency and enhanced quality throughout the national network of governmental public health agencies at the federal, state, and local levels.

Public health infrastructure funding was channeled to the states and several large cities (including New York, Chicago, Los Angeles, and Washington, DC) through CDC. Each state received a minimum award of $5 million plus an additional amount based on a population formula. Activities supported by these funds were to be consistent with federal guidance. In several funding cycles, additional priorities were added, some without additional resources. In 2003 federal guidance incorporated specific smallpox preparedness and response capacities and allowed for costs associated with smallpox preparedness to be covered by grant funds. In 2006, pandemic flu preparedness became a priority with some additional one time funding provided. Amidst the evolution of broader federal policies on national security, CDC guidance since 2011 has focused on increasing specific capabilities at the state and local level.

State and Local Emergency Preparedness Capabilities

In 2011, CDC implemented a systematic process for defining a set of public health preparedness capabilities to assist state and local health departments with their strategic planning. The resulting public health preparedness capabilities established national standards for public health preparedness capability-based planning in order to assist state and local planners in identifying gaps in preparedness, determining the specific jurisdictional priorities, and developing plans for building and sustaining capabilities.

CDC identified 15 public health preparedness capabilities (shown below in their corresponding domains) as the basis for state and local public health preparedness:

Biosurveillance

- Public Health Laboratory Testing
- Public Health Surveillance and Epidemiological Investigation

Community Resilience

- Community Preparedness
- Community Recovery

Countermeasures and Mitigation

- Medical Countermeasure Dispensing
- Medical Materiel Management and Distribution
- Non-Pharmaceutical Interventions
- Responder Safety and Health

Incident Management

- Emergency Operations Coordination

Information Management

- Emergency Public Information and Warning
- Information Sharing

Surge Management

- Fatality Management
- Mass Care
- Medical Surge
- Volunteer Management[12]

The basic strategy was for each jurisdiction to determine the order of the capabilities it would pursue based upon the jurisdictional risk assessment completed as part of the community preparedness capability. Jurisdictions were strongly advised to ensure that they first were able to demonstrate capabilities within the biosurveillance, community resilience, countermeasures and mitigation, incident management, and information sharing domains.

In order to delineate the public health aspects for each capability, CDC adopted the terminology and definitions from the DHS Target Capabilities List, content from the Pandemic and All-Hazards Preparedness Act, and capabilities from the National Health Security Strategy (NHSS) as a baseline. Aligning across national programs, the Pandemic and All-Hazards Preparedness Act emphasizes the need to maintain consistency with other key national programs, specifically the NHSS preparedness goals. PAHPA also directs that the NHSS be consistent with the DHS National Preparedness Guidelines, a major component of which is the Target Capabilities List. The National Preparedness Guidelines represent a standard for preparedness based on establishing national priorities through a capabilities-based planning process. In addition to aligning with the National Preparedness Guidelines, CDC determined that the public health preparedness capabilities should also be aligned with the essential public health services framework. CDC conducted a mapping process which determined that several of the public health preparedness capabilities aligned with multiple essential public health services. Thus, the state and local preparedness capabilities align with both the DHS target capabilities and the HHS essential public health services, with a focus on public health capabilities critical to preparedness (see **Figure 6-7**).

The public health preparedness capabilities represent a national public health standard for state and local preparedness that better prepares state and local health departments for responding to public health emergencies and incidents, and supports the accomplishment of the essential public health services. Each of the public health preparedness capabilities identifies priority resource elements that are relevant to both routine public health activities and essential public health services. While demonstrations of capabilities can be achieved through different means (e.g., exercises, planned events, and real incidents), jurisdictions are encouraged to use routine public health activities to demonstrate and evaluate their public health preparedness capabilities.

The content of each public health preparedness capability is based on evidence-informed documents, applicable preparedness literature, and subject matter expertise gathered from across the federal government and the state and local practice community. Each capability includes a definition of the capability and list of the associated functions, performance measures, tasks, and resource considerations.

FIGURE 6-7 Public Health Emergency Preparedness Capabilities

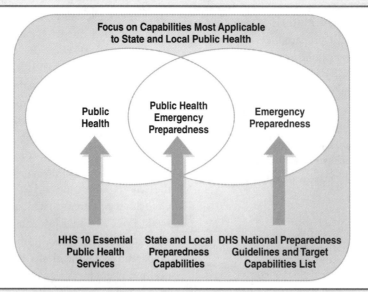

OUTSIDE-THE-BOOK THINKING 6-4

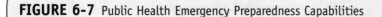

© Alfred Bondarenko/Shutterstock.

What is meant by the term "surge capacity," and how is this addressed in public health emergency response plans?

Early Lessons

Effective state and local preparedness programs require hazard and vulnerability analyses, forecasts of the probable health effects, analyses of the availability of needed resources, identification of vulnerable populations, and development of detailed plans for both preparedness and response. Many factors influence the ability of states and localities to complete these tasks. Public health preparedness is particularly challenging because public health and public safety roles differ for federal, state, and local governments. The federal government has primary responsibility for national security, while state and local governments carry the responsibility and financial burden for most other public health responsibilities.

At the local level, public health preparedness must be well coordinated with hospital preparedness. Virtually all states now recognize the importance of exercises and drills and there have been a number of national exercises involving the top officials of federal and state government.

Ideally, the infusion of resources to shore up the sagging public health infrastructure would foster positive structural changes in public health systems at the state and local level. The early evidence supports this contention. Yet federal funding is slowly eroding, with the average awards to LHDs in 2013 providing only $1.15 per capita and with smaller LHDs receiving larger per capita awards than LHDs serving more populous communities.[5]

Despite fears that the increased focus on emergency preparedness would weaken other public health duties, this has not occurred. Preparedness is now viewed as an important quality or attribute of an effective public health system rather than as another priority program operating within its own silo. This is the essence of the philosophy that has come to be known as the "dual use," "multiple use," or "all-hazards" strategy. Although still early in the process, some things are clear.

The price for public health preparedness is high, regardless of how it is calculated. In crude dollar terms, its costs reflect a significant increase in the federal investment in governmental public health services provided through governmental public health agencies. This increase will need to be sustained indefinitely, because it primarily supports information, communications, and workforce development systems that are ongoing in nature. And it will require commensurate commitment and investment on the part of state and local governments. Otherwise, supplanting will occur in one form or another and the opportunity for federal preparedness funds to leverage other resources will be lost.

The price in terms of federalism and intergovernmental relationships will also be high. States will need to encourage and accept stronger federal leadership on the one hand and generate a better understanding of local needs and priorities on the other. These will need to be fashioned into effective local, regional, state, and multistate efforts in ways that will challenge states to live up to their primary responsibility for the health of their citizens. All this must be done while navigating through a treacherous obstacle course laden with political, economic, and bureaucratic impediments to sustained progress.

The federal government must avoid the pitfall of merely throwing money at the problem, without fostering a national vision of public health preparedness and nurturing the state-local public health systems that must carry out that vision. This will require the federal agencies to be accountable for meaningful capacity and performance standards, consistent credibility as to ends and means, integration both across focus areas and across federal agencies, and leadership rather than either regulatory or advisory approaches to dealing with state-local public health system issues.

Although these are formidable challenges, the opportunities are unprecedented. The boost in federal funding and potential for federal leadership provide a unique opportunity to fashion a more coordinated national public health system. Certainly, the public now expects this, and the price of not being prepared will be even higher.

OUTSIDE-THE-BOOK THINKING 6-5

© Alfred Bondarenko/Shutterstock.

Choose a public health discipline or occupational group (either your own or one that you are somewhat familiar with) and describe the range of tasks that this discipline may be asked to perform in disaster preparedness and response.

CONCLUSION

Preparing for and responding to emergencies is a well-established role for public health agencies and their workers. This role, highlighted in the Public Health in America statement[1] as one of six critical responsibilities, has often been viewed as one of responding to an occasional natural disaster such as an earthquake, hurricane, or flood. Large-scale events that threaten public health and safety have seldom been intentionally inflicted, until recent examples to the contrary, such as the anthrax mailings in 2001 and the bombings of the federal building in Oklahoma City in the 1990s and the Boston Marathon in 2013. Geopolitical events in the international theater now raise the specter of increased risk for terrorist acts, including bioterrorism, directed against the American population, underscoring the need for sustained preparedness and response capacities at all levels of government.

The cycle of progress in public health preparedness has been remarkably consistent over several centuries in the United States. A terrible epidemic or another form of health-related disaster or threat occurs. Public expectations call for such an event to never occur again. Significant new resources are deployed to raise the level of preparedness and protection. There is no immediate recurrence and the threat seems to dissipate over time. Preparedness, though still important, becomes relatively less important. Eventually, a new threat or event appears, and the cycle repeats itself.

This recurring scenario raises the question as to whether current preparedness efforts represent a new and different strategy that could interrupt this chain of events. Past preparedness efforts focused on a specific threat and diminished as that specific threat diminished. Perhaps a more broadly focused preparedness campaign, one that is valued because it battles many different threats, will fare differently.

REFERENCES

1. Public Health Functions Steering Committee. *Public Health in America*. Washington, DC: U.S. Public Health Service; 1995.
2. Landesmann LY. *Public Health Management of Disasters: The Practice Guide*. Washington, DC: American Public Health Association; 2001.
3. Presidential Homeland Security Directive No. 5, February 28, 2003.
4. The Center for Law and the Public's Health. *The Model State Emergency Health Powers Act*. Baltimore, MD: Georgetown and Johns Hopkins Universities; 2001.
5. National Association of County and City Health Officials. *2013 Profile of Local Health Departments*. Washington, DC: NACCHO; 2014.
6. National Association of County and City Health Officials. *Elements of Effective Local Bioterrorism Preparedness: A Planning Primer for Local Health Departments*. Washington, DC: National Association of County and City Health Officials; 2001.

7. National Association of County and City Health Officials. *Local Centers for Public Health Preparedness: Models for Strengthening Local Public Health Capacity.* Washington, DC: National Association of County and City Health Officials; 2001.

8. Centers for Disease Control and Prevention. *Local Emergency Preparedness and Response Inventory: A Tool for Rapid Assessment of Local Capacity to Respond to Bioterrorism, Outbreaks of Infectious Disease, and Other Public Health Threats and Emergencies.* Atlanta, GA: Centers for Disease Control; 2001.

9. Columbia University School of Nursing, National Association of County and City Health Officials, and Centers for Disease Control and Prevention. 2003. Bioterrorism and Emergency Readiness Competencies for All Public Health Workers. https://training.fema.gov/EMIWeb/downloads/BioTerrorism%20and%20Emergency%20Readiness.pdf. Accessed October 7, 2014.

10. Lake, Snell, Perry. & Associates. *Americans Speak Out on Bioterrorism and U.S. Preparedness to Address Risk.* Princeton, NJ: Robert Wood Johnson Foundation; December 2002.

11. Centers for Medicare and Medicaid Services. National Health Accounts.

12. Centers for Disease Control and Prevention, Office of Public Health Preparedness and Response. *Public Health Preparedness Capabilities: National Standards for State and Local Planning, March 2011.* CDC; Atlanta, GA; 2011.

CHAPTER **7**

Public Health Workforce

Public health is important work, and the people who carry out that work contribute substantially to the health status and quality of life of the individuals, families, and communities they serve. Yet public health is not among the best known or most highly respected careers, in part because when public health efforts are successful, nothing happens. Events that don't occur don't attract attention. For example, the remarkable record of declining mortality rates and ever increasing spans of healthy life, due in large part to public health efforts, draws little public attention. Indeed, the vast majority of those who will ultimately benefit from the efforts of past and present public health workers are yet to be born. With the work of public health not widely recognized and valued for its accomplishments and contributions, it is not surprising that careers in public health are among the least understood and appreciated in the health sector.

Nonetheless, even if the public views public health as poorly defined and abstract, public health workers are real and tangible. These workers make up a public health workforce that can be defined and described in several important dimensions, including its size, distribution, composition, skills, and career pathways. Unfortunately, there is less information on these vital statistics of the public health workforce than for many other professional and occupational categories working in the health sector today.

For too long, too little attention has been directed to the public health workforce and its needs. Despite ample warnings in the 1988 Institute of Medicine (IOM) report, there were few efforts between 1980, when the Health Resources and Services Administration (HRSA) produced crude estimates of the size and composition for the United States Congress and 2000, when Kristine Gebbie and colleagues completed their landmark enumeration report on the public health workforce at the turn of the century.[1-3] Two decades of inattention provide eloquent testimony to the low priority given to the public health system's most important asset—its workforce.

Beginning in the year 2002, funding for public health workforce preparedness and training increased dramatically. This influx of funding also brought increased expectations for positive change and greater accountability for results. As a result, the public health system is now under the microscope, with federal, state, and local governments needing to show that the vital signs of the public health infrastructure, including its workforce, are improving. Unfortunately, decades of inattention left little information to serve as a basis for comparison.

A central challenge for public health workforce development efforts today is to provide more and better information about key dimensions of the public health workforce in terms of its size, distribution, composition, and competency, as well as its impact on public health goals and community health. This chapter, like the *Public Health Workforce Enumeration 2000* report, seeks to advance this important agenda.

Subsequent chapters focus on various public health occupations and careers in order to assist individuals seeking to make career decisions. This chapter sets the stage for an appreciation of what specific categories of public health workers do and how they contribute to societal well-being in the 21st century by examining the following questions:

- What is the public health workforce?
- How large is this workforce and how is it distributed?
- What professions and occupations are included?
- How does the public health workforce impact the health of populations?
- Will the public health workforce continue to grow? What trends in the overall economy, the health sector, or the public sector will impact public health jobs and career opportunities in the future?

PUBLIC HEALTH WORK AND PUBLIC HEALTH WORKERS

From a functional perspective, it is the individuals involved in carrying out the core functions and essential services of public health who constitute the public health workforce. Critical to an understanding of this characterization of the public health workforce are the terms *core functions* and *essential public health services*. These terms are examined in depth in other chapters with a useful summary of these concepts provided in the "Public Health in America" statement.[4] In it, the practice of public health is described in terms of both its ends (vision, mission, and six broad responsibilities) and how it accomplishes those ends (essential public health services). These essential public health services constitute an aggregate job description for the entire public health workforce, with the workload divided among the many different professional and occupational categories comprising the total public health workforce.

This functional perspective clearly links public health workers to public health practice. Unfortunately, this does not simplify the practical task of determining who is, and who is not, part of the public health workforce. There has never been any specific academic degree, even the master's of public health (MPH) degree, or unique set of experiences that distinguish public health's workers from those in other fields.

Many public health workers have a primary professional discipline in addition to their attachment to public health. Physicians, nurses, dentists, social workers, nutritionists, health educators, anthropologists, psychologists, architects, sanitarians, economists, political scientists, engineers, epidemiologists, biostatisticians, managers, lawyers, and dozens of other professions and disciplines carry out the work of public health. This multidisciplinary workforce, with somewhat divided loyalties to multiple professions, blurs the distinctiveness of public health as a unified profession. At the same time, however, it facilitates the interdisciplinary approaches to community problem identification and problem solving, which are hallmarks of modern public health practice.

OUTSIDE-THE-BOOK THINKING 7-1

© Alfred Bondarenko/Shutterstock.

What distinguishes a public health professional from a clinical professional working for a public health organization?

SIZE AND DISTRIBUTION OF THE PUBLIC HEALTH WORKFORCE

There is little agreement as to the size of the public health workforce in the United States except that it is only a small subset of the more than 15 million persons employed in the health sector of the American economy. Enumerations and estimates of public health workers suffer from one central limitation—the definition of a public health worker is unclear. An influential 2003 IOM report on public health education offered a seemingly straightforward definition of a public health professional as "a person educated in public health or a related discipline who is employed to improve health through a population focus".[5] Yet even this definition lacks precision and impedes enumeration; many public health professionals were not educated in public health or related disciplines; many others are not employed in organizations seeking to improve health through a population focus. Public health workers employed outside governmental public health agencies are especially difficult to identify; and not all employees of public health organizations and agencies have population health responsibilities associated with their jobs. Identifying specific types of public health workers is also difficult, since many have other professional affiliations.

Because of these limitations, a precise picture of the public health workforce is not available. But it is clear that efforts to identify and categorize public health workers must take into account three important aspects of public health practice:[6]

- Work setting: Public health workers work for organizations actively engaged in promoting, protecting, and preserving the health of a defined population group. The organization may be public or private, and its public health objectives may be secondary or subsidiary to its principal objectives. In addition to governmental public health agencies, other public and private organizations employ public health workers. For example, school health nurses working for the local school district and health educators employed by the local Red Cross chapter are part of the public health workforce.

- Work content: Public health workers perform work addressing one or more of the essential public health services. Relatively few job descriptions for public health workers are tailored from the essential public health services, and even when they are, the scope of tasks can be very broad. A focus on populations, as opposed to individuals, is often a distinguishing characteristic of these job descriptions. For example, an individual trained as a health educator who works for a community-based teen pregnancy prevention program is clearly a public health worker. But the same can't be said of a health educator working for a commercial advertising firm promoting cosmetics.

- Worker: The individual must occupy a position that conventionally requires at least 1 year of postsecondary specialized public health training and that is (or can be) assigned a professional, administrative, or technical occupational title (to be defined later in this chapter). This distinction may seem artificial but rests on the notion that public health practice relies on a foundation of knowledge, skills, and attitudes that, in most circumstances, cannot be completely acquired through work experiences alone.[6]

The relationships among these three aspects are illustrated in **Figure 7-1**, although there is no attempt to draw this modified Venn diagram to scale. Nonetheless, the total area captured with this composite represents all workers who would meet one or more of the definitions established for the individual workers, work content, and work settings using these three dimensions. For example, workers could be defined at some level of educational attainment and/or

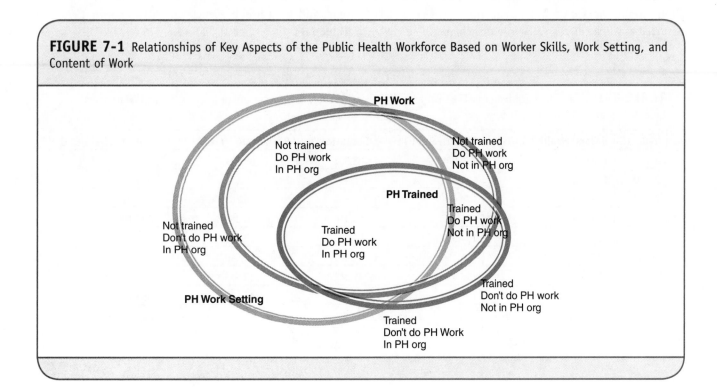

FIGURE 7-1 Relationships of Key Aspects of the Public Health Workforce Based on Worker Skills, Work Setting, and Content of Work

work experience. Perhaps an undergraduate or graduate level degree in public health and/or 5 years of experience could be elements of this definition.

Similarly, the definition of the work setting could call for working in an organization or entity whose mission focused on achieving public health goals. A more restrictive definition might focus on public or voluntary sector organizations or perhaps only on governmental health agencies. A definition for the content of the work could require consistency with the public health core functions/essential public health services framework. For example, if more than 50% of the work effort encompassed core functions or essential public health services, this could meet the definition.

Once definitions for the worker, work setting, and work content are established, the universe of public health workers would be established and seven different sectors within that universe could be identified. Whether everyone meeting any of the three definitions would be considered a public health worker, or whether some combination of categories (e.g., trained, doing public health work, within a governmental health agency) would be used to establish a conceptual definition of the public health workforce requires discussion and eventual consensus. With a rational definition of who is and who is not a public health worker, strategies to enumerate and capture key information on public health workers can be devised and implemented. Without a common frame of reference, widely varying estimates of the current and past public health workforce will proliferate. This has in fact occurred as will be discussed later in this chapter.

Despite these uncertainties as to the size of the public health workforce, there is information documenting general trends over recent decades. For example, the number of workers in the health sector of the U.S. economy has been steadily increasing while the proportion of total national health expenditures attributed to public health activity has remained fairly constant.[1] This evidence suggests the number of public health workers has grown at a rate generally consistent with that of all health workers and that the public health workforce likely includes 500,000–750,000 workers (and perhaps even more if public health workers in industries outside the governmental and health industry sectors are included).

This range is consistent with the crude enumeration of the public health workforce conducted for the year 2000, which identified 450,000 public health workers.[3] The year 2000 enumeration did not include most public health workers employed by nongovernmental agencies as well as many public health workers employed by government agencies other than official public health agencies. As a result the actual total exceeded the 450,000 number reported in the enumeration.

Another indication that the public health workforce has been increasing over recent decades comes from data collected in the ongoing employment and payroll census of federal, state, and local governments by the U.S. Bureau of the Census.[7] Data from this source indicated that there were 103,000 more full-time equivalent (FTE) workers of federal, state, and local health agencies in 2012 than in 1995 (see **Table 7-1**).

TABLE 7-1 Full-Time Equivalent (FTE) Workers of Federal, State, and Local Governmental Health* Agencies, Selected Years, 1995–2012, U.S.

Year	Federal Health Full Time	State Health FTE	Local Health FTE	State + Local FTE	Total (F+S+L) FTE
1995	125,048	160,061	208,558	368,619	493,667
2000	120,362	172,678	236,496	409,174	529,536
2005	125,163	178,465	246,300	424,765	549,918
2008	140,026	185,667	260,416	446,083	586,109
2009	141,713	184,539	254,005	438,544	580,257
2010	147,165	193,456	254,463	447,919	595,084
2011	152,347	196,424	249,242	445,666	598,013
2012	153,578	199,508	243,319	442,827	596,405

*Health: public health services, emergency medical services, mental health, alcohol and drug abuse, outpatient clinics, visiting nurses, food and sanitary inspections, animal control, other environmental health activities (e.g., pollution control), etc.

Data from U.S. Bureau of the Census. Federal, State, and Local Governments, Public Employment and Payroll Data. Available at www.census.gov/govs/apes. Accessed June 10, 2014.

Between 1995 and 2008 the number of workers employed in federal, state, and local government health agencies increased steadily, with the greatest gains at the local government level. The economic recession of 2008/2009 temporarily slowed the increase for workers in federal and state health agencies, but the pattern of steady increases reappeared when the recession ended. The number of workers in health agencies of local government fell both during and after the recession through 2012. It is likely that the influx of financial support for state and local governments associated with the American Recovery and Reinvestment Act of 2009 minimized the loss of local government employees through 2010, when this funding was discontinued. Fiscal and political pressures on local governments persisted after 2010 accounting for continuing losses of local government workers. This downward trend persisted through 2012, after which stabilization and small increases reappeared. **Figure 7-2** traces the ratio of state and local government health agency workers to population between 1995 and 2012 further illustrating these trends. By 2012 the ratio of state and local government health agency workers to population had reverted to levels not seen since the late 1990s.

Similar to other health sector workers, public health workers are more likely to be found in urban and suburban settings rather than rural communities. The public health worker to population ratio, however, is often higher in rural areas than in urban areas. States show significant variation

OUTSIDE-THE-BOOK THINKING 7-2

© Alfred Bondarenko/Shutterstock.

Choose a recent (within the last 3 years) outbreak or other public health emergency situation that has drawn significant media attention. Describe how specific occupational categories in the public health infrastructure contributed to either the emergency situation or its solution. The *Morbidity and Mortality Weekly Report* contents for recent weeks would be a good place to look for recent outbreaks; various print and electronic media may also be useful sources of information.

as well, with higher ratios in many of the smaller and less urban states in the East and West and lower ratios in the Central states.

The national public health workforce enumeration study completed in 2000 found that one-third of the public health workforce were employed by state agencies and another one-third by local governmental agencies.[3] This enumeration also reported that 20% worked for federal agencies and 14% worked for nongovernmental organizations

FIGURE 7-2 Full-Time Equivalent (FTE) Workers for State and Local Health* Agencies per 10,000 Population, Selected Years 1995–2012, United States

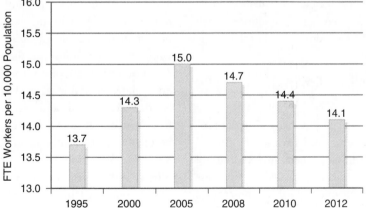

Data from U.S. Bureau of the Census. Federal, State, and Local Governments, and Public Employment and Payroll Data. Available at www.census.gov/govs/www/apes. Accessed June 15, 2014.

in the voluntary and private sectors. Government employment census data, which excludes nongovernmental workers, also classify one-third as state workers but 44% as employees of local government and 24% as working for federal agencies. Some of these differences can be attributed to state public health systems in which state employees work at the local level but are counted as state employees in the employment census data and as local health department (LHD) employees in the public health enumeration study. These differences may also be partly attributed to the inclusion of workers in state and local governmental agencies other than the local public health agency in the government employment census data; these were not captured in the year 2000 public health enumeration study. For example, substance abuse and mental health prevention services, school health services, or restaurant inspections may operate from local mental health agencies, school districts, or consumer affairs agencies rather than from the LHD. The National Association of County and City Health Officials (NACCHO) estimated that LHDs employed 162,000 workers (146,000 FTEs) in 2013.[8]

Although recent decades have witnessed an increase in the number of public health workers employed by nongovernmental agencies because of expanded partnerships for public health priorities, governmental public health workers are often considered the primary public health workforce. Their number, composition, distribution, and competence are issues of public concern.

Government employment census data provide useful insights into overall trends at the national level and among the various levels of government. The year 2000 public health enumeration study, together with periodic surveys of state and local public health agencies, provide richer information on the composition of the public health workforce, such as the proportion and types of professional occupational categories within that workforce. Together these sources enrich our understanding of the size and composition of the public health workforce today.

COMPOSITION OF THE PUBLIC HEALTH WORKFORCE

Public health is multidisciplinary, with many different professions and occupations involved in its work. The Bureau of Labor Statistics (BLS) tracks workers in hundreds of standard occupational classifications (SOCs) regardless of the industry (such as government, health care, etc.) in which they are employed. In recent years, there has been an effort to link standard occupational classifications for public health worker titles and positions, although this effort has been challenging. Because the overall universe of

public health workers is poorly defined, the precise proportion of the various occupational categories within it cannot be determined. It is clear that nurses and environmental health practitioners constitute the largest subgroups of public health workers. Managers, epidemiologists, health educators, nutritionists, and laboratory workers are also significant subgroups. **Figure 7-3** provides general information on occupational categories and titles from the public health workforce enumeration completed in 2000. Specific categories and titles were not reported for one-fourth of the workers in this study.

Despite the lack of precise information, it appears that professional occupational categories comprise more than one-half of the estimated 500,000–800,000 workers in the public health workforce. For comparison purposes, there were 2.7 million nurses, 900,000 physicians, 200,000 pharmacists, 170,000 dentists, and 90,000 dietitians/nutritionists employed in the United States in 2012.[9]

Ongoing surveys of local health departments (LHDs) document that three positions are found in more than 80% of all LHDs—public health nurse, administrator, and sanitarian/environmental health specialist.[8,10] These positions are present in large and small agencies alike. The next most frequent positions (emergency preparedness coordinator, health educator, dietitian/nutritionist, and physician) are found in only 40–60% of LHDs. There is considerable variation in the median FTEs in these positions, largely associated with agency size (**Figure 7-4**).

Two general patterns of LHD staffing exist around a core set of employees. One pattern focuses on clinical services, the other on more population-based programs.[11] The core employees consist of dietitian/nutritionists, sanitarians/environmental specialists, administrators, lab specialists, and health educators. The clinical pattern adds physicians, nurses, and dental health workers. The population-based pattern includes epidemiologists, public health nurses, social workers, and program specialists.

The availability of information on public health workers at the state and local level varies from state to state and is often inconsistent and incomplete. Detailed information from the official state health departments has only recently become available, although this does not include public health workers employed by state agencies other than the official state health department. The periodic profiles of LHDs completed by NACCHO before 2005 provide only general data on the proportion of responding agencies that employ specific public health job titles, either directly or through contracted services. The national profiles of LHDs completed after 2005 provide national estimates on the total

FIGURE 7-3 Percentage of Public Health Workers in Selected Occupational Categories and Titles, United States, 2000

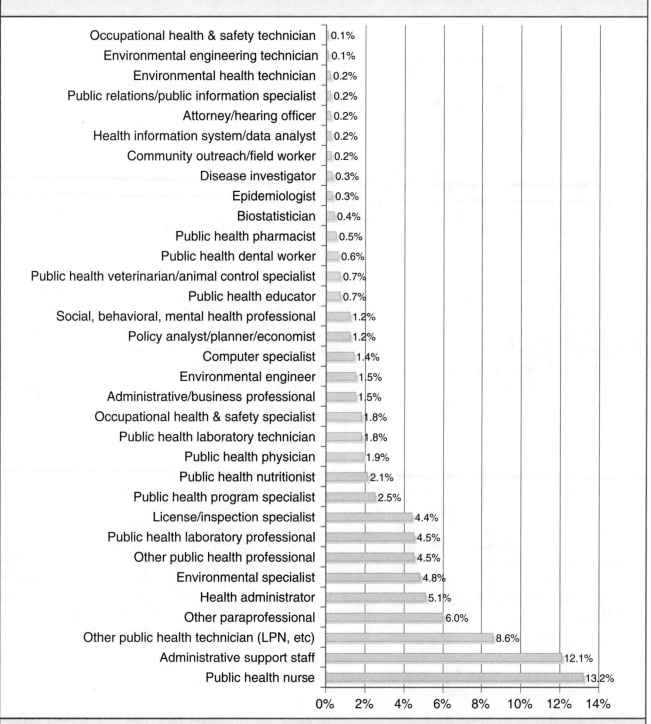

Occupational Category	Percentage
Occupational health & safety technician	0.1%
Environmental engineering technician	0.1%
Environmental health technician	0.2%
Public relations/public information specialist	0.2%
Attorney/hearing officer	0.2%
Health information system/data analyst	0.2%
Community outreach/field worker	0.2%
Disease investigator	0.3%
Epidemiologist	0.3%
Biostatistician	0.4%
Public health pharmacist	0.5%
Public health dental worker	0.6%
Public health veterinarian/animal control specialist	0.7%
Public health educator	0.7%
Social, behavioral, mental health professional	1.2%
Policy analyst/planner/economist	1.2%
Computer specialist	1.4%
Environmental engineer	1.5%
Administrative/business professional	1.5%
Occupational health & safety specialist	1.8%
Public health laboratory technician	1.8%
Public health physician	1.9%
Public health nutritionist	2.1%
Public health program specialist	2.5%
License/inspection specialist	4.4%
Public health laboratory professional	4.5%
Other public health professional	4.5%
Environmental specialist	4.8%
Health administrator	5.1%
Other paraprofessional	6.0%
Other public health technician (LPN, etc)	8.6%
Administrative support staff	12.1%
Public health nurse	13.2%

Data from Health Resources and Services Administration, Bureau of Health Professions, National Center for Health Workforce Information and Analysis and Center for Health Policy, Columbia School of Nursing. *The Public Health Workforce Enumeration 2000*. Washington, DC: HRSA; 2000.

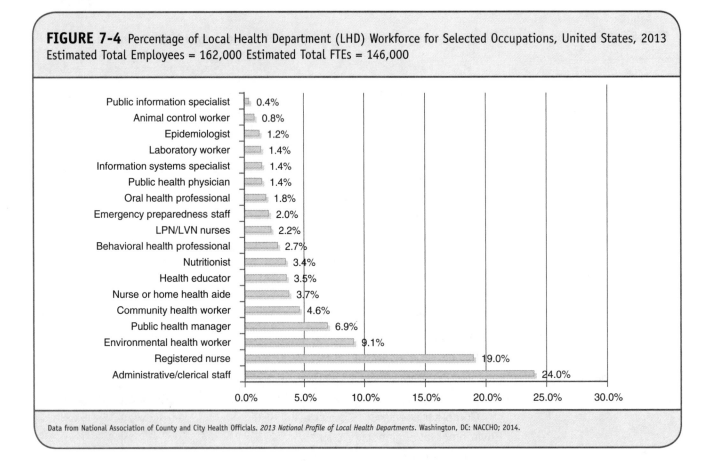

FIGURE 7-4 Percentage of Local Health Department (LHD) Workforce for Selected Occupations, United States, 2013 Estimated Total Employees = 162,000 Estimated Total FTEs = 146,000

Data from National Association of County and City Health Officials. *2013 National Profile of Local Health Departments*. Washington, DC: NACCHO; 2014.

number of full time equivalent (FTE) workers as well as FTEs for 10–15 specific titles.

Gaps in information on the public health workforce extend to some of the most basic and important characteristics of that workforce. For example, there is very little information available on the racial and ethnic characteristics of the overall public health workforce. Although important, information on cultural competency is virtually nonexistent.

PUBLIC HEALTH WORKER ETHICS AND EDUCATION

Public health workers may come from different academic, professional, and experiential backgrounds, but they share a common bond. All are committed to a common mission and share common ethical principles, as exemplified by the following list advanced by the American Public Health Association:

- Public health should address principally the fundamental causes of disease and requirements for health, aiming to prevent adverse health outcomes.

- Public health should achieve community health in a way that respects the rights of individuals in the community.

- Public health policies, programs, and priorities should be developed and evaluated through processes that ensure an opportunity for input from community members.

- Public health should advocate and work for the empowerment of disenfranchised community members, aiming to ensure that the basic resources and conditions necessary for health are accessible to all.

- Public health should seek the information needed to implement effective policies and programs that protect and promote health.

- Public health institutions should provide communities with the information they have that is needed for decisions on policies or programs and should obtain the community's consent for their implementation.

- Public health institutions should act in a timely manner on the information they have within the resources and the mandate given to them by the public.

- Public health programs and policies should incorporate a variety of approaches that anticipate and respect diverse values, beliefs, and cultures in the community.
- Public health programs and policies should be implemented in a manner that most enhances the physical and social environment.
- Public health institutions should protect the confidentiality of information that can bring harm to an individual or community if made public. Exceptions must be justified on the basis of the high likelihood of significant harm to the individual or others.
- Public health institutions should ensure the professional competence of their employees.
- Public health institutions and their employees should engage in collaborations and affiliations in ways that build the public's trust and the institution's effectiveness.[12]

Information from national and state surveys indicates that the majority of public health workers lack formal education and training in public health. In 1980, HRSA determined that only 20% of the 250,000 professionals in the primary public health workforce had formal training in public health.[2] More than three decades later, there is little evidence that this situation has improved. While the proportion of those who have formal training varies by category of worker, the lack of formal training is striking in even some of the most critical categories. For example, NACCHO surveys from the early 1990s through 2013 found that only 20–25% of local health department leaders had formal public health education or training.[13]

This is not surprising in view of the small number of undergraduate, graduate, and doctoral degrees in public health that are awarded each year. Public health degrees at the undergraduate level represent only 0.2% of all undergraduate degrees, and public health doctoral degrees comprise the same percentage of all doctoral degrees. Master's degrees in public health, however, comprise about 1.3% of all master's-level degrees.[14]

Formal training for many public health workers focuses only on a specific aspect of public health practice, such as environmental health or community or school health nursing. Environmental health practitioners, nurses, administrators, and health educators account for the majority of public health workers with formal training in public health. Even among those with formal training in public health, public health workers with graduate degrees from schools of public health or other graduate public health programs represent only a small fraction of the total. The total number of master's-level graduates of schools of public health and other graduate-level public health degree programs was about 12,000 in 2010.

OUTSIDE-THE-BOOK THINKING 7-3

© Alfred Bondarenko/Shutterstock.

Are public health professionals viewed as change agents in their communities today? Why or why not? Do you hold the same opinion for public health organizations? Why or why not?

Evidence of the lack of formal training within this workforce, however, does not necessarily lead to the conclusion that public health workers are unprepared.[15] Instead, public health workers enter the field having earned a wide variety of degrees and professional training credentials from academic programs and institutions unrelated to public health. Often overlooked, these institutions produce the bulk of the public health workforce and represent major assets for addressing unmet needs.

On-the-job training and work experience contribute substantially to the overall competency and preparedness of the public health workforce. For example, public health workers are frequently involved in responses to earthquakes, floods, and other disasters and have increasingly acquired and demonstrated skills in assessing community health needs and devising community health improvement plans. These are skills that most public health workers acquired through real-world work experience rather than through their formal training.

Continuing education and career development for public health workers has long been a cottage industry involving many different parties. Academic institutions certainly are contributors, but public health agencies at the state and local level, public health associations and institutes (national, state, and local), and other voluntary-sector health organizations participate as well. Many different entities offer credits for continuing education, including professional organizations, academic institutions, and hospitals, among others. Public health workers value continuing education credits as a means to satisfy requirements of their core disciplines in order to maintain some level of credentialing status (such as licensed physicians and nurses, certified health education specialists, and so on). Very few states enforce continuing education requirements for the public health disciplines licensed by that state. There is no formal system of public health-specific continuing education units (CEUs) and only fledgling efforts toward credentialing public health workers. The notable development in this area is the Certified in Public Health (CPH) credential offered since 2008 by the National Board of Public Health Examiners for graduates of master's degree programs accredited by the Council on Education in Public Health. As of 2014, more than 3,000 public health workers had earned the CPH credential.[16]

CHARACTERISTICS OF PUBLIC HEALTH OCCUPATIONS

The remaining sections of this chapter define and describe several key dimensions of public health occupations and organizations that provide the framework for examining specific positions and careers for public health workers in later chapters. Information on the full spectrum of occupations in the public health workforce is available from a variety of sources, including federal health and labor agencies and national public health organizations. **Table 7-2** previews the public health titles, occupational categories, and careers examined in the occupation-focused chapters that follow. The first column identifies the public health job titles and careers addressed in each chapter. The second column lists specific BLS standard occupational categories (SOCs) included in each chapter. SOCs are explained more fully later in this chapter.

TABLE 7-2   Public Health Occupations and Careers Addressed in Subsequent Chapters

Chapter Number	Career Category with Examples of Titles Used in Public Health Organizations	Bureau of Labor Statistics Standard Occupational Categories Related to Public Health
8	**Public Health Administration** • Health Services Manager • Public Health Agency Director • Health Officer • Emergency Preparedness and Response Director	Professional Occupations • Emergency Management Directors • Medical and Health Services Managers • Social and Community Services Managers
9	**Environmental and Occupational Health** • Environmental Engineer • Environmental Health Specialist (entry level) • Environmental Health Specialist (midlevel) • Environmental Health Specialist (senior level) • Occupational Health and Safety Specialist	Professional Occupations • Environmental Engineers • Environmental Scientists and Specialists (including Health) • Health and Safety Engineers (except Mining Safety Engineers and Inspectors) • Occupational Health and Safety Specialists Technical Occupations • Environmental Engineering Technicians • Environmental Science and Protection Technicians (including Health) • Occupational Health and Safety Technicians
10	**Public Health Nursing** • Public Health Nurse (entry level) • Public Health Nurse (senior level) • Licensed Practical/Vocational Nurse	Professional Occupations • Nurse Practitioners • Registered Nurses Technical Occupations • Home Health Aides • Licensed Practical and Licensed Vocational Nurses • Nursing Assistants

TABLE 7-2 Public Health Occupations and Careers Addressed in Subsequent Chapters (*continued*)

Chapter Number	Career Category with Examples of Titles Used in Public Health Organizations	Bureau of Labor Statistics Standard Occupational Categories Related to Public Health
11	**Epidemiology and Disease Control** • Disease Investigator • Epidemiologist (entry level) • Epidemiologist (senior level)	Professional Occupations • Epidemiologists • Statisticians
12	**Public Health Education and Information** • Public Health Educator (entry level) • Public Health Educator (senior level) • Public Information Officer • Community Health Workers (and other Outreach Occupations)	Professional Occupations • Health Educators • Public Relations Specialists Technical Occupations • Community Health Workers
13	**Other Public Health Professional and Technical Personnel** • Public Health Nutritionist/Dietician • Public Health Social, Behavioral and Mental Health Worker • Public Health Laboratory Worker • Public Health Physician • Public Health Veterinarian • Public Health Pharmacist • Public Health Oral Health Professional • Administrative Law Judge/Hearing Officer • Public Health Program Specialist/Coordinator • Public Health Policy Analyst • Public Health Information Specialist	Professional Occupations • Audiologists • Administrative Law Judges, Adjudicators, and Hearing Officers • Dental Hygienists • Dentists (General Dentist) • Dieticians and Nutritionists • Healthcare Social Workers • Medical and Clinical Laboratory Technologists • Mental Health Counselors • Mental Health and Substance Abuse Social Workers • Microbiologists • Optometrists • Pharmacists • Physician Assistants • Physicians (Family or General Practitioners) • Substance Abuse and Behavioral Disorder Counselors • Veterinarians Technical Occupations • Animal Control Workers • Emergency Medical Technicians and Paramedics • Medical and Clinical Laboratory Technicians

There are many aspects of an occupation or career that are important to current and prospective public health workers. The framework used in this book includes

- Occupational classification: these are based on job titles and whether the duties of the job are primarily administrative, professional, technical, or supportive in nature. Many positions in public health practice have a variety of job titles associated with them.

Similarly, the same job title can have a variety of regular duties and day-to-day responsibilities.

- Public health practice profile: The public health functions and essential public health services addressed by each occupational grouping are presented in a public health practice profile.
- Important and essential duties: These are the defining characteristics of any position describing what the

worker does on a daily basis. Examples are derived from a sampling of job and position descriptions from a variety of sources.

- Minimum qualifications: Some positions require a specific academic degree or credential; many do not. Some require previous experience, while others do not. All require some particular minimum level of knowledge, skills, and abilities. Many also require specific physical capabilities. These characteristics will be identified for each public health occupation.
- Workplace considerations: This description will identify levels of government that employ significant numbers of workers in each occupational category as well as important nongovernmental work settings for public health workers. This section will also highlight considerations related to physical demands, work schedules, travel, and general working conditions.
- Salary estimates: Salary levels for public health workers are estimated based on information from current job postings and the May 2013 survey of employment and wages coordinated by the Labor Department's BLS.
- Career prospects: Estimates as to current need and future demand for specific public health occupations and career paths are provided, based on the analyses performed by public health organizations and the BLS' projections for various occupations.
- Additional information: Sources of additional information for each occupation or career are identified, including education and training opportunities.

The following sections briefly describe the type and source of information included for each of these characteristics.

Occupational Classifications

Throughout the economy, including the health sector, occupations are broadly classified as either white collar or blue collar, depending on the degree of education and experience normally required. White collar occupations include five major occupational categories (professional, administrative, technical, clerical, and other), based on the subject matter of work, the level of difficulty or responsibility involved, and the educational requirements established for each occupation. Blue collar occupations are composed of the trades, crafts, and manual labor (unskilled, semiskilled, skilled), including foreman and supervisory positions entailing trade, craft, or laboring experience and knowledge as the paramount requirement.

The U.S. Office of Personnel Management tracks occupations in various industries using four general categories—professional, administrative, technical, and support.

- Professional occupations are those that require knowledge in a field of science or learning characteristically acquired through education or training equivalent to a bachelor's or higher degree with major study in or pertinent to the specialized field, as distinguished from general education. The work of a professional occupation requires the exercise of discretion, judgment, and personal responsibility for the application of an organized body of knowledge that is continuously studied to make new discoveries and interpretations, and to improve the data, materials, and methods. Professionals require specialized and theoretical knowledge. Well-known examples of professional job titles include physicians, registered nurses (RNs), dietitians, health educators, social workers, psychologists, lawyers, accountants, economists, system analysts, and personnel and labor relations workers. Professionals comprise the majority (56%) of public health workers (see **Figure 7-5**).
- Administrative occupations are those that involve the exercise of analytical ability, judgment, discretion, personal responsibility, and the application of a substantial body of knowledge of principles, concepts, and practices applicable to one or more fields of administration or management. Although these positions do not require specialized educational majors, they do involve the type of skills (analytical, research, writing, judgment) typically gained through a college-level general education, or through progressively responsible experience. Administrators set broad policies, oversee overall responsibility for the execution of these policies, direct individual departments or special phases of the agency's operations, or provide specialized consultation on a regional, district, or area basis. Common job titles for administrators include department heads, bureau chiefs, division chiefs, directors, deputy directors, and similar titles. Administrators and managers comprise 5% of all public health workers.
- Technical occupations are those that involve work that is not routine in nature and is typically associated with, and supportive of, a professional or administrative field. Such occupations involve extensive practical knowledge gained through on-the-job experience, or specific training less than that represented by college

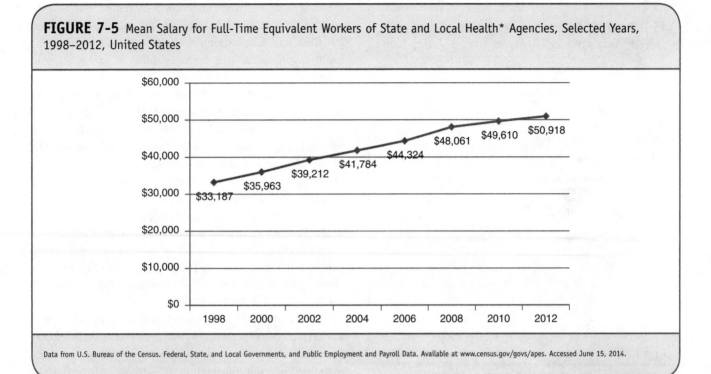

FIGURE 7-5 Mean Salary for Full-Time Equivalent Workers of State and Local Health* Agencies, Selected Years, 1998–2012, United States

Data from U.S. Bureau of the Census. Federal, State, and Local Governments, and Public Employment and Payroll Data. Available at www.census.gov/govs/apes. Accessed June 15, 2014.

graduation. Work in these occupations may involve substantial elements of the work of the professional or administrative field but requires less than full competence in the field involved. Technical occupations require a combination of basic scientific or technical knowledge and manual skills. Titles include computer specialists, licensed practical nurses (LPNs), inspectors, programmers, and a variety of technicians (environmental, laboratory, medical, nursing, dental, and so on). The technical occupations category also includes paraprofessionals who perform some of the duties of a professional or technician in a supportive role usually requiring less formal training and experience than that normally required for professional status. Included are community health workers, outreach workers, research assistants, medical aides, child support workers, home health aides, emergency medical technicians, among others. Workers in technical occupations account for 20% of all public health workers.

• Administrative support occupations are those that involve structured work in support of office, business, or fiscal operations; duties are performed according to established policies or techniques and require training, experience, or working knowledge related to the tasks to be performed. Clerical titles are often responsible for internal and external communication as well as recording and retrieval of data, information, and other paperwork required in an office. This category includes bookkeepers, messengers, clerk typists, stenographers, court transcribers, hearing reporters, statistical clerks, dispatchers, license distributors, payroll clerks, office machine and computer operators, telephone operators, legal assistants, and so on. In addition, workers in any of the blue-collar occupational categories are considered support workers within the public health workforce. About 19% of public health workers are in the administrative support category.

As documented in **Figure 7-6**, 81% of public health workers fall into the professional, administrative, and technical categories. More than one half (56%) are classified as professionals, similar to the proportion of professionals among all 15 million health workers. Nursing and environmental health activities account for the largest number of public health workers when both professional and technical occupations are considered. RNs represent the largest professional category within the public health workforce.

The U.S. Department of Labor collects information on occupations throughout the economy, including the public sector. An official taxonomy for occupations allows the

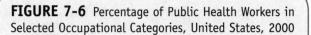

FIGURE 7-6 Percentage of Public Health Workers in Selected Occupational Categories, United States, 2000

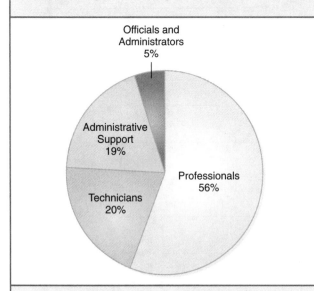

Data from Health Resources and Services Administration, Bureau of Health Professions, National Center for Health Workforce Information and Analysis and Center for Health Policy, Columbia School of Nursing. *The Public Health Workforce Enumeration 2000.* Washington, DC: HRSA; 2000.

Department of Labor's BLS to track information on hundreds of SOCs in terms of the number and location of jobs, salaries, and duties performed. BLS also develops projections for the number of future positions for these occupational categories based on economic and employment trends. Occupations generally can be found in a variety of industries, making it difficult to pinpoint trends and needs specific to the public health system. For example, RNs are the largest occupational category in the overall health workforce, with 2.7 million workers, but only a small percentage of all RNs (about 75,000) work in public health agencies. Many more work in hospitals and other healthcare organizations. This is also true for physicians, health services administrators, health educators, nutritionists, and many other occupations. Public health agencies, however, are the largest employers of several SOCs, such as environmental health specialists and epidemiologists. For those occupational categories, BLS information is especially useful.

SOCs relevant for public health are identified in the second column of Table 7-2, with nearly 40 specific categories listed.[17] Each of these categories is addressed in subsequent chapters, with the greatest attention on those with the largest numbers of workers in the public health workforce. These 39 occupational categories clearly do not cover all titles found in public health organizations. Nor do they capture the entire scope of work undertaken by public health workers. For these reasons, each chapter will focus specifically on job titles and job descriptions commonly found in public health organizations (see the first column of Table 7-2), with information on titles, duties, public health roles, and qualifications. Related job titles are addressed in the same chapter in order to illustrate links and possible career pathways.

Estimates of the number of current workers in each occupational category are synthesized from two sources. The BLS conducts surveys of all standard occupational categories twice yearly, including information on the industries and levels of government that employ workers in each SOC.[17] This source allows for estimates of the total number of workers in a particular SOC who work for federal, state, and local agencies.

Projections for the number of positions for each occupational title in the year 2022 are also provided by the BLS, allowing for estimates of total job openings expected to occur between the years 2012 and 2022.

A second important source of estimates for public health workers in relevant SOCs is the *Public Health Workforce Enumeration 2000* study commissioned by HRSA.[3] This enumeration collected information on workers of federal, state, and local public health agencies in the year 2000 based on existing data, reports, and surveys. As such, it was as much a qualitative and descriptive enumeration as a quantitative one. The year 2000 public health workforce enumeration identified a total of 450,000 public health workers, including 15,000 workers in voluntary sector organizations and 15,000 public health students. Occupational categories could not be established for 112,000 public health workers, making it difficult to project the actual number of workers in specific categories, such as public health nurses or epidemiologists. Both sources provide insights useful for estimating the number of existing positions for each occupational category and title.

Public Health Practice Profile

Individual workers, as well as occupational categories, produce work important to achieving public health goals and objectives. As described in previous chapters, key public health goals and objectives address preventing disease and injury, promoting healthy behaviors, protecting against health risks and threats, responding to emergencies, and ensuring the quality of health services.[4] This overall public health practice framework provides the basis for channeling contributions both by individuals and organizations toward common goals. The specific public health practice tasks of different occupations and individuals generally fall into one or more of the 10 essential public health services. Earlier chapters characterized the essential public health services as how the work of public health is accomplished and its ends are achieved. It is useful to view these functions and essential public health services as an aggregate job description for the entire public health workforce, with the workload then shared among the many different professional and occupational categories composing the total public health workforce.

The chapters that follow will each identify several purposes and essential public health services that form the core of the duties and job descriptions for each occupational category and public health career. An example of this format is provided in **Table 7-3**. A similar summary,

in checklist format, appears in each occupation-focused chapter.

In this example, the public health occupational category is primarily involved in addressing three public health goals: preventing epidemics, preventing injuries, and promoting healthy behaviors. This public health occupational category works to address these goals largely through performing five essential public health services—monitoring health status, investigating health problems, educating people about health, evaluating effectiveness, and researching new solutions to health problems.

For this example, and those in later chapters, the assignment of specific public health purposes and essential public health services may appear somewhat arbitrary. In each case, however, judgments are made as to which purposes and essential services are most closely associated with each occupational category. Some occupational categories may appear to have a relatively limited focus (e.g., public health laboratory workers) in comparison with others (e.g., public health nurses) that may have very broad roles that could conceivably cover all purposes and services. For each occupational category and title, however, the number of purposes and essential services identified for each occupational category is limited to no more than one half the number possible (3 of 6 purposes, 5 of 10 essential public health services). **Table 7-4** provides a composite profile that aggregates information from selected public health occupations examined in subsequent chapters.

Characterizing the work of an occupational category in this manner provides a functional view of the work performed. It also facilitates an understanding of how the work of one occupational category relates to the work of other categories and how the overall workload is distributed across the various public health occupational categories.

Important and Essential Duties

The most important aspect of any job or career is what workers do day in and day out. It is those basic and routine duties that best define positions in public health or any other field of endeavor. This list varies considerably from one position to another and often from one level of the same position to a higher level (e.g., from an entry-level environmental health specialist to a midlevel environmental health specialist). Important and essential duties for various titles within subsequent chapters are based on information from a sampling of job and position descriptions from a variety of public health organizations. In order to illustrate these routine duties, each of these chapters also provides an example of a daily schedule for the occupational category addressed in that chapter.

TABLE 7-3 Public Health Profile Example
(Example) **Public Health Practitioners** **Make a Difference by:**
Public Health Purposes
✓ Preventing epidemics and the spread of disease
Protecting against environmental hazards
✓ Preventing injuries
✓ Promoting and encouraging healthy behaviors
Responding to disasters and assisting communities in recovery
Ensuring the quality and accessibility of health services
Essential Public Health Services
✓ Monitoring health status to identify community health problems
✓ Diagnosing and investigating health problems and health hazards in the community
✓ Informing, educating, and empowering people about health issues
Mobilizing community partnerships to identify and solve health problems
Developing policies and plans that support individual and community health efforts
Enforcing laws and regulations that protect health and ensure safety
Linking people with needed personal health services and ensuring the provision of health care when otherwise unavailable
Ensuring a competent public health and personal healthcare workforce
✓ Evaluating effectiveness, accessibility, and quality of personal and population-based health services
✓ Researching new insights and innovative solutions to health problems

TABLE 7-4 Composite Public Health Practice Profile for Public Health Occupations and Titles Addressed in Subsequent Chapters

Selected Public Health Professional Occupations Make a Difference by:	Adm	EH	PHN	Epi	HE	Nutr	BH	Lab	Docs	Oral	Law	Prog	Pol
Public Health Purposes													
Preventing epidemics and the spread of disease	✓	✓	✓	✓	✓	✓		✓	✓	✓	✓		✓
Protecting against environmental hazards		✓		✓				✓			✓	✓	✓
Preventing injuries		✓		✓	✓							✓	
Promoting and encouraging healthy behaviors		✓			✓	✓	✓		✓	✓		✓	
Responding to disasters and assisting communities in recovery	✓						✓						
Assuring the quality and accessibility of health services	✓		✓			✓	✓	✓	✓	✓	✓		✓
Essential Public Health Services													
Monitoring health status to identify community health problems		✓		✓		✓		✓	✓	✓		✓	
Diagnosing and investigating health problems and health hazards in the community		✓	✓	✓				✓	✓			✓	
Informing, educating, and empowering people about health issues		✓			✓	✓	✓			✓			✓
Mobilizing community partnerships to identify and solve health problems	✓				✓		✓						✓
Developing policies and plans that support individual and community health efforts	✓				✓		✓				✓	✓	✓
Enforcing laws and regulations that protect health and ensure safety	✓	✓						✓			✓	✓	
Linking people with needed personal health services and assuring the provision of health care when otherwise unavailable			✓		✓	✓	✓		✓	✓			
Assuring a competent public health and personal healthcare workforce	✓			✓							✓		
Evaluating effectiveness, accessibility, and quality of personal and population-based health services	✓	✓	✓	✓		✓	✓	✓	✓	✓	✓	✓	✓
Researching new insights and innovative solutions to health problems			✓	✓		✓		✓	✓		✓		✓

Notes: Adm: public health managers; EH: environmental health workers; PHN: public health nurses; Epi: epidemiologists; HE: health educators; Nutr: nutritionists and dieticians; BH: behavioral health professionals; Lab: public health laboratory workers; Docs: physicians, veterinarians, optometrists, pharmacists; Oral: oral health professionals; Law: administrative judges and hearing officers: Spec; public health program specialists/coordinators; Pol: policy analysts.

Minimum Qualifications

Another key dimension of a position is a statement of the minimum qualifications necessary for that job. Often these minimum qualifications must be met in order for a worker to apply for a particular position. Minimum qualifications may emphasize experience or education or both. In any event, there is a battery of skills or competencies that are expected of those applying for and those working in public health positions. Minimum levels of knowledge, skills, and abilities are presented for public health job titles addressed in the subsequent occupation-specific chapters. Additional qualifications, such as physical capabilities appropriate for specific jobs or job locations, are also presented. These qualifications are synthesized from a sampling of current position descriptions.

The range of public health occupations and careers extends from those requiring considerable education and training to those that require relatively little. For example, some state and local health officials may hold several degrees, such as a bachelor's degree in science, an MPH, and a doctoral degree in medicine. At the same time, key staff performing investigations of communicable disease or environmental threats may have only an associate or bachelor's degree at the undergraduate level. It is not uncommon for some technical and clerical staff to have attained no more than a high school diploma with on-the-job training. Because this book largely targets undergraduate and graduate-degree students, particular emphasis is on occupations and careers requiring at least an undergraduate degree.

Workplace Considerations

Public health work takes place in many organizations and settings other than governmental public health agencies such as state health agencies or local public health departments. Many community and voluntary organizations collaborate with governmental public health agencies and employ staff whose work parallels that of workers in governmental public health agencies. This is true both for nongovernmental public health efforts here in the United States and those on the international level.

Another important workplace consideration relates to special physical capabilities, travel requirements, and other unique aspects of specific jobs. For example, some positions may require the ability to lift and move items weighing up to 50 pounds. Other jobs may require the ability to walk great distances or to have normal vision or hearing. Others may require the ability to work outside in cold and inclement weather, or to work unusual hours.

Salary Estimates

Detailed and specific salary information is not widely available. Information will be provided based on limited sources, including BLS data and current job postings. This information should not be considered to be definitive, timely, or completely accurate. Salary scales vary widely from agency to agency depending on a variety of circumstances and conditions. Figure 7-5 indicates that the overall average salary of a full-time workers employed by a state or local health agency increased by 50% to more than $50,000 between 1998 and 2012.

Career Prospects

Current and future opportunities for public health careers, as do careers in all fields, are a function of relationships among the population, the labor force, the overall economy, and the demand for public health programs and services.[17] The size and composition of the population strongly influence both the size of the workforce and the types of services needed by the population.

The U.S. population continues to increase, although at a slower rate than in recent decades. The average age of the population continues to increase as well, and the proportion of the population in the older age categories will continue to increase. As older workers near retirement, replacement of workers will create job opportunities and career advancement possibilities in addition to those created by the continued growth of the overall population.

Among the various sectors of the U.S. economy, the health sector is projected to grow faster and add more jobs than other sectors. About one in every four new jobs will be in the health sector, with professional and technical occupational categories exhibiting the greatest growth and offering the greatest opportunities for new jobs and career advancement. In sum, the overall outlook for professional and technical occupations in public health is very bright for those now in or about to enter the job market.

The optimal number of public health workers is controversial and uncertain. There is widespread concern within the public health community that there will soon be a shortage of public health workers. Several key public health occupational categories are currently in short supply, such as public health nurses and epidemiologists. The information provided in the career prospect section will identify specific occupational categories that are projected to be in greatest need. Despite the uncertainties, the BLS provides projections for the number of positions likely to be needed in 2022 and the number of job openings that will occur through new positions and retirements.

Subsequent chapters focus on specific public health occupations and careers. But careers in public health, like those in many fields, are not always straightforward. Individual workers can begin in one career pathway and then shift into another. For example, administrators of public health agencies could come up through the ranks of program and agency management or from one of the public health professional categories, such as environmental health, nursing, or health education. This section will identify some of these paths and career ladders for public health workers.

Additional Information

Only basic information is offered in the chapters that follow. Most public health occupational categories and careers, however, have excellent sources for more detailed information. Several sources, often professional associations or organizations, will be identified whenever possible. Career development opportunities through education, training, and credentialing are also identified for each public health workforce category.

OUTSIDE-THE-BOOK THINKING 7-4

© Alfred Bondarenko/Shutterstock.

How have the needs for different public health occupations changed over the past century? How will the need for various public health occupations change over the next two decades?

PUBLIC HEALTH WORKFORCE GROWTH PROSPECTS

Will the public health workforce increase or decrease in size over the next several decades? There should be little debate over this question, but there is. One reason for controversy derives from the general lack of information on the public health workforce between 1980 and 2000. Another relates to the many complex forces within public health and the broader economy that influence the number of public health workers needed.

In hindsight, it is clear that HRSA's estimate as to the size of the public health workforce in 1980 lacked precision. This is unfortunate, because the 500,000 figure from 1980 is frequently cited as documentation that the public health workforce must be shrinking because only 450,000 public health workers were enumerated in 2000. On closer examination, however, the HRSA 1980 estimate actually indicated that only 250,000 of the 500,000 public health workers were in the primary public health workforce consisting of federal, state, and local public health agency workers and selected others who devoted most of their work efforts to public health activities.[2] Even within this 250,000 figure were faculty and researchers at academic institutions; occupational health physicians and nurses working for various private companies; health educators teaching in schools; and administrators working in hospitals, nursing homes, and other medical care settings. The actual number of public health professionals working for federal, state, and local public health agencies in 1980, after adjusting for these inclusions, was closer to 140,000. The total for the comparable categories from the *Public Health Workforce Enumeration 2000* was 260,000, a figure that indicates the public health workforce grew rather than shrank between 1980 and 2000. Data from the employment census of governmental agencies support this conclusion, showing there has been a steady increase in FTE workers of governmental health agencies over the past several decades.

Together this evidence suggests that the public health workforce has been increasing throughout the 1990s, and into the first and second decades of the new century. This is consistent with the documented expansion of the health sector within the overall economy, which continues to grow at a more rapid rate than the rest of the economy. If public health activities continue to maintain even their current small share of total health spending, funding for public health activities and public health workers will grow commensurately. It is conceivable that public health activities could even increase their share of overall health spending, fostering even more rapid growth of employment opportunities. Several prevention and public health provisions of the Affordable Care Act suggest that this is possible.

There are mounting concerns, however, that the growth of the public health workforce may be slowing, at least in the public sector. It was somewhat surprising that the infusion of bioterrorism preparedness funding after 2001 didn't result in even greater numbers of state and local public health workers than are reflected in Table 7-1. It appears that state and local governments initially shifted some workers onto federal bioterrorism grant payrolls, thereby saving state and local resources or possibly shifting resources from public health to other priorities such as education. The severe national economic downturn in 2008/2009 forced many states and localities to suspend hiring and subject workers to furloughs and layoffs. The massive infusion of funding to state and local governments through the American Recovery and Reinvestment Act of 2009 also served to temporarily support positions in public health agencies until this funding ended in 2010. The long-term impact of the recession on the national public health workforce remains uncertain, although surveys conducted by the Association of State and Territorial Health Officials and NACCHO suggest that state and local health departments suffered significant staff reductions between 2008 and 2012.[18]

Recent history indicates that federal funding to states and localities for bioterrorism preparedness served as a temptation to replace or supplant state and local support for public health with federal money. The funding of epidemiologists further illustrates this phenomenon. In 2004, federal bioterrorism funds paid the salaries of 460 epidemiologists; among 390 epidemiologists working on bioterrorism and emergency response activities, 62% were funded by the federal government. Infectious disease epidemiologists did not increase between 2001 and 2004, but in 2004 nearly 20% were paid through federal bioterrorism funds.[19] This scenario likely affected several other public health occupational categories, such as laboratory workers and emergency response coordinators. It underscores the important role of the underlying fiscal environment of state and local governments in determining the size of the public health workforce.

OUTSIDE-THE-BOOK THINKING 7-5

© Alfred Bondarenko/Shutterstock.

What factors determine the optimum size of the public health workforce in a community? Are these the same factors that would determine the optimum size of the public health workforce at the state or national level?

Two additional modern forces affect public health workforce size. These are the expansion of information technology and the resulting increase in worker productivity. Public health practice, by its very nature, is information dependent and information driven. Enhanced information technology tools and increased individual worker productivity mean fewer workers are needed to support the work of administrators, professionals, and technical staff. This trend would tend to increase the proportion of professionals within the public health workforce; however, these trends also mean fewer professionals are needed to perform the same volume of work. The net effect is therefore difficult to forecast in terms of the number and type of workers needed.

Trends within the health sector will also continue to affect public health workers. Health is highly valued both as a personal and societal goal. The economic value placed on health exceeds $3 trillion annually, or nearly $10,000 per person in the United States.[9] There is no indication that health will assume a lower priority within the American social value system. In recent years, for example, expenditures for health purposes have grown faster than the rate for the overall economy. In effect, health is becoming an even greater priority. Between the two general strategies to achieve health—preventive and therapeutic approaches—the balance may be slowly shifting toward more prevention. There is still a notable imbalance, with a 20 to 1 ratio; however, this shift is likely to continue. Taken together with an increased priority on health itself, public health activities, including those carried out by public health agencies and workers, should continue to increase in size, importance, and value to society.

The value placed on public health activities can be measured in economic terms, such as funding levels for programs, services, and the workers who implement public health programs and services. To sustain or even enhance public health funding, national leadership is necessary. Federal health agencies such as CDC and HRSA are especially important in the area of public health workforce development. Complementing sustained national leadership, state and local governments must remain committed to and invested in public health objectives. However, states and local governments across the United States face difficult economic circumstances and tough choices as they look to cut back services that are either low priority or that have other funding sources.

Beyond funding, administrative and bureaucratic obstacles challenge public health workforce development efforts in the public sector. State and local agencies are often the locus of some of the most significant recruitment and retention problems facing the public health workforce. These include slow hiring by governmental agencies, civil service systems, hiring freezes, budget crises affecting state and local government, and the lack of career ladders, competitive salary structures, and other forms of recognition that value workers for their skill and performance.

Despite the uncertainties inherent in these influences, past trends and current forces suggest that professional and administrative jobs and careers in public health are likely to grow over the next decade. Unfortunately, it will be difficult to measure progress without deployment of a standard taxonomy for public health occupations and more comprehensive enumeration strategies and tools that provide better information on the key dimensions of the public health workforce.[20,21]

Job opportunities generally track with population density and demographic shifts. Within the health sector, job opportunities cluster around metropolitan areas. Public health positions also follow this pattern. There are more positions, and therefore more opportunities, in metropolitan areas than there are in rural areas. General demographic trends indicate a continuing shift of population from the Northeast and Midwest regions of the United States to the South, Southwest, and West Coast. It is likely that health sector jobs and public health positions will also follow this pattern.

The ratio of positions to population, however, is higher in rural areas (and states that have higher proportions of their population living in nonmetropolitan areas). This occurs because there is a basic core staffing that must be present regardless of the size of the population and because rural and remote communities often lack other public health resources and assets. Higher public health worker to population ratios in rural areas raise questions as to whether scarce resources, in the form of public health professionals, are used efficiently in state-local public health systems. Given limited resources, this finding argues in favor of further consolidation of small local public health agencies into larger ones.

The demand for many public health professional occupations is growing steadily. In recent decades, an increasing number of LHDs employed epidemiologists, health educators, health information specialists, emergency response coordinators, and public health information officers. The aftermath of terrorist events of 2001, including the series of anthrax spore attacks through the postal system, spotlighted the need for two professional positions in particular. The first, emergency response coordinators, is new to the list

of public health occupations; the second, epidemiologists, is one of the oldest public health professional occupations. State and local public health agencies are rapidly hiring emergency response coordinators. These people come to these new positions with a wide range of academic and experiential qualifications. Epidemiologists, on the other hand, have more restrictive qualifications in terms of academic preparation such as master's and doctoral degrees. Concerns over the past few decades that epidemiologists were in short supply and great demand are now heightened as agencies seek to hire more of these specialists. The number of epidemiologists coming out of graduate programs does not appear to be keeping pace with the need, despite an increase in interest as measured by the number of applications for epidemiology training programs.

Prior to 2001, health educators and community health planners were steadily growing professional categories in the public health workforce. Expansion of health education and promotion programs, and an increase in community health planning and community health improvement activities account for this trend. More recently, the Affordable Care Act has focused increased attention on the potential roles for community health workers. If the U.S. health system shifts even slightly toward a greater emphasis on public health and prevention activities, other public health occupations may benefit as well.

PUBLIC HEALTH PRACTITIONER COMPETENCIES

Beyond workforce size, distribution, and composition are issues related to the essential competencies and skills that will be most important in public health practice and how these skills are best acquired. Establishing and promoting competencies for public health workers is tricky business. For one thing, public health workers come from a variety of professional backgrounds, many of which have their own core competencies. For example, public health nursing has a set of core competencies and health educators use a sophisticated competency framework for purposes of certification. The same is true for public health physicians, administrators, epidemiologists, and several other public health professional occupations. Identifying a common core for these various professional categories generally leads to a framework with very general and nonspecific competencies that are difficult to relate to a specific situation or problem. The Council on Linkages between Academia and Public Health Practice spent two decades grappling with this problem before arriving at the set of core competencies for public health professionals summarized in **Table 7-5** for entry-level workers.

TABLE 7-5   Core Competencies for Tier 1 (Entry-Level) Public Health Workers

Analytical/Assessment Skills

 1. Describes factors affecting the health of a community (e.g., equity, income, education, environment)
 2. Identifies quantitative and qualitative data and information (e.g., vital statistics, electronic health records, transportation patterns, unemployment rates, community input, health equity impact assessments) that can be used for assessing the health of a community
 3. Applies ethical principles in accessing, collecting, analyzing, using, maintaining, and disseminating data and information
 4. Uses information technology in accessing, collecting, analyzing, using, maintaining, and disseminating data and information
 5. Selects valid and reliable data
 6. Selects comparable data (e.g., data being age-adjusted to the same year, data variables across datasets having similar definitions)
 7. Identifies gaps in data
 8. Collects valid and reliable quantitative and qualitative data
 9. Describes public health applications of quantitative and qualitative data
10. Uses quantitative and qualitative data
11. Describes assets and resources that can be used for improving the health of a community (e.g., Boys & Girls Clubs, public libraries, hospitals, faith-based organizations, academic institutions, federal grants, fellowship programs)
12. Contributes to assessments of community health status and factors influencing health in a community (e.g., quality, availability, accessibility, and use of health services; access to affordable housing)
13. Explains how community health assessments use information about health status, factors influencing health, and assets and resources
14. Describes how evidence (e.g., data, findings reported in peer-reviewed literature) is used in decision making

Policy Development/Program Planning Skills

 1. Contributes to state/Tribal/community health improvement planning (e.g., providing data to supplement community health assessments, communicating observations from work in the field)
 2. Contributes to development of program goals and objectives
 3. Describes organizational strategic plan (e.g., includes measurable objectives and targets; relationship to community health improvement plan, workforce development plan, quality improvement plan, and other plans)
 4. Contributes to implementation of organizational strategic plan
 5. Identifies current trends (e.g., health, fiscal, social, political, environmental) affecting the health of a community
 6. Gathers information that can inform options for policies, programs, and services (e.g., secondhand smoking policies, data use policies, HR policies, immunization programs, food safety programs)
 7. Describes implications of policies, programs, and services
 8. Implements policies, programs, and services
 9. Explains the importance of evaluations for improving policies, programs, and services
10. Gathers information for evaluating policies, programs, and services (e.g., outputs, outcomes, processes, procedures, return on investment)
11. Applies strategies for continuous quality improvement
12. Describes how public health informatics is used in developing, implementing, evaluating, and improving policies, programs, and services (e.g., integrated data systems, electronic reporting, knowledge management systems, geographic information systems)

(continues)

TABLE 7-5   Core Competencies for Tier 1 (Entry-Level) Public Health Workers (*continued*)

Communication Skills

1. Identifies the literacy of populations served (e.g., ability to obtain, interpret, and use health and other information; social media literacy)
2. Communicates in writing and orally with linguistic and cultural proficiency (e.g., using age-appropriate materials, incorporating images)
3. Solicits input from individuals and organizations (e.g., chambers of commerce, religious organizations, schools, social service organizations, hospitals, government, community-based organizations, various populations served) for improving the health of a community
4. Suggests approaches for disseminating public health data and information (e.g., social media, newspapers, newsletters, journals, town hall meetings, libraries, neighborhood gatherings)
5. Conveys data and information to professionals and the public using a variety of approaches (e.g., reports, presentations, email, letters)
6. Communicates information to influence behavior and improve health (e.g., uses social marketing methods, considers behavioral theories such as the Health Belief Model or Stages of Change Model)
7. Facilitates communication among individuals, groups, and organizations
8. Describes the roles of governmental public health, health care, and other partners in improving the health of a community

Cultural Competency Skills

1. Describes the concept of diversity as it applies to individuals and populations (e.g., language, culture, values, socioeconomic status, geography, education, race, gender, age, ethnicity, sexual orientation, profession, religious affiliation, mental and physical abilities, historical experiences)
2. Describes the diversity of individuals and populations in a community
3. Describes the ways diversity may influence policies, programs, services, and the health of a community
4. Recognizes the contribution of diverse perspectives in developing, implementing, and evaluating policies, programs, and services that affect the health of a community
5. Recognizes the contribution of diverse perspectives in developing, implementing, and evaluating policies, programs, and services that affect the health of a community
6. Describes the effects of policies, programs, and services on different populations in a community
7. Describes the value of a diverse public health workforce

Community Dimensions of Practice Skills

1. Describes the programs and services provided by governmental and nongovernmental organizations to improve the health of a community
2. Recognizes relationships that are affecting health in a community (e.g., relationships among health departments, hospitals, community health centers, primary care providers, schools, community-based organizations, and other types of organizations)
3. Suggests relationships that may be needed to improve health in a community
4. Supports relationships that improve health in a community
5. Collaborates with community partners to improve health in a community (e.g., participates in committees, shares data and information, connects people to resources)
6. Engages community members (e.g., focus groups, talking circles, formal meetings, key informant interviews) to improve health in a community
7. Provides input for developing, implementing, evaluating, and improving policies, programs, and services
8. Uses assets and resources (e.g., Boys & Girls Clubs, public libraries, hospitals, faith-based organizations, academic institutions, federal grants, fellowship programs) to improve health in a community
9. Informs the public about policies, programs, and resources that improve health in a community
10. Describes the importance of community-based participatory research

TABLE 7-5   Core Competencies for Tier 1 (Entry-Level) Public Health Workers (*continued*)

Public Health Sciences Skills

1. Describes the scientific foundation of the field of public health
2. Identifies prominent events in the history of public health (e.g., smallpox eradication, development of vaccinations, infectious disease control, safe drinking water, emphasis on hygiene and hand washing, access to health care for people with disabilities)
3. Describes how public health sciences (e.g., biostatistics, epidemiology, environmental health sciences, health services administration, social and behavioral sciences, and public health informatics) are used in the delivery of the 10 Essential Public Health Services
4. Retrieves evidence (e.g., research findings, case reports, community surveys) from print and electronic sources (e.g., PubMed, *Journal of Public Health Management and Practice*, *Morbidity and Mortality Weekly Report*, *The World Health Report*) to support decision making
5. Recognizes limitations of evidence (e.g., validity, reliability, sample size, bias, generalizability)
6. Describes evidence used in developing, implementing, evaluating, and improving policies, programs, and services
7. Describes the laws, regulations, policies, and procedures for the ethical conduct of research (e.g., patient confidentiality, protection of human subjects, Americans with Disabilities Act)
8. Contributes to the public health evidence base (e.g., participating in Public Health Practice-Based Research Networks, community-based participatory research, and academic health departments; authoring articles; making data available to researchers)
9. Suggests partnerships that may increase use of evidence in public health practice (e.g., between practice and academic organizations, with health sciences libraries)

Financial Planning and Management Skills

1. Describes the structures, functions, and authorizations of governmental public health programs and organizations
2. Describes government agencies with authority to impact the health of a community
3. Adheres to organizational policies and procedures
4. Describes public health funding mechanisms (e.g., categorical grants, fees, third-party reimbursement, tobacco taxes)
5. Contributes to development of program budgets
6. Provides information for proposals for funding (e.g., foundations, government agencies, corporations)
7. Provides information for development of contracts and other agreements for programs and services
8. Describes financial analysis methods used in making decisions about policies, programs, and services (e.g., cost-effectiveness, cost-benefit, cost-utility analysis, return on investment)
9. Operates programs within budget
10. Describes how teams help achieve program and organizational goals (e.g., the value of different disciplines, sectors, skills, experiences, and perspectives; scope of work and timeline)
11. Motivates colleagues for the purpose of achieving program and organizational goals (e.g., participating in teams, encouraging sharing of ideas, respecting different points of view)
12. Uses evaluation results to improve program and organizational performance
13. Describes program performance standards and measures
14. Uses performance management systems for program and organizational improvement (e.g., achieving performance objectives and targets, increasing efficiency, refining processes, meeting *Healthy People* objectives, sustaining accreditation)

(continues)

TABLE 7-5   Core Competencies for Tier 1 (Entry-Level) Public Health Workers (*continued*)

Leadership and Systems Thinking Skills

1. Incorporates ethical standards of practice (e.g., Public Health Code of Ethics) into all interactions with individuals, organizations, and communities
2. Describes public health as part of a larger interrelated system of organizations that influence the health of populations at local, national, and global levels
3. Describes the ways public health, health care, and other organizations can work together or individually to impact the health of a community
4. Contributes to development of a vision for a healthy community (e.g., emphasis on prevention, health equity for all, excellence and innovation)
5. Identifies internal and external facilitators and barriers that may affect the delivery of the 10 Essential Public Health Services (e.g., using root cause analysis and other quality improvement methods and tools, problem solving)
6. Describes needs for professional development (e.g., training, mentoring, peer advising, coaching)
7. Participates in professional development opportunities
8. Describes the impact of changes (e.g., social, political, economic, scientific) on organizational practices
9. Describes ways to improve individual and program performance

Note: Tier 1 competencies apply to public health professionals who carry out the day-to-day tasks of public health organizations and are not in management positions. Responsibilities of these professionals may include data collection and analysis, fieldwork, program planning, outreach, communications, customer service, and program support.

Reproduced from Council on Linkages between Academia and Public Health Practice; 2014. Available at http://www.phf.org/resourcestools/Pages/Core_Public_Health_Competencies.aspx. Accessed July 11, 2014.

CONCLUSION

Recent decades witnessed an increase in the number of public health workers employed by both governmental and nongovernmental agencies. This expansion of the workforce, however, leaves many questions unanswered as to the appropriate number, distribution, training, and preparedness of the public health workforce, making these issues of public concern. Some of these concerns have persisted since the late 1800s, as suggested by an editorial appearing in the *Journal of the American Medical Association* more than a century ago:

> It is unfortunate that in the absence of epidemics or pestilence, too little attention is paid to the protection of the public health, and as a necessary consequence, to the selection of those whose duties require them to guard the public health.[22(p189)]

Other concerns are of more recent vintage. The economic recession of 2008/2009 displaced millions of workers in both the public and private sectors of the economy. State and local governments were especially hard hit, and are recovering slowly. Sources point to the aging of the public health workforce, current shortages of public health nurses and epidemiologists, and the imminent retirement of many public health professionals. On the other hand, national health reform legislation enacted in 2010 included several provisions for stabilizing and strengthening the public health workforce and an increased emphasis on population-focused prevention.

The public health workforce is growing and will continue to grow for years to come. Many public health occupational categories will see a steady increase; others will grow even more rapidly. Core public health practice competencies will increasingly influence education and training programs and hopefully find their way into the human resource activities and personnel systems of governmental public health agencies. Worker recognition initiatives based on relevant competencies, such as credentialing and certification programs, will also grow in order to address the need for both heightened accountability and expanded career pathways.

Although strategies that focus on the pipeline are necessary and useful, they will never be sufficient to ensure an effective public health workforce over the long term. Comprehensive workforce development strategies must focus not only on current and future workers, but also on the organizations in which the work of public health is performed. In the decades that lie ahead, the most important resource and asset of the public health system—its workforce—faces as many challenges as opportunities.

REFERENCES

1. Institute of Medicine, National Academy of Sciences. *The Future of Public Health.* Washington, DC: National Academy Press; 1988.

2. Health Resources and Services Administration, U.S. Department of Health and Human Services. *Public Health Personnel in the United States, 1980: Second Report to Congress.* Washington, DC: U.S. Public Health Service; 1982.

3. Health Resources and Services Administration, U.S. Department of Health and Human Services. *Public Health Workforce Enumeration 2000.* Washington, DC: Government Printing Office; December 2000.

4. Public Health Functions Steering Committee. *Public Health America.* I. Washington, DC: U.S. Public Health Service; 1995.

5. Institute of Medicine, National Academy of Sciences. *Who Will Keep the Public Healthy? Education Public Health Professionals for the 21st Century.* Washington, DC: National Academy Press; 2003.

6. Kennedy VC, Moore FI. A systems approach to public health workforce development. *J Public Health Manage Pract.* 2001; 7: 17–22.

7. U.S. Bureau of the Census. *Federal, State, and Local Governments, Public Employment and Payroll Data.* www.census.gov/govs/apes/. Accessed June 16, 2014.

8. National Association of County and City Health Officials. *2013 National Profile of Local Health Departments.* Washington, DC: National Association of County and City Health Officials; 2014.

9. Centers for Disease Control and Prevention, National Center for Health Statistics. *Health United States, 2013.* Hyattsville, MD: National Center for Health Statistics; 2014.

10. National Association of County and City Health Officials. *2008 National Profile of Local Health Departments.* Washington, DC: National Association of County and City Health Officials; 2009.

11. Gerzoff RB, Baker EL. The use of scaling techniques to analyze U.S. local health department staffing structures, 1992–1993. *Proceedings of the Section on Government Statistics and Section on Social Statistics of the American Statistical Association.* 1998: 209–213.

12. Thomas JC, Sage M, Dillenberg J, Guillory VJ. A code of ethics for public health. *Am J Public Health.* 2002; 92: 1057–1059.

13. Gerzoff RB, Richards TB. The education of local health department top executives. *J Public Health Manage Pract.* 1997; 3: 50–56.

14. U.S. Department of Education, National Center for Education Statistics, Integrated Postsecondary Education Data System (IPEDS), Fall 2010, Completions component. 2011.

15. Turnock BJ. Roadmap for public health workforce preparedness. *J Public Health Manage Pract.* 2003; 9: 471–480.

16. National Board of Public Health Examiners. http://www.nbphe.org. Accessed June 9, 2014.

17. Bureau of Labor Statistics, U.S. Department of Labor. www.bls.gov. Accessed June 15, 2014.

18. National Association of County and City Health Officials. Local health department job looses and program cuts: Findings from the 2013 Profile study. Washington, DC: NACCHO; 2013.

19. Council of State and Territorial Epidemiologists. *2004 National Assessment of Epidemiologic Capacity: Findings and Recommendations.* Washington, DC: Council of State and Territorial Epidemiologists; 2004. http://www.cste.org/Assessment/ECA/pdffiles/ECAfinal05.pdf. Accessed October 8, 2014.

20. Tilson H, Gebbie KM. The public health workforce. *Ann Rev Public Health.* 2004; 25: 341–356.

21. Gebbie KM, Turnock BJ. The public health workforce, 2006: new challenges. *Health Aff (Millwood).* 2006; 25: 923–933.

22. American Medical Association. Editorial. *JAMA.* 1893; 20: 189.

CHAPTER **8**

Public Health Administration

Public health organizations require leaders, managers, and administrators at various levels throughout the organization to plan, organize, direct, control, and coordinate health services, education, or policy. The people serving in these positions come from a wide variety of educational, professional, and work experience backgrounds. Many lack formal training and previous experience in public health. Nonetheless, they constitute the third largest occupational category within the public health workforce, behind only nurses and environmental health workers, and they represent a force even larger than their numbers. **Table 8-1** offers a snapshot of an average day in the life of a public health administrator.

OCCUPATIONAL CLASSIFICATION

There is no standard occupational category (SOC) specific to public health administrators and managers. There is a generic

standard occupational category for medical and health services managers that encompasses administrative positions in any healthcare or health services organization. This SOC is one of the administrative occupations within the white collar grouping of occupations.

Public health administrators are health services managers leading a public health agency, program, or major subunit. Public health administrators plan, analyze, organize, direct, coordinate, and evaluate the use of resources to deliver health services, education, or policy; they often manage or regulate health agencies and facilities. The category includes such job titles as director, administrator, chief, manager, or one of the many titles indicating chief public health official of a jurisdiction (e.g., secretary of health, health officer, health commissioner, administrator, or health official). Titles that include the term coordinating or senior are generally not classified as public health administrators but are included with the profession referenced (e.g., coordinating nutritionist with public health nutritionist, senior public health nurse with public health nurse).

Data from the Bureau of Labor Statistics (BLS) indicate there were 300,000 health services administrators in the United States in 2013, with 25,000 working for federal, state, and local health agencies,[1] The *Public Health Workforce Enumeration 2000* study suggests there were about 21,000 working in governmental public health agencies in the year 2000.[2] Recent surveys of local and state public health agencies indicate that more than 16,000 of these positions are in local health departments (LHDs) and official state health agencies.[3,4] Data and information from these various sources are used throughout this chapter.

TABLE 8-1   A Typical Day for a Public Health Administrator

7:30 a.m.	Breakfast with local hospital administrator and staff regarding diabetes screening
8:30 a.m.	In office, follow-up call with state epidemiologist regarding recent outbreak of foodborne illness
9:00 a.m.	Weekly meeting with senior staff
10:15 a.m.	Meet with epidemiology, health education, and planning staff regarding completion of community needs assessment
10:45 a.m.	Meet with county commissioner regarding West Nile Virus concerns in her area
11:15 a.m.	Review and update electronic slide presentation for today's lunch meeting
11:45 a.m.	Meet with local Chamber of Commerce leadership before lunch, which includes public health presentation to business community
1:00 p.m.	Discuss budget amendment proposal with fiscal and program staff
1:30 p.m.	Media interview regarding West Nile Virus concerns
2:00 p.m.	Give welcoming remarks and overview for new employee orientation
3:00 p.m.	Conference call for committee of National Association of County and City Health Officials task force on workforce and leadership development
4:00 p.m.	Review information suggested by senior staff for presentation to board of health
4:30 p.m.	Drop by the clinic to see how things went today
5:15 p.m.	Prepare remarks for board of health meeting
7:00 p.m.	Attend monthly meeting of board of health

In addition to medical and health services managers, there are several other standard occupational classifications that may be involved with public health administration. These include the SOCs for social and community services managers and emergency management directors, as well as administrative business professionals and support staff.

Social and community services managers plan, direct, or coordinate the activities of a social service program or community outreach organization. These positions generally oversee a program or organization's budget and policies regarding participant involvement, program requirements, and benefits. This work may involve directing health and social workers, counselors, or probation officers. In 2013 there were 115,000 workers in this occupational category with nearly 25,000 employed in the public sector.

As with medical and health services managers, titles for social and community services managers vary considerably. Common titles include Program Director, Social Services Director, Program Manager, Vocational Rehabilitation Administrator, Adoption Services Manager, Children's Service Supervisor, Clinical Services Director, Community Services Block Grant/Outreach Social Worker, Director of Child Welfare Services, and Director of Social Services. Social and community services organizations frequently collaborate with a variety of public and voluntary sector organization

to achieve public health objectives for a community, often through participating in community health improvement initiatives and activities.

Emergency management directors provide oversight to organizations or units involved with preparing for and responding to a spectrum of emergency situations and threats. Within public health agencies, such managers may supervise the public health emergency preparedness and response activities of the organization. Since the turn of the century, positions such as emergency response coordinator or manager have experienced steady growth in state and local public health agencies.

Administrative business professionals are trained at a professional level in their field of expertise prior to entry

OUTSIDE-THE-BOOK THINKING 8-1

© Alfred Bondarenko/Shutterstock.

What will be the most important new or expanded roles for public health administrators in the 21st century?

in public health and perform work in business, finance, auditing, management, and accounting. Data extrapolated from the *Public Health Workforce Enumeration 2000* study identified 7,500 administrative business professionals working in governmental public health agencies in the year 2000. Administrative business support staff, including bookkeepers, accounting clerks, and auditing clerks, work with administrative business professionals in areas of business and financial operations. In addition, there were another 80,000 administrative support workers (such as receptionists, typists, and stenographers) who perform nontechnical support work in all areas of agency management and program administration. Administrative business professionals and administrative support staff titles fall within the administrative chain of command of an agency but are not classified within the administrator and manager category. Nonetheless, these titles can serve as steps along a career development path leading to a public health administrator position.

PUBLIC HEALTH PRACTICE PROFILE

Public health managers and administrators work at a level within an organization that often bears responsibility for achieving organizational goals and objectives. This means they may be involved with addressing any or all six public health responsibilities, although their background and experience may provide greater expertise in some of these roles than others. For example, administrators of local public health agencies who worked their way to the top of the organization through the ranks of environmental health may continue to be directly involved in protecting against environmental hazards or responding to disasters. An administrator from the ranks of the nursing staff may remain more directly involved in disease prevention and quality assurance of health services. For most public health administrators, managing responses to public health emergencies and ensuring the quality of health services require their personal attention. If these administrators also have professional training in

epidemiology, disease and injury prevention, environmental health, or health education, they may be directly involved in these duties as well. Otherwise, the professional and program staff of the organization guide activities for these roles.

Similarly, among the 10 essential public health services, administrators may have more personal expertise in some services than others. There are several essential public health services, however, that all administrators must address. These include developing and mobilizing collaborative relationships and partnerships within the community, developing policies and plans, enforcing laws and regulations, ensuring a competent workforce, and evaluating the effectiveness, accessibility, and quality of health services. **Table 8-2** summarizes

TABLE 8-2 Public Health Practice Profile for Public Health Administration

Public Health Administrators Make a Difference by:
Public Health Purposes
✓ Preventing epidemics and the spread of disease
Protecting against environmental hazards
Preventing injuries
Promoting and encouraging healthy behaviors
✓ Responding to disasters and assisting communities in recovery
✓ Ensuring the quality and accessibility of health services
Essential Public Health Services
Monitoring health status to identify community health problems
Diagnosing and investigating health problems and health hazards in the community
Informing, educating, and empowering people about health issues
Mobilizing community partnerships to identify and solve health problems
✓ Developing policies and plans that support individual and community health efforts
✓ Enforcing laws and regulations that protect health and ensure safety
Linking people with needed personal health services and ensuring the provision of health care when otherwise unavailable
Ensuring a competent public health and personal healthcare workforce
✓ Evaluating effectiveness, accessibility, and quality of personal and population-based health services
Researching new insights and innovative solutions to health problems

OUTSIDE-THE-BOOK THINKING 8-2

© Alfred Bondarenko/Shutterstock.

What are the most important contributions to improving the health of the public that public health managers and administrators make today?

public health purposes and essential public health services at the core of positions for public health administrators.

IMPORTANT AND ESSENTIAL DUTIES

There are many possible job titles and positions for public health administrators. The focus in this chapter will be on four positions: (1) health services manager; (2) local health department (LHD) director; (3) health officer; and (4) public health emergency preparedness and response coordinator. Each of these positions and a representative panel of their important and essential duties are described in this section.

Health Services Manager

This is an administrative and management position that directs, plans, analyzes, and coordinates health, public health, and regulatory programs and services. A worker in this or a similar title (such as health administrator) is often responsible for directing or assisting in the overall planning, directing, and coordinating of assigned health, public health, and regulatory programs and services, including the identification of program priorities and the development and implementation of new programs and services. This position could be located at a variety of managerial levels. Responsibilities may be in areas such as chronic disease prevention; environmental health and communicable disease prevention; health standards and licensure; maternal, child, and family health; nutritional health and services; health information; regulation; senior services; health improvement; emergency response; or closely related areas. Positions have program management and decision-making authority and usually have policy, assessment, planning, budget, and supervisory responsibilities. Direction is received from a designated administrative superior who reviews work through conferences, reports, and evaluation of operational results. The health services manager, however, is expected to exercise considerable initiative and judgment in planning and carrying out assignments.

Important and essential duties for health services managers may include

- Directs or assists in the overall planning, development, and administration of assigned health, public health, and regulatory programs and services in such areas as chronic disease prevention; maternal, child, and family health; environmental health and communicable disease prevention; nutritional health and services; health standards and licensure; health information; regulations; health improvement; or emergency response

- Develops and coordinates comprehensive public health systems for a specific geographic area, such as a county, city, or district
- Provides consultation to physicians, healthcare providers, hospitals, LHDs, and other agencies linked with health care in the effective delivery of health, public health, and regulatory programs and services
- Ensures individuals receive program services appropriate to their needs and program eligibility
- Oversees or assists in the development of community-based coalitions and works with coalitions, advocacy groups, and others interested in program issues to develop plans and outcomes on how to address specific health, public health regulatory, and senior programs and services concerns
- Prepares new or revises existing legislation and develops standards, regulations, and policies to implement the legislation
- Directs or assists administrative personnel in general management aspects of policy development and program planning and coordination as related to assigned responsibilities; assists in the evaluation of the effect of policy and organizational changes and new programs
- Reviews and revises programs in area of responsibility to ensure compliance of operations with laws, regulations, policies, plans, and procedures
- Supervises staff to carry out the strategies of the organization or program
- Participates in meetings with agency administrators to develop, coordinate, implement, and interpret new or revised initiatives
- Participates in conferences and meetings relating to areas of assigned responsibility
- Participates in the development of budget requests and the monitoring of expenditures according to budget allocations and appropriations
- Conducts research, institutes special studies, and prepares or reviews reports and related information to evaluate existing organizations, policies, procedures, and practices as related to the assigned program
- Maintains contact, cooperates with, and addresses local and community organizations and other interested groups pertaining to the assigned programs

Local Health Department Director

Under administrative direction, LHD directors plan, organize, direct, manage, and supervise public health programs for their jurisdiction; direct the enforcement of federal, state, and local health laws and regulations; direct staff providing public health and education programs; represent agency activities, programs, and services with community organizations and other governmental agencies; perform special assignments as directed; and provide administrative support for its governing bodies (such as a board of health or a city or county board of supervisors). LHD directors often serve as agency head with general responsibility for the administration of the jurisdiction's public health programs and functions and may serve as the health officer for the jurisdiction. Many of the nonmedical duties of health officers are also performed by LHD directors. This position may report to a municipal or county board of health or board of supervisors (or perhaps a city council) through the municipal or county administrative officer or chief elected official. As agency head, this position often directly supervises positions such as director of nursing, fiscal officer, director of environmental health, director of health education, and sometimes a medical health officer.

Important and essential duties for a LHD director may include

- Plans, organizes, directs, coordinates, and administers public health programs for the jurisdiction, such as communicable disease control, immunization, environmental health, health education, maternal and child health, vital statistics, and health programs for adults, children, handicapped children, and schools
- Enforces public health laws and regulations within the jurisdiction
- Develops and recommends agency goals, objectives, and policies
- Provides strategic direction and leadership in identifying community health needs and developing and implementing community health improvement plans that meet identified needs
- Prepares and administers agency budgets recommended by the jurisdiction's executive officer and approved by the governing board or entity
- Controls fiscal expenditures and revenues
- Monitors and evaluates overall agency and program performance and directs change to improve quality and effectiveness
- Hires, supervises, evaluates, and ensures proper training of agency staff in accordance with personnel rules
- Administers a variety of categorical programs
- Provides direction and develops policies for clinical services through protocol development

- Develops policies and protocols for the control and prevention of communicable diseases
- Plans and develops new program efforts
- Develops and administers grants
- Initiates appropriate epidemiologic investigations of communicable disease outbreaks
- Provides health information to the public, community organizations, and other county staff
- Maintains contact with the press and community organizations
- Interprets policies and regulations for the public
- Supervises administration, program development, fiscal management, and provision of direct client services at agency clinic sites
- Represents the agency with other government agencies

Health Officer

Health officers, often physicians, plan, organize, direct, and provide medical oversight over public health programs for their local public health jurisdictions; provide technical consultation to citizens, public officials, staff, and community organizations and agencies on public health and preventive medicine issues; and serve as the designated health officers. A health officer provides medical supervision for the LHD by coordinating public healthcare services with external agencies and healthcare providers and providing ongoing communication with the local medical community. This position is also responsible for providing medical oversight and enforcement of public health regulations for a variety of public health programs and services including environmental health, vital records, communicable disease control, public health nursing, emergency and disaster medical planning, public health education, and state maternal and child health services. This title is distinguished from the LHD director in that the latter has overall management responsibility for the LHD's programs and services, whereas the health officer directs the medical oversight for all public health programs. In some instances, the health officer also serves as LHD director; in others, this position reports to the public health director or to the director of a higher-level health and human services agency. Some states (about one half) require the health officer to be a licensed physician; the other one half allows non-physicians to serve as health officers or sets no requirements. Health officers often supervise titles such as the director of public health nursing, the director of environmental health, director of health education, and other professional and program directors.

Important and essential duties for health officers may include

- Plans, organizes, directs, and evaluates the medical oversight of public health programs
- Ensures enforcement of applicable public health, environmental health, and sanitation orders, ordinances, and statutes
- Analyzes legislative changes; evaluates and develops medical and public health policies, programs, and procedures; and formulates improvements
- Serves as an advocate to promote statewide public health policies, which also benefit the local jurisdiction
- Disseminates and interprets policies, laws, regulations, and state and federal directives regarding medical and public health issues to physicians, department staff, and representatives of hospitals, nursing homes, medical clinics, and schools by written means and personal contacts; acts as medical epidemiologist for public health diseases
- Consults and coordinates with federal and state officials and representatives of local public and private health agencies in the enforcement of health laws and the development of programs to meet public health needs
- Plans, organizes, directs, coordinates, and administers public health programs for the jurisdiction, such as communicable disease control, immunization, environmental health, health education, maternal and child health, vital statistics, and programs for adults, children, handicapped children, and schools
- Provides direction and advice regarding policies and procedures directed by the state immunization board
- Works closely with the agency director and health services managers to monitor performance and effect changes in practice to improve quality of services
- Confers with members of the public and representatives of federal, state, and local agencies regarding health department programs; cooperates with federal and state public health groups in the enforcement of health and sanitary matters
- Supervises, directs, and evaluates assigned staff, to include assigning work, handling employee concerns and problems, and counseling
- Reviews technical requirements, reports, and procedures generated by the health department
- Prepares public health information materials and news releases

- Consults with physicians, nurses, patients, staff members, other governmental agencies, or other individuals in the diagnosis of, and investigation of, cases of suspected communicable diseases and exchanges information or provides recommendations; takes measures to prevent and control epidemics
- Serves on emergency medical services and public health emergency preparedness committees
- Represents the jurisdiction on committees, boards, at meetings, or otherwise as assigned

Public Health Emergency Preparedness and Response Coordinator

Public health emergency preparedness and response coordinators perform planning functions for a local public health agency, ensuring compliance with federal and state planning guidelines and regulations. These positions coordinate response plans with the state health department as well as other federal, state, and local government entities; perform all hazard, bioterrorism, and emergency planning; and coordinate plans with various response agencies, volunteer organizations, businesses, and private industries.

Massive federal bioterrorism preparedness funding for state and local public health agencies stimulated a rapid increase in the number of emergency preparedness and response positions in the United States, making this title one of the fastest growing within the public health workforce. There was no information on public health emergency response coordinators available in the *Public Health Workforce Enumeration 2000* report.

Important and essential duties for a public health emergency response coordinator include

- Performs administrative, technical, and planning duties to integrate bioterrorism and public health emergency preparedness and response plans with activities for other emergency management programs
- Develops and maintains the local public health agency's various emergency operations plans
- Reviews and maintains bioterrorism response appendices to meet Centers for Disease Control and Prevention (CDC) planning guidance and local standard operating guidelines
- Assists with coordination, integration, and implementation of emergency response plans and procedures from various jurisdictions, governmental entities, private industries, utility companies, among others

- Reviews specialized studies and reports, formulates comments and summarizes content, and provides emergency planning recommendations
- Coordinates with the local jurisdiction's emergency management agency and the state health emergency management agency in continual development and review of effective emergency preparedness and response activities
- Identifies unique planning considerations for bioterrorism threats
- Assists the public health community in developing jurisdictional emergency plans by attending meetings and facilitating discussions, reviewing concepts and procedures, and coordinating emergency response efforts of various agency units
- Acts as a resource for the public health community and governmental public health agencies in documenting their standard operating guidelines and operational checklists
- Coordinates overall emergency planning activities
- Conducts regular review of local, state, federal, and private industry emergency response plans, employing standard emergency management concepts and strategic methodologies
- Works in conjunction with the executive director, environmental health supervisor, risk communicator, epidemiologist, and public information officer to promote awareness of local public health agency emergency response plans and procedures
- Provides requisite planning activity reports, budget submissions, and other required documentation for federal and state emergency response funding sources
- Assists with the development of operational drills and exercise scenarios designed to train, test, and evaluate emergency response concepts or standard operating guidelines
- Adjusts emergency plans, procedures, or protocols to reflect changes and improve efficiency as appropriate
- Demonstrates continuous effort to improve operations, decrease turnaround times, streamline work processes, and work cooperatively and jointly to provide quality seamless customer service

MINIMUM QUALIFICATIONS

Public health administrators can emerge from either a professional occupational category or from a career in other management positions. Those arising from the professional ranks may acquire management skills either as part of their education, such as in a relevant master's degree program. Relevant degrees include the master's of public health (MPH), master's of public administration (MPA), master's of health administration (MHA), or master's of business administration degree (MBA) or, less commonly, a public health doctoral degree program. Schools of public health commonly target the doctor of public health degree (DrPH) for leaders and other high-level public health practitioners. Doctor of philosophy (PhD) and doctor of science (ScD) degrees in public health sciences and disciplines are also offered by many institutions.

More commonly, however, public health administrators and managers lack formal training at the master's or doctoral level in public health. For example, only 20–25% of chief administrators of LHDs reported formal training in public health in recent surveys of LHDs.[3] This includes administrators whose public health training was in their primary profession (such as nursing, environmental health, medicine, or health education), suggesting that few received public health training in programs preparing administrators. Many public health administrators acquire public health practice management skills on a nondegree basis through a variety of means including management academies and leadership development institutes. Several dozen states have developed such institutes for workers in their own and collaborating states. There are also national public health leadership institutes for state and local public health officials and a national public health management academy.

Public health administrators represent a significant portion of the public health workforce for which career pathways are particularly unclear. Efforts to establish a greater professional identity for public health administrators are receiving increased attention. Management and leadership development programs are one example. Credentialing of public health administrators is another option under consideration. Several states license public health administrators, and one program credentials public health administrators through an independent review board. Some public health administrators view degrees from programs accredited by the Accrediting Commission on Education for Health Services Administration (ACHESA) or subsequent recognition from the American College of Healthcare Executives as meaningful credentials.

To be considered as qualified for a position as a public health administrator, both experience and education are important. Typical minimum qualifications for health services managers, local public health administrators, health officers, and emergency response coordinators are detailed in the following section.

Typical Minimum Qualifications for Health Services Manager

Knowledge, Skills, and Abilities

A health services manager generally has knowledge of:

- Principles and practices involved in the administration of health, public health, and regulatory programs and services
- The organization and operation of public agencies at the national, state, and local levels that are involved in health, public health, and regulatory programs and services
- The philosophy and objectives of state health and public health regulatory programs and services
- Programs and objectives of state and local public health agencies and of the interprofessional relationships in the implementation of their programs
- Current human service issues and theories
- The organization and functions of advocacy groups, voluntary agencies, civic organizations, and similar groups interested in health, public health, and regulatory programs and services and activities
- Managerial techniques and administrative practices

A health services manager generally has the skills and ability to:

- Plan, promote, and direct complex public health programs or services at the state level
- Analyze complex health data and formulate plans for coordinating and establishing new or improved health services and programs
- Secure active cooperation from other public and private agencies in developing and guiding health, public health, regulatory, and senior programs and services
- Develop, implement, and administer assigned programs or services to achieve positive program and client outcomes
- Establish and maintain working relationships with departmental officials, legislators, staff associates, the general public, and others
- Analyze and evaluate policies and operations and formulate recommendations
- Communicate effectively
- Provide leadership and supervision to professional, technical, and related program staff
- Manage change, provide program management, and achieve results

- Develop short- and long-range plans that meet established objectives and contribute to the overall goals and mission of the agency

Experience and Education

In many personnel systems, any combination of training and experience that provides the required knowledge and abilities qualifies an individual for this position. A typical career pathway for health services managers is through 3 or more years of professional experience in public health, healthcare delivery, environmental health or regulation, protective services for adults or the disabled, in-home services, or long-term care. In addition, a qualified applicant would have graduated from an accredited 4-year college or university with specialization in public health; healthcare administration; public, personnel, or business administration; biological, physical, environmental, or social sciences; nursing; nutrition/dietetics; social work; human services; gerontology; physical rehabilitation; education; or closely related areas. Graduate work in specified educational areas may sometimes be substituted on a year-for-year basis for 1 or more years of the required experience. Additional qualifying experience in the specified areas may be substituted on a year-for-year basis for any deficiencies in the stated education.

Typical Minimum Qualifications for Local Health Department Director

Knowledge, Skills, and Abilities

The LHD director generally has knowledge of:

- Basic principles of medical science and their application to local public health programs
- Public health problems and issues and their relationship to the development and operations of public health programs and services
- Federal, state, and local laws, ordinances, and regulations applicable to public health programs and communicable disease control
- Clinical skills and procedures
- Grant development and administration
- Principles, techniques, and practices of business and public health administration
- Budget development and expenditure control
- Principles and techniques of effective employee supervision, training, and development
- Public personnel management

The LHD director generally has the skills and ability to:

- Plan, organize, supervise, and administer the functions and programs of the local public health agency
- Ensure proper enforcement of public health statutes, laws, and regulations
- Provide direction, supervision, and training for agency staff
- Develop and administer budgets and control expenditures
- Develop and administer grants
- Review the work of agency staff and resolve problems
- Oversee the development, maintenance, and preparation of public health statistics, medical records, and reports
- Direct the preparation of and prepare clear, concise reports
- Effectively represent the local public health agency in contact with the public, community organizations, and other government agencies
- Establish and maintain cooperative working relationships
- Coordinate assigned activities with community organizations and other government agencies

Experience and Education

Any combination of training and experience that provides the required knowledge and abilities can qualify an individual for this position. A typical pathway to obtain the required knowledge and abilities is through broad and extensive experience in the development, analysis, and administration of public health programs and services with 3 years of the background and experience in a management or full supervisory capacity. Ideally this experience includes work in the areas of fiscal management, personnel management, and program development. In addition, a master's degree in public health, public administration, or healthcare administration is highly desirable.

Typical Minimum Qualifications for Health Officer
Knowledge, Skills, and Abilities

The health officer generally has knowledge of:

- Principles, practices, and responsibilities of medicine and of contemporary public health programs and service needs
- Applicable federal and state laws and regulations

- Organization, purpose, and function of federal and state health agencies
- Local medical associations and community health groups
- Principles and methods of public and community relations, and public information practices and techniques
- Principles and methods of determining and servicing public health needs
- Socioeconomic and psychological factors that can impact the effectiveness of health services delivery
- Communicable diseases and methods of control of sexually transmitted diseases
- Basic principles of budgeting
- Principles and practices of management necessary to plan, analyze, develop, evaluate, and direct diverse and complex activities of major health programs

The health officer generally has the skills and ability to:

- Plan, organize, and direct public health programs within professional standards, legal requirements, and financial constraints
- Direct and supervise professional and technical personnel
- Analyze situations accurately and take effective actions
- Interpret laws, regulations, and standards pertaining to public health
- Prepare clear and comprehensive records and reports
- Maintain accurate records
- Communicate effectively, both orally and in writing
- Speak effectively in public
- Establish and maintain effective working relationships with staff members, other departments, agencies, public groups, and organizations

Education and Experience

Any combination of training and experience that provides the required knowledge and abilities will qualify an individual for this position. A typical pathway to obtain the required knowledge and abilities is through 3 years of administrative or supervisory public health medical experience or possession of an MPH from an accredited school of public health and one year of public health medical experience. In some states, health officers must be a graduate of a medical school in good standing and possess a valid license to practice medicine in that state.

Typical Minimum Qualifications for Emergency Preparedness and Response Coordinator

Knowledge, Skills, and Abilities

Relevant knowledge, skills, and abilities for public health emergency response coordinators include

- Skill in organization and planning techniques
- Skill in public relations and public speaking
- Skill in computer and communication equipment operation
- Knowledge of basic budget development and fiscal management
- Knowledge of public health and epidemiology
- Ability to establish and maintain effective working relationships with other government and public health officials, employees, agencies, volunteers, and the public
- Ability to communicate effectively, verbally and in writing
- Ability to learn the principles, practices, and techniques involved in emergency management
- Knowledge of principles and practices of governmental and public health agency structures and resources
- Minimum qualifications call for the equivalent of a master's degree in public health, biologic sciences, community health, emergency management, planning, hazard assessment, business or public administration, or other related field; and 2 years of emergency management, community planning, or other related work experience. Selected applicants are subject to, and must pass, a full background check. In addition, emergency response coordinators generally are required to possess a valid state driver's license. Other organizations may require 5 years of responsible experience in public administration, research and finance, including 3 years of emergency management experience and a master's degree in public or business administration, government management, industrial engineering, or a related field. Other combinations of experience and education that meet the minimum requirements may be substituted.

WORKPLACE CONSIDERATIONS

Every organization has a management structure with various levels of management positions. Larger and more complex organizations have greater numbers of managers and administrators, although their scope of responsibility is often limited to a specific program or constellation of programs. Smaller organizations are more likely to be dominated by professionals, with administrative positions often filled by workers with professional backgrounds and credentials. For example, more than one half of the directors of the approximately 3,000 local public health agencies in the United States hold a health professional degree but no degree in public health.[3] For several decades, there has been a general trend toward more nonprofessional managers rather than elevating professionals into top management positions. This has been occurring at all governmental levels but somewhat more frequently among state and federal health agencies than for local public health agencies.

Work settings also influence the typical physical requirement for positions in this occupational category. Similar to administrators and managers throughout the health sector, public health administrators work long and irregular hours. Most public health administration positions call for workers to be able to sit for extended periods and to frequently stand and walk short distances. Normal manual dexterity and eye-hand coordination, hearing, and vision corrected to within the normal range are also important considerations. Normally, public health administrators will be able to communicate verbally and use office equipment including computers, telephones, calculators, copiers, and fax machines. Although much of the work is performed in an office environment, frequent and/or continuous contact with staff and the public is also necessary. In many situations, administrators may be required to possess a valid driver's license.

Special requirement for public health emergency preparedness and response manager positions may include the ability to travel and to be on call 24 hours a day, 7 days a week. Emergency preparedness and response managers may be required to complete training courses a recommended and made available through federal or state public health and emergency management agencies. In some instances, emergency preparedness and response managers may be required to complete the Certified Emergency Manager program through the National Coordinating Council on Emergency Management within some specified period of time after employment.

Working conditions for these positions include most work being performed in an office, library, computer room, or other environmentally controlled room. Emergency response activities may require work in a full-body protective suit with respirator protection from potential biologic, chemical, or nuclear material hazards

POSITIONS, SALARIES, AND CAREER PROSPECTS

In 2013, there were 300,000 medical and health services managers employed in the United States, with 25,000 working for federal, state, and local governmental agencies. Federal agencies employed 11,000 health administrators and managers, while state and local governments employed another 14,000 (**Table 8-3** and **Table 8-4**). Although the total number of medical and health services managers has been increasing faster than most other occupational categories in recent decades, a trend projected to continue through this decade, the number working in the public sector has been steady. This trend is projected to continue through 2022. *Public Health Enumeration 2000* data suggests there were 21,200 public health administrators at the turn of the century.

The median annual salary for all public sector medical and health managers was $95,000 in 2013 with the middle 50% earning between $76,000 and $118,000 (Table 8-4). Entry-level salaries were in the $60,000–$70,000 range. Small LHDs have notoriously lower salary scales (often in the $50,000–$70,000 range), making it difficult to attract administrators with graduate degrees or with extensive previous experience. Larger governmental agencies can often offer salaries that are competitive with those found in private and voluntary sector agencies. Administrators with professional credentials, especially physicians, dentists, veterinarians, epidemiologists, and nurses, may be able to attract salaries in the six-figure category.

The number of positions for medical and health services managers is expected to grow to nearly 390,000 by the year 2022, but with only 26,000 employed by government agencies

TABLE 8-3   Number of Workers in 2013 and Projected for 2022 for All Industries and Government and Number of Positions to Be Filled 2012–2022 for All Industries

Occupational Category	Workers in All Industries			Workers in Government	
	2013	Projected 2022	2012–2022 Positions To Be Filled	2013	Projected 2022
Medical and Health Services Managers	300,210	388,800	149,900	25,430	25,700
Social and Community Services Managers	115,330	160,600	55,100	24,620	26,800
Emergency Management Directors	9,800	10,700	2,200	6,380	7,000

Data from Bureau of Labor Statistics, U.S. Department of Labor. Selected Occupational Projections Data. Available at www.bls.gov/data/. Accessed June 15, 2014.

TABLE 8-4   Number and Salary Profile for Federal and State/Local Workers for Selected Occupations, 2013

Occupational Category	2013 Government Workers			
	Federal Workers	State / Local Workers	Median Annual Salary	25th–75th Percentile Salary Range
Medical and Health Services Managers	11,140	14,290	$95,460	$76,020-$117,800
Social and Community Services Managers	870	23,760	$71,340	$54,900-$90,490
Emergency Management Directors	30	6,350	$55,680	$40,350-$76,620

Notes: Federal: excludes postal service; State/Local: excludes hospitals and education

Data from Bureau of Labor Statistics, U.S. Department of Labor. Employment and Wages from Occupational Employment Statistics (OES) Survey. Available at www.bls.gov/data/. Accessed June 15, 2014.

(Table 8-3). Job growth in the government sector will lag behind the growth rate for medical and health administrator positions in the overall economy. Based on the growth in the number of positions and the need to fill other positions due to job changes and retirement, nearly 150,000 positions for medical and health administrators will be filled between 2012 and 2022 but with relatively few of these in the government sector.

Similar data and information for social and community services managers and for emergency management directors are provided in Tables 8-3 and 8-4. Numbers and trends for social and community services managers working for government closely parallel those for medical and health services managers. There were 25,000 public sector social and community services managers in 2013 with little growth forecasted through 2022. A greater proportion of social and community services managers work in the public sector compared with medical and health services managers. Salaries for social and community services managers are well below those for medical and health services managers.

Most emergency management directors are employed in the public sector, most frequently in emergency management agencies. Some, however, work for state health agencies and LHDs serving large populations. The number of these positions has been increasing over the past decade and some growth is anticipated through 2022. Average salaries for emergency preparedness and response managers fall in the $80,000–$110,000 range.[4] Salaries for emergency management directors in general, however, are somewhat below those for social and community services managers, and well below those for medical and health services managers.

Turnover among health managers is relatively frequent and, in addition to the wide range of qualifications required by potential employers, often results in vacant administrative and management positions being filled even when there are not many applicants with the optimal desired qualifications. This is easy to appreciate, because organizations must have people in leadership and management positions.

It is not uncommon to hear public health officials express concerns over difficulties in filling administrative positions with qualified candidates. It is not clear, however, whether this is a supply and demand issue or whether there are not adequate systems in place to recognize, reward, and value competent performance. Lack of succession planning within public health organizations may also be an important factor. Because administration and management require fairly nonspecific and generic skills, these positions are many times filled with individuals who are new to the field of public health. Public health professionals within such organizations often view such administrators as not necessarily committed to the same values and ethics as the professional staff. In any event, overall demand for public health administrators appears to be relatively steady and stable.

Public health administrators often have a general academic degree at the bachelor's or associate degree level and rise through the ranks of public service in the governmental sector. It is also common for an experienced public health professional such as an environmental health practitioner or public health nurse to be promoted into an agency leadership position. In sum, career pathways are many and varied for public health administration positions.

OUTSIDE-THE-BOOK THINKING 8-4

© Alfred Bondarenko/Shutterstock.

In which organizations and geographic regions will the need for public health administrators expand most rapidly in the next two decades?

ADDITIONAL INFORMATION

There are many good sources of information on public health administration as a career. Several sources are available for information on educational programs for health administration as well as for continuing education and leadership development for practicing public health administrators.

The Association of University Programs in Health Administration (AUPHA) web site (www.aupha.org) provides information on approximately 150 undergraduate and graduate degree programs in health administration in the United States. AUPHA works closely with the Commission on Accreditation of Healthcare Management Education (www.cahme.org/) and ACHESA, the organization that accredits master's-level programs. Only ACHESA-accredited programs can become a full member of AUPHA.

Both AUPHA and ACHESA are linked with the American College of Healthcare Executives (www.ache.org), which credentials health administrators. A similar, but considerably smaller, program that certifies public health administrators is operated by the Public Health Practitioner Certification Board (www.phpcb.org).

Schools of public health are among the institutions offering graduate degrees in health administration. The

TABLE 8-5   Health Administration Competency Expectations for Graduates of MPH Degree Programs

1. Identify the main components and issues of the organization, financing, and delivery of health services and public health systems in the United States.
2. Describe the legal and ethical bases for public health and health services.
3. Explain methods of ensuring community health safety and preparedness
4. Discuss the policy process for improving the health status of populations.
5. Apply the principles of program planning, development, budgeting, management, and evaluation in organizational and community initiatives.
6. Apply principles of strategic planning and marketing to public health.
7. Apply quality and performance improvement concepts to address organizational performance issues
8. Apply "systems thinking" for resolving organizational problems.
9. Communicate health policy and management issues using appropriate channels and technologies
10. Demonstrate leadership skills for building partnerships.

Reproduced from the Association of Schools of Public Health (ASPH). MPH Core Competency Development Process, Version 2.3. Washington, DC: ASPH. 2006. Available at http://www.aspph.org. Accessed June 15, 2014.

Association of Schools and Programs of Public Health (www.aspph.org) has identified a battery of core health administration competencies appropriate for all students receiving the MPH degree (**Table 8-5**). These competencies provide a useful baseline for professional public health administration and indicate what, upon graduation, a student with an MPH should be able to do.

The American Public Health Association's (APHA) Health Administration Section is another good source of information for public health administration. Its web site can be accessed through the main APHA site (www.apha.org). The Health Administration Section has a nearly 100-year history, beginning as a section for medical health officers but expanding to include a broader spectrum of public health administrators.

The Public Health Leadership Society (www.phls.org) includes graduates of the National Public Health Leadership Institute (www.phli.org), operating from the University of North Carolina School of Public Health, as well as alumni of approximately 20 state and regional public health leadership development institute. These programs serve public health practitioners through an intensive leadership development curriculum undertaken on a continuing education basis. The University of North Carolina also offers a Management Academy for Public Health, serving public health managers and administrators from states in the southeast region of the United States.

CONCLUSION

Public health administrators are one of the largest and most important of the professional occupational categories in the public health workforce. There are more than 25,000 health administrators working in governmental health settings. This group is also one of the most diverse in terms of academic credentials and previous work experiences. Public health administration offers a variety of work settings, especially at the local level, and a broad range of career pathways that are open to both individuals trained in public health and those new to the field. Because of the diverse backgrounds and skill levels, ongoing education and training are especially relevant issues for this occupational category. Demand for these positions in the private and voluntary sectors is steady to slightly increasing and likely to remain so over the near term. Prospects in the public sector are not so bright.

REFERENCES

1. Bureau of Labor Statistics, U.S. Department of Labor. Databases and tables. www.bls.gov/data/. Accessed June 15, 2014.
2. Health Resources and Services Administration, Bureau of Health Professions, National Center for Health Workforce Information and Analysis and Center for Health Policy, Columbia School of Nursing. *Public Health Workforce Enumeration 2000*. Washington, DC: HRSA; 2000.
3. National Association of County and City Health Officials. *2013 National Profile of Local Health Departments*. Washington, DC: NACCHO; 2014.
4. Association of State and Territorial Health Officials. *Profile of State Public Health, Volume Three, 2012*. Washington, DC: ASTHO; 2014.

CHAPTER **9**

Environmental and Occupational Health

Environmental and occupational health is an expansive field that has been an important part of public health practice for more than 150 years. The exploits of John Snow in battling cholera in England in the 1850s elucidated the link between communicable disease and sanitary conditions. As described in our review of public health history, the pioneering efforts of Chadwick in England and Shattuck in the United States resulted in blueprints for early public health responses and systems. Many public health successes in the latter part of the 1800s and the early decades of the 20th century were the direct result of environmental engineering and sanitation advances. The people carrying out these duties have been an integral part of the public health workforce and remain so. These workers are employed in public health and environmental protection agencies at all levels of government and throughout the private sector as well. The Bureau of Labor Statistics (BLS) reported nearly 193,000 workers in environmental engineering, specialist, and technician positions and another 100,000 in occupational and industrial health and safety positions in 2013.[1] There were nearly 90,000 environmental and occupational health workers employed by federal, state, and local governmental agencies. *Public Health Workforce Enumeration 2000* data identified 40,000 working for federal, state, and local public health agencies in the year 2000.[2] Surveys conducted in 2012 and 2013 reported about 20,000 environmental health workers in state and local public health agencies.[3,4] Data from these key sources are used throughout this chapter. Differences among these various sources indicate that many environmental and occupational health personnel work in nonhealth agencies at all levels of government, such as environmental protection agencies, departments of natural resources, and sanitation agencies. In any event, environmental and occupational health workers are one of the largest occupational groupings within the public health workforce today. Environmental and occupational public health workers are increasingly finding positions in private sector organizations that offer a wide variety of environmental and occupational health services. **Table 9-1** provides a snapshot of an average day in the life of an environmental health practitioner.

OCCUPATIONAL CLASSIFICATION

There are seven specific standard occupational categories (SOCs) for environmental health workers. These include environmental engineer, environmental engineering technician, environmental scientist/specialist, environmental

TABLE 9-1   A Typical Day for an Environmental Health Practitioner

7:30 a.m.	Visit septic field inspection site to assist environmental health specialists on site
8:30 a.m.	Office time for paperwork and information sharing with staff
9:00 a.m.	Staff meeting to review priorities for week
10:15 a.m.	Interview candidates for vacant entry-level environmental health specialist position
10:45 a.m.	Meet with communicable disease control, epidemiology, and public health nursing staff regarding community concerns over West Nile Virus threat
11:45 a.m.	Brown bag lunch with other environmental health staff; today's guest is a professor from a state university undergraduate degree program in environmental health
1:00 p.m.	Brief agency director regarding status of West Nile Virus threat
1:30 p.m.	Supervise inspection of food services, swimming pools, and septic systems at county fair site
3:00 p.m.	Conference call meeting with epidemiology and environmental health staff of neighboring jurisdictions and state health department regarding current status of West Nile Virus
4:00 p.m.	Review information suggested by staff for tonight's community meeting
4:30 p.m.	More paperwork related to permit approvals
5:15 p.m.	Prepare remarks for tonight's community meeting
7:00 p.m.	Represent agency at community meeting regarding West Nile Virus concerns

science and protection technician, health and safety engineer, occupational health and safety specialist, and occupational health and safety technician. Four of these titles are professional occupations (environmental engineer, environmental scientist/specialist, health and safety engineer, and occupational health and safety specialist). The others are technical occupations.

- Environmental engineers (e.g., water supply or wastewater engineers, solid waste engineers, air pollution engineers, sanitary engineers) apply engineering principles to control, eliminate, ameliorate, and/or prevent environmental health hazards. There were 53,000 environmental engineers in the United States in 2013. Private-sector companies (architectural and engineering companies, management and technical consulting firms) employ the largest numbers of environmental engineers. Federal, state, and local government agencies employed 15,000 environmental engineers in 2013. *Public Health Workforce Enumeration 2000* data suggest that about 7,000 were working in governmental public health agencies in 2000.

- Environmental engineering technicians (e.g., water or wastewater plant operators, water or wastewater testing technicians, air pollution technicians) assist environmental engineers and other environmental

health professions in controlling, eliminating, ameliorating, and/or preventing environmental health hazards. There were 18,000 environmental engineering technicians working in the United States in 2013. Architectural and engineering companies employ the largest number of environmental engineering technicians, followed by local government and scientific research and development companies. Governmental agencies employed only 3,200 environmental engineering technicians in 2013, 600 of whom were identified in the *Public Health Workforce Enumeration 2000* study.

- Environmental scientists or specialists (e.g., environmental researchers, environmental health specialists, food scientists, soil and plant scientists, air pollution specialists, hazardous materials specialists, toxicologists, water or wastewater or solid waste specialists, sanitarians, entomologists) apply biological, chemical, and public health principles to control, eliminate, ameliorate, and/or prevent environmental health hazards. There were 87,000 environmental specialists working in the United States in 2013. State governments are the leading source of employment for environmental specialists. Local government and private sector companies also employ large numbers of environmental specialists. Governmental agencies employed 38,000 environmental specialists in 2013; the *Public Health Workforce Enumeration 2000* study identified 23,000 in federal, state, and local public health agencies in 2000.

- Environmental science and protection technicians (e.g., air pollution technicians, vector control workers) assist environmental scientists and specialists and other environmental health professionals in the control, elimination, and/or prevention of environmental health hazards. There were nearly 35,000 workers in the United States in environmental science and engineering technician positions in 2013. Local governments are the largest employer of environmental science technicians. Private companies and state governments are other important employment sources. Nearly 9,000 environmental science and protection technicians worked for government agencies in 2013. The *Public Health Workforce Enumeration 2000* study identified 700 working in governmental public health agencies in 2000.

- Health and safety engineers (e.g., aerospace safety engineers, fire prevention and protection engineers, product safety engineers, and systems safety engineers) develop procedures and design systems to prevent people from getting sick or injured and to keep property from being damaged. They combine knowledge of systems engineering and of health or safety to make sure that chemicals, machinery, software, furniture, and consumer products will not cause harm to people or property. Health and safety engineers also investigate industrial accidents, injuries, or occupational diseases to determine their causes and to determine whether the incidents could have been or can be prevented. They interview employers and employees to learn about work environments and incidents that lead to accidents or injuries. They also evaluate the corrections that were made to remedy violations found during health inspections. There were nearly 24,000 health and safety engineers in 2013 with only 3,000 working for public sector agencies. Health and safety engineers were not one of the categories included in the *Public Health Workforce Enumeration 2000* study.

- Occupational health and safety specialists (e.g., industrial hygienists, occupational health specialists, radiologic health inspectors, safety inspectors) review, evaluate, and analyze workplace environments and exposures. These workers design programs and procedures to control, eliminate, ameliorate, and/or prevent disease and injury caused by chemical, physical, biological, and ergonomic risks to workers. There were 63,000 occupational health and safety specialists in the United States in 2013. Local and state governments are the largest employment sources for occupational safety and health specialists; hospitals are another large employer. Government agencies employed nearly 19,000 occupational health and safety specialists in 2013. The *Public Health Workforce Enumeration 2000* study identified nearly 9,000 working in governmental public health agencies.

- Occupational health and safety technicians collect data on workplace environments and exposures for analysis by occupational safety and health specialists; they also implement programs and conduct evaluation of programs designed to limit chemical, physical, biologic, and ergonomic risks to workers. There were 14,000 occupational health and safety technicians in the United States in 2013, with 2,700 working for federal, state, and local governmental agencies. The *Public Health Workforce Enumeration 2000 study* identified only 150 working in governmental public health agencies in 2000.

OUTSIDE-THE-BOOK THINKING 9-1

© Alfred Bondarenko/Shutterstock.

What will be the most important new or expanded roles for environmental and occupational health workers in the 21st century?

As is apparent from these occupational categories, both professional and technical positions are common in the environmental health component of the public health workforce. Among the 40,000 environmental and occupational health positions identified in the *Public Health Workforce Enumeration 200* study, more than one half were professional titles. Among professional positions, environmental health ranks second only to nursing within the public health workforce. Professional titles include engineers, scientists, and specialists. Technical titles include technicians and technologists.

PUBLIC HEALTH PRACTICE PROFILE

Environmental and occupational health workers generally function at a program or unit level within public health agencies at all levels of government, but especially those at the local and state level. They are most frequently involved in public health responsibilities that focus on protecting against environmental hazards, preventing injuries, and preventing epidemics and the spread of disease. Environmental and occupational health workers may also be key components of efforts to prepare and respond to public health emergencies, especially natural disasters for which protection of water and food supplies can be critical.

Among the 10 essential public health services, environmental and occupational health workers are most likely to be involved in diagnosing and investigating health problems and health hazards in the community, enforcing laws and regulations that protect health and ensure safety, monitoring health status to identify community health status, and evaluating the effectiveness and quality of environmental and occupational health services in the community. With much of their work done in community settings, environmental and occupational health workers also inform, educate, and empower people about important health issues. **Table 9-2** summarizes public health purposes and essential public health services at the core of positions for environmental and occupational health workers.

OUTSIDE-THE-BOOK THINKING 9-2

© Alfred Bondarenko/Shutterstock.

What are the most important contributions to improving the health of the public that environmental and occupational health workers make today?

IMPORTANT AND ESSENTIAL DUTIES

There are many different job titles and positions used for environmental and occupational health workers. This chapter will focus on five representative positions: (1) environmental engineer; (2) entry-level environmental health specialist; (3) midlevel environmental health specialist; (4) senior-level environmental health specialist; and (5) midlevel occupational health and safety specialist. Each of these positions and a representative panel of their important and essential duties are described in this section.

TABLE 9-2   Public Health Practice Profile for Environmental Health

Environmental and Occupational Health Workers Make a Difference by:
Public Health Purposes
✓ Preventing epidemics and the spread of disease
✓ Protecting against environmental hazards
✓ Preventing injuries
Promoting and encouraging healthy behavior
Responding to disasters and assisting communities in recovery
Ensuring the quality and accessibility of health services
Essential Public Health Services
✓ Monitoring health status to identify community health problems
✓ Diagnosing and investigating health problems and health hazards in the community
✓ Informing, educating, and empowering people about health issues
Mobilizing community partnerships to identify and solve health problems
Developing policies and plans that support individual and community health efforts
✓ Enforcing laws and regulations that protect health and ensure safety
Linking people with needed personal health services and ensuring the provision of health care when otherwise unavailable
Ensuring a competent public health and personal healthcare workforce
✓ Evaluating effectiveness, accessibility, and quality of personal and population-based health services
Researching new insights and innovative solutions to health problems

Environmental Engineer

This is a professional environmental engineering position with duties within an assigned environmental program involving the protection of public health and/or the protection or restoration of the environment. There are often several grades for this position. Entry-level titles generally do not have any supervisory responsibilities. Higher level environmental engineer titles may supervise or lead assigned engineers and/or other staff. Workers in this title are responsible for the performance of professional engineering duties in performing field surveys and investigations of water supplies, sewage systems, streams, industrial waste facilities, solid and hazardous waste facilities, air pollution control systems, and/or dams and reservoirs. Work includes preparing reports of findings, and making recommendations to improve the public health, safety, and the environment. Environmental engineers work under general technical supervision and receive work assignments from a designated superior. There may be several levels of positions with this title.

Important and essential duties for environmental engineers include

- Participates in the engineering review of the hydraulics and details of water supply systems and plants, industrial and domestic waste treatment systems, solid and hazardous waste management systems, air pollution control systems, dams and reservoirs, etc.
- Gathers and interprets data on pollution, contamination, and construction and design features relevant for environmental engineering projects
- Reviews engineering plans and specifications for sewage and industrial waste treatment plants, water supply systems, solid and hazardous waste disposal areas, air pollution control systems, and dams and reservoirs for compliance with approved standards
- Confers with officials and owners/operators of plants and establishments with regard to laws, regulations, and engineering requirements of appropriate state and local agencies
- Collects samples of water and sewage for bacteriologic, chemical, or biologic analysis
- Examines and prepares charts, tables, and maps for the interpretation of engineering data, and prepares reports of findings and analysis
- Prepares papers and lectures on subjects relating to the environment and/or dam safety
- Prepares technical and detailed reports of engineering surveys

- Participates in special investigations of fish kills and unusual stream conditions with representatives of other agencies
- Supervises, assigns, and assists in the work of a unit composed of a small group of professional personnel
- Trains subordinate engineers and other technical staff

Environmental Specialist (Entry Level)

This position serves as an entry-level environmental specialist performing one or more of the following functions under close direction and supervision: conducting routine compliance and enforcement activities; assisting in the development of draft legislation, policies, and regulations; conducting routine scientific analyses and technical services on assigned office or field projects; providing regulatory assistance; providing project administration and environmental technical assistance for grants, contracts, or loans; interpreting policy and technical assistance; conducting less complex surveys and analyses; recording field conditions; gathering and analyzing information to assist in developing recommendations and decision making; and assisting in permit development. The number of levels for this position varies from one personnel system to another. In many personnel systems there are three to five levels of environmental health specialist positions that allow for career advancement.

Important and essential duties for entry-level environmental health specialists include

- Assists in the installation, operation, and maintenance of environmental monitoring/sampling equipment; assists in performing field and office surveys and studies; performs surveillance and other special projects
- Assists in routine repairs and calibrations of environmental monitoring/sampling equipment, in accordance with specifications and standard operating procedures; performs basic sampling data review for precision and accuracy
- Assists in responding to complaints, routine inspections/surveillance, and permit review to meet compliance requirements
- Assists in the research and compilation of basic information for use in regulation or policy development
- Enters and maintains basic databases or inventories
- Assists in preparing for public meetings, hearings, and workshops
- Assists with routine inspections or investigations of facilities or project sites that require specialized knowledge of industry processes, pollutant sources, or natural processes

- Responds to routine inquiries or requests for technical assistance regarding the scientific background and technical implementation of agency programs
- Reviews plans for technical accuracy and makes recommendations to higher-level staff
- Conducts routine sampling and testing; analyzes, evaluates, and interprets data; writes reports; and assists higher-level staff
- Maintains and utilizes computerized environmental databases in support of technical projects
- Reviews routine permit applications for technical accuracy and makes recommendations regarding the scientific merit of proposals
- Provides technical and administrative assistance to grant, contract, or loan recipients in the planning, design, construction, and implementation of environmental protection projects

Environmental Specialist (Midlevel)

This position serves as a staff environmental specialist performing one or more of the following functions independently with little direction and supervision: conducting compliance and enforcement activities; developing draft legislation; developing, performing, coordinating, implementing, and evaluating scientific analyses, plans, or services involving office or field projects; conducting surveys, analyses, and recording field conditions; providing project administration and environmental technical assistance for grants, contracts, and loans; gathering and analyzing information to develop recommendations for decision making and permit development, review, and oversight. This position may lead or supervise assigned staff.

Important and essential duties for midlevel environmental specialists include

- Independently performs the installation, operation, and maintenance of environmental monitoring/sampling equipment; on an area or site list basis performs and/or provides guidance for surveys, field studies, or other special data-gathering activities
- Performs complex equipment repair and calibrations; reviews monitored data for evaluation of equipment performance
- Responds to and investigates complex or highly technical complaints or violations; performs complex inspections or field investigations; coordinates complaint and enforcement priorities, schedules, and assists in negotiating agreements and settlements;

prepares final permit evaluation or report for approval; may impose on-site enforcement action; performs follow-up inspections to ensure corrective action is implemented

- Plans, develops, researches, and conducts or oversees technical data collection and analyzes, evaluates, and interprets data; analyzes or interprets information requirements and coordinates information gathering for a team or other assignment outside of a team; writes reports and reviews draft reports
- Determines database or inventory requirements; works with agency and nonagency sources on data submittals; evaluates databases or inventories for analysis, reporting, or compliance purposes; may design and/or develop databases or inventories to be utilized in support of technical projects
- Reviews permit applications for technical accuracy, negotiates permit conditions, conducts conflict resolution, and makes decisions regarding the scientific merit of proposals; serves as a senior permit writer or historical/institutional memory for geographic area or complex site
- Develops and/or implements project plans, consent decrees, orders, or scientific studies for cleanups, resource management, or policy/regulation development; conducts research for technical projects; reviews project plans for technical accuracy and makes decisions on the scientific merit of proposals
- Oversees contractor or consultant services for compliance and certifies performance; provides assistance to other staff, agencies, and the public
- Makes recommendations to senior staff regarding new or modified sampling and analytical testing methods, best management practices, and technical operating procedures
- Makes technical and scientific recommendations regarding the development, coordination, and implementation of environmental technical assistance programs involving pollution prevention, pollution control, or natural resource management
- Evaluates data to determine technical compliance with regulatory requirements
- Plans, facilitates, and represents the program or agency in public meetings, hearings, and workshops
- Conducts literature evaluations to assess evidence-based practice; formulates grant proposals; proposes and designs assessment and research projects
- Develops evidence-based protocols for specific program interventions and services

- Independently provides technical and administrative assistance to grant, contract, or loan recipients in the planning, design, construction, or implementation of environmental protection projects
- Coordinates the development of policies, procedures, statutes, and regulations of a high degree of complexity
- Directs or coordinates nonagency employees at large spills or complex sites

Environmental Specialist (Senior Level)

This position serves as a senior program expert in one or more program subject areas as designated in writing by a program manager, agency director, or higher. A senior environmental specialist performs, directs, implements, and evaluates activities that are of critical agency, regional, statewide or national interest, sensitivity, or complexity. Such activities may include planning and directing surveys and analyses of projects that are a high priority for the agency or involve participation in the resolution of major environmental questions. In most circumstances, this position supervises five or more professional environmental staff.

Important and essential duties for senior-level environmental specialists include

- Advises program management on monitoring and sampling policies, priorities, effectiveness, and cross-media or agency issues and requirements
- Evaluates equipment inventories for material readiness, amortization, and technology transfer; management of contracted services and equipment utilization; conducts equipment needs assessments
- Advises program management on violations of critical or controversial agency interest; evaluates rule effectiveness and recommends enforcement/compliance rule making; may represent the program on multimedia or highly complex or controversial enforcement/compliance actions involving other programs or agencies
- Works with other programs and agencies in identifying information required for policy development, legislation, regulations, and recommended priorities, scheduling requirements, and information parameters for program management
- Evaluates databases and inventories for policy or regulation development; determines new, changing, or emerging requirements for databases and inventories; may work with other programs or agencies on database/inventory requirements

- Conducts literature evaluations to assess evidence-based practice; formulates grant proposals; proposes and designs assessment and research projects
- Develops evidence-based protocols for specific program interventions and services
- Coordinates controversial or critical plans for resource management, policy or regulation development, or statewide cleanup priorities
- Advises program or agency management on the need for contractor or consultant services versus agency staff and expertise
- Identifies critical or emerging issues and recommends preventive or corrective measures
- Represents agency and testifies at legal or public hearings or conferences and before legislative bodies
- Provides expertise or historical background not otherwise available to the agency that is used as a basis for agency management decisions
- Serves as an agency representative to regional and national commissions and environmental or professional organizations relevant to assigned responsibilities with the agency

Occupational Health and Safety Specialist

This is midlevel professional scientific work in evaluating work and indoor environments for safety and health hazards. Occupational health and safety specialists make comprehensive safety and health hazard evaluations, including the more difficult evaluations, of all general industry and indoor environments, involving office buildings and factories. A comprehensive safety and health hazard evaluation may consist of the following: conducting a physical survey; establishing appropriate sampling techniques; collecting samples as necessary to assess the presence of chemical, physical, and microbial agents in accordance with the requirements of the Occupational Safety and Health Act; analyzing the data generated by sampling and making a professional judgment using accepted industrial hygiene practices and federal standards to determine the degree of hazard present; interviewing employers and employees and other potentially exposed individuals to determine possible sources of safety and health hazards; preparing a technical report of the safety and health hazard evaluation that can be understood and followed by lay personnel; and making recommendations within this report that will reduce or correct the health hazard. Occupational health and safety specialists receive minimal supervision from an administrative superior.

Important and essential duties for midlevel occupational health and safety specialists include

- Conducts initial conferences with employers to introduce the services offered by the agency
- Consults with employers on the existence, utilization, and operating condition of powered mechanical ventilation devices, personal safety equipment and procedures, noise abatement equipment and procedures, material safety data sheets, hazardous chemical correction, and safety and health programs
- Performs difficult safety and health hazard evaluations requiring literature research, analysis, and scientific design
- Determines the magnitude of exposure or nuisance to workers and the public; selects or devises methods and instruments suitable for measurements; studies and tests materials associated with the work operation
- Collects samples from office buildings and other workplaces to determine the presence of toxic substances and other potential hazards; evaluates building ventilation systems for possible deficiencies; and provides technical advice on remedial action
- Interprets results of the examination of the work environment in terms of the potential of causing a community nuisance or damage or impairing worker safety, health, and efficiency; and presents specific conclusions to appropriate interested parties by means of a technical report
- Determines the need for, or effectiveness of, control measures, and when necessary, recommends procedures that will be suitable and effective in achieving those measures
- Interprets occupational safety and health laws, rules, and regulations; determines compliance with safety and health laws; holds conferences with management to discuss identified violations and deficiencies and recommends corrections
- Reviews facility safety and health programs required by the federal Occupational Safety and Health Administration

MINIMUM QUALIFICATIONS

Environmental and occupational health includes a mix of professional and technical occupations, both of which generally have several levels of positions. This provides a natural career pathway and allows environmental and occupational health workers to remain in this field for many years. Comparable positions exist in local public agencies of all sizes, making career advancement from a small to larger employer a common pathway for these workers.

Although environmental and occupational health professionals are produced by schools of public health, there are also many undergraduate and graduate degree programs specializing in environmental sciences. It is these programs that are even larger producers of environmental and occupational health practitioners. Many workers in technical positions have less than a bachelor degree; some have no more than a high school degree.

As with virtually all public health positions, both experience and education are important considerations for hiring and promotion. Experience and education both contribute to necessary knowledge, skills, and abilities required for workers in this field. Typical minimum qualifications for environmental engineers, three levels of environmental health specialists, and occupational health and safety specialists are detailed below.

Typical Minimum Qualifications for Environmental Engineer

Knowledge, Skills, and Abilities

An environmental engineer will generally have knowledge of:

- Principles and practices of environmental engineering and/or environmental sanitation
- Design, construction, and operation of air quality control, water supply and treatment, and sewage and industrial waste disposal systems
- Laws and regulations governing sanitation
- Physical and biologic sciences, including chemistry, bacteriology, and physical properties of ambient air, water, sewage, and liquid waste as related to environmental engineering
- Mathematics, geometry, calculus, and engineering formulas

An environmental engineer will generally have the skills and ability to:

- Develop designs involving environmental engineering theory and judgment
- Establish and maintain cooperative working relationships with public officials and community groups
- Perform investigations involving the application of professional theory and interpretation of laws, regulations, and requirements
- Plan, promote, and conduct engineering projects

- Analyze significant environmental engineering and sanitation data
- Consult with and advise plant owners and operators on proper design, construction, and operation of plants
- Prepare engineering reports and papers and lectures related to the environment

Experience and Education

Any combination of training and experience that provides the requisite knowledge and abilities will qualify an individual for this position. A typical way to obtain the required knowledge and abilities is through acquisition of a master's degree with major study in one of the engineering fields (such as sanitary, water resource, civil, geotechnical, environmental, chemical, or mechanical engineering) and 1 year of experience in environmental engineering. Another path is through acquisition of an engineer-in-training certificate or a bachelor degree with a major study in one of the engineering fields listed above and 2 years of environmental engineering experience. Some jurisdictions may require registration as a professional engineer within the state or another state with equivalent requirements for registration or an engineer-in-training certificate. In some instances, a doctoral degree in an engineering field may substitute for 1 or more years of environmental engineering experience. Requirements for professional registration as an engineer in some states may require up to 8 years of professional experience (which may include up to 4 years of college-level engineering education) and successful completion of professional licensing exams.

Typical Minimum Requirements for Entry-Level Environmental Specialist

Knowledge, Skills, and Abilities

An entry-level environmental health specialist will generally have knowledge of:

- Field investigative techniques, including data gathering and basic research
- Practices and methods of environmental problem solving
- Soil, water, or air sampling methods and techniques
- Characteristics of pollutants
- Principles, practices, and methods of environmental science, natural resource management, pollution prevention, and pollution control

- Applicable federal, state, and local environmental regulations

An entry-level environmental health specialist will generally have the skills and ability to:

- Use sound judgment in performing assigned tasks
- Understand and apply environmental regulations and related laws
- Write clearly and concisely, and prepare maps, plans, charts, and graphs
- Communicate effectively with agency staff, other agencies, industry, and the general public

Experience and Education

Entry-level environmental health specialists come from a wide range of educational levels and previous work experiences, which generally include:

- A bachelor degree involving major study in environmental, physical, or one of the natural sciences; environmental planning; or other allied field
- Experience at or above the environmental technician level, or equivalent will substitute, year for year, for education

Typical Minimum Requirements for Midlevel Environmental Specialist

Knowledge, Skills, and Abilities

A midlevel environmental health specialist will generally have knowledge of:

- Principles, practices, and methods of environmental or resource management and environmental pollution prevention and pollution control
- Methods and techniques of field sampling, testing, data gathering, basic research, and field investigations
- Soil science, geology, hydrology, hydrogeology, metrology, and toxicology
- Applicable federal, state, and local environmental regulations and policies
- Characteristics and health effects of pollutants
- Technical report writing methods

A midlevel environmental health specialist will generally have the skills and ability to:

- Use sound, independent judgment in making decisions on environmental problems and completing assigned tasks

- Understand and interpret plans, maps, and equipment specifications
- Prepare clear and concise written reports and make oral presentations
- Analyze and prepare plans and reports
- Understand and communicate complex environmental regulations and statutes
- Communicate effectively with agency staff, other agencies, industry, and the general public

Experience and Education

Any combination of training and experience that provides the requisite knowledge and abilities will qualify an individual for this position. A typical pathway to obtain the required knowledge and abilities is through acquisition of a bachelor degree involving major study in environmental, physical, or one of the natural sciences; environmental planning; or other allied field; and 2 years of professional-level experience in environmental analysis, control, or planning. Additional qualifying experience may substitute, year for year, for education. A master's degree in one of the above fields may also substitute for 1 year of the required experience. Another way to meet these qualifications is through acquisition of a doctoral degree in one of the above fields or through 1 year of experience in the next lower-level environmental specialist position.

Typical Minimum Qualifications for Senior-Level Environmental Specialist

Knowledge, Skills, and Abilities

A senior-level environmental specialist will generally have knowledge of:

- Applicable federal, state, and local environmental regulations and policies
- Soil science, geology, hydrology, hydrogeology, metrology, and toxicology
- Methods for the development of an environmental program or complex study
- Multimedia environmental principles and practices

A senior-level environmental specialist will generally have the skills and ability to:

- Identify and assess program or agency service delivery needs and requirements
- Recognize emerging issues and conduct advanced planning to address those issues
- Represent program or agency management on complex or controversial issues with other agencies, jurisdictions, or interest groups

- Effectively negotiate and resolve conflict
- Effectively communicate technical information clearly, both orally and in writing
- Demonstrate a high degree of technical expertise in a particular field or specialty as shown through the publication of papers in peer-reviewed, scientific, or technical journals or the presentation of papers at professional conferences

Experience and Education

Any combination of training and experience that provides the requisite knowledge and abilities will qualify an individual for this position. A typical pathway to obtain the required knowledge and abilities is through a bachelor degree involving major study in environmental, physical, or one of the natural sciences; environmental planning; or other allied field; and 6 years of professional-level experience in environmental analysis, control, or planning, which includes 2 years equal to the midlevel environmental specialist position. Additional qualifying experience may substitute, year for year, for education. Another pathway to satisfy these qualifications is through acquisition of a master's degree in one of the preceding fields and 4 years of professional-level experience that include 2 years equal to a midlevel environmental specialist. Yet another way to satisfy these requirements is through acquisition of a doctoral degree in one of the preceding fields and 3 years of professional-level experience that include 2 years equal to a midlevel environmental specialist.

Typical Minimum Qualifications for Occupational Health and Safety Specialist

Knowledge, Skills, and Abilities

An occupational health and safety specialist generally has knowledge of:

- Sampling and direct measuring techniques for gas, vapor, dust, noise, and radiation
- Microbiology, radiology, physiology, and chemistry
- Common diseases and health hazards related to indoor environments and industrial occupations and of their possible sources
- The standard types of machinery and equipment used in industrial and commercial establishments
- The Occupational Safety and Health Act and the applicable regulations of the U.S. Environmental Protection Agency (EPA) that relate to workplace safety and health

An occupational health and safety specialist generally has the skills and ability to:

- Analyze complex problems of environmental hazard reduction and arrive at sound decisions regarding actions to be taken
- Develop, organize, and present training through a comprehensive company-specific safety program
- Analyze and interpret technical reports and criteria documents on exposure limits
- Operate and maintain detection and measurement apparatus
- Communicate thoughts and ideas clearly and concisely
- Establish and maintain effective working relationships with plant managers, safety directors, employees, and the public

Experience and Education

Any combination of training and experience that provides the requisite knowledge and abilities will qualify an individual for this position. A typical way to obtain the required knowledge and abilities is through 1 year of experience as an entry-level occupational safety and health specialist or 1 year of professional experience in safety and health consultation in a governmental agency or program or in private industry as an industrial hygienist, industrial safety professional, safety manager, or other closely related position in the occupational safety or health field, and graduation from an accredited 4-year college or university with specialization in industrial hygiene or safety or a closely related area. In some instances, graduate work in industrial hygiene or safety may be substituted on a year-for-year basis for the stated experience. Certification as a certified industrial hygienist (CIH) by the American Board of Industrial Hygiene or as a certified safety professional (CSP) by the Board of Certified Safety Professionals (BCSP) may be substituted for 6 months of the stated experience. Some states may require specific certifications and licensing.

WORKPLACE CONSIDERATIONS

Federal, state, and local governmental agencies employ nearly 90,000 environmental and occupational health workers (both professional and technical titles), making governmental agencies the largest sources of jobs for environmental and occupational health workers.

Work settings and working conditions influence the typical physical requirement for positions in environmental and occupational health categories. For example, entry-level and midlevel environmental and occupational health specialists spend considerable time outside the office. Environmental health specialists often find themselves at various environmental sites; occupational health specialists often do their work at business sites. Environmental engineers and higher-level environmental and occupational health specialists spend somewhat more time in an office setting.

Most positions call for workers to be able to sit for extended periods and to frequently stand and walk extended distances. Normal manual dexterity and eye-hand coordination, hearing, and vision corrected to within the normal range are also important considerations. This work requires good vision to peruse and review correspondence, statutes, and related material and to perform visual inspections required for work activities conducted on site. Also important are the ability to stand, walk, and have full use of upper and lower extremities to effect investigations and collection efforts in business establishments and in the field. At times, this work may require climbing ladders and entering confined areas for investigations.

Normally, environmental and occupational health workers can communicate verbally and use office equipment including computers, telephones, calculators, copiers, and fax machines. For work performed in an office environment, frequent or continuous contact with staff and the public is also necessary. In many situations, environmental and occupational health workers must be mobile and may be required to possess a valid driver's license. Important attributes are verbal and reasoning ability in order to read and understand a variety of written matter; to process directives, reports, and correspondence; and to initiate action required. These positions require emotional stability and good judgment to deal with the public and personnel whose business activities are being inspected or investigated.

OUTSIDE-THE-BOOK THINKING 9-3

© Alfred Bondarenko/Shutterstock.

What features make public health environmental and occupational health a career worth pursuing?

POSITIONS, SALARIES, AND CAREER PROSPECTS

In 2013, there were 300,000 environmental and occupational health professionals and technicians employed in the United States, with nearly 90,000 working for federal, state, and local governmental agencies. **Table 9-3** identifies the number of total workers and the number employed by government for the seven standard occupational categories considered in this chapter. Projections for the year 2022 are also provided. Each of the four professional categories (environmental engineers, environmental scientists and specialists, health and safety engineers, and occupational health and safety specialists) grew significantly over the past decade. The technical categories (environmental engineering technicians, environmental health and safety technicians, and occupational health and safety technicians) also grew but not nearly as rapidly as the professional occupational categories. Job growth was somewhat less for government employment than outside government. This trend is expected to continue for at least the next decade.

The total number of positions for environmental and occupational health workers is expected to grow to 334,000 by the year 2022 with about one fourth employed by government agencies. Based on the growth in the number of positions and the need to fill other positions because of job changes and retirement, nearly 125,000 positions will be filled between 2012 and 2022. Environmental scientists and

specialists and occupational health and safety specialists represent the largest categories of positions to be filled.

Salaries vary considerably across environmental and occupational health categories, depending on whether they are professional or technical titles as well as on educational attainment and previous work experience. Median salaries in 2013 for public sector environmental engineers averaged $81,000, with the middle 50% earning between $63,000 and $97,000 (**Table 9-4**). Average salaries were lower for environmental engineers working in state and local governmental agencies and higher for those in the private sector (architectural and engineering companies and management and technical consulting companies). Entry-level salaries were in the $47,000–$55,000 range.

The median salary for environmental engineering technicians employed by government agencies in 2013 was $51,000, with the middle 50% earning between $41,000 and $63,000. Entry-level salaries were in the $30,000–$35,000 range.

The median salary for environmental health scientists and specialists employed by government agencies in 2013 was $63,000, with the middle 50% earning between $48,000 and $80,000. Average salaries were lower for environmental health scientists and specialists working in governmental agencies and higher for those working in the private sector. Entry-level salaries were in the $40,000–$45,000 range.

TABLE 9-3   Number of Workers in 2013 and Projected for 2022 for All Industries and Government and Number of Positions to Be Filled 2012–2022 for All Industries

Occupational Category	Workers in All Industries			Workers in Government	
	2013	Projected 2022	2012–2022 Positions To Be Filled	2013	Projected 2022
Environmental Engineers	53,020	61,400	21,100	14,570	14,100
Environmental Engineering Technicians	18,020	22,500	7,400	3,160	3,600
Environmental Scientists and Specialists (including Health)	87,380	103,200	39,700	37,750	38,700
Environmental Science and Protection Technicians (including Health)	34,510	38,900	19,000	8,810	9,800
Health and Safety Engineers (except Mining Safety Engineers and Inspectors)	23,850	26,700	9,700	3,000	2,900
Occupational Health and Safety Specialists	62,830	67,100	21,300	18,840	19,600
Occupational Health and Safety Technicians	13,660	13,900	4,800	2,660	2,700

Data from Bureau of Labor Statistics, U.S. Department of Labor. Selected Occupational Projections Data. Available at www.bls.gov/data/. Accessed June 15, 2014.

TABLE 9-4 Number and Salary Profile for Federal and State/Local Workers for Selected Occupations, 2013

Occupational Category	2013 Government Workers			
	Federal Workers	State / Local Workers	Median Annual Salary	25th–75th Percentile Salary Range
Environmental Engineers	3,420	11,150	$80,720	$63,020–$96,320
Environmental Engineering Technicians	20	3,140	$50,690	$40,970–$62,450
Environmental Scientists and Specialists (including Health)	5,580	31,970	$62,100	$48,170–$79,500
Environmental Science and Protection Technicians (including Health)	240	8,580	$43,370	$33,940–$55,810
Health and Safety Engineers (except Mining Safety Engineers and Inspectors)	720	2,280	$87,370	$58,770–$103,290
Occupational Health and Safety Specialists	7,040	11,810	$66,300	$51,610–$79,870
Occupational Health and Safety Technicians	180	2,480	$47,830	$38,860–$56,940

Notes: Federal: excludes postal service; State/Local: excludes hospitals and education

Data from Bureau of Labor Statistics, U.S. Department of Labor. Employment and Wages from Occupational Employment Statistics (OES) Survey. Available at www.bls. gov/data/. Accessed June 15, 2014.

The median salary for environmental engineering technicians employed by government agencies in 2013 was $44,000, with the middle 50% earning between $34,000 and $56,000. Entry-level salaries were in the $28,000–$34,000 range.

The median salary for public sector health and safety engineers in 2013 was $87,000 with the middle 50% earning between $59,000 and $103,000. Entry-level salaries were in the $60,000–$75,000 range.

The median salary for occupational health and safety specialists employed by government agencies in 2013 was $66,000, with the middle 50% earning between $51,000 and $80,000. Average salaries were lower for occupational health and safety specialists working in governmental agencies and were similar to those working in the private sector. Entry-level salaries were in the $40,000–$50,000 range.

The median salary for occupational health and safety technicians employed by government agencies in 2013 was $48,000, with the middle 50% earning between $39,000 and $57,000. Entry-level salaries were in the $30,000–$35,000 range.

Over the next 10 years, the Bureau of Labor Statistics projects that job growth will be greater than average for environmental engineers, environmental health specialists, occupational health and safety specialists, and environmental technicians. There are several reasons for these projections. There is increasing recognition of environmental engineering as a specialty distinct from civil and other engineering

fields of endeavor. In addition, there has been an increasing recognition of the importance of regulatory compliance for industries and businesses in order to protect and maintain the environment and ensure the safety of workers. An increasing emphasis on prevention as an overall strategy to safeguard environmental and human resources also fosters new job opportunities for these occupations. Opportunities in the public sector, however, will be limited in comparison to those in other industries.

Although environmental and occupational health is a broad category, career pathways can be somewhat limited. Specific academic preparation and experience are necessary for environmental engineers. For example, there is little opportunity for a technician in this field to advance to engineer status without completing the academic degrees required for the field. The academic requirements for environmental and occupational health and safety specialists are somewhat less restrictive. It is possible for technicians to advance into some of these professional positions through continuing education and work experience.

Technicians often begin work as trainees in routine positions under the direct supervision of a professional title or a more experienced senior technician. Technicians with previous hands-on experience with equipment used in that field usually require shorter periods of on-the-job training. As they become more experienced and proficient, technicians progress to become more independent in carrying out their duties. Their ability to move beyond technical titles, however, may be limited unless they acquire additional education or secure specific professional certifications.

Most of these occupational categories do provide a reasonable job ladder with several levels of titles for entry-level to midlevel to senior-level positions. Over a span of several decades, these can comprise a satisfactory framework for a career. At higher levels, professional titles can lead to appointments into management and leadership positions. A substantial number of local public health agency directors, for example, come from the ranks of environmental health professionals.

OUTSIDE-THE-BOOK THINKING 9-4

© Alfred Bondarenko/Shutterstock.

In which organizations and geographic regions will the need for environmental and occupational health workers expand most rapidly in the next two decades?

ADDITIONAL INFORMATION

There are many good sources of information on environmental and occupational health as a career. Several sources are available for information on educational programs for environmental and occupational health as well as for continuing education and leadership development for practitioners.

The National Environmental Health Association (NEHA) (www.neha.org) offers several nationally recognized credentials within the environmental health profession. Each credential signifies a level of expertise and competence based on education and experience. Eligibility to sit for these credentialing exams is determined by the NEHA. Certifications and credentials available through NEHA include

- Onsite wastewater system installers: This credential was developed through a cooperative agreement with the EPA. Credentialing and licensing is one of the goals of the EPA Voluntary Management Guidelines and is also recommended by the National Onsite Wastewater Recycling Association Model Code.
- Registered environmental health specialist/registered sanitarian (REHS/RS): The REHS/RS is the premiere NEHA credential. It is available to a wide range of environmental health professionals. Individuals holding the REHS/RS credential show competency in environmental health issues, direct and train personnel to respond to routine or emergency environmental situations, and frequently provide education to their communities on environmental health concerns. The advantages of NEHA's REHS/RS registration program are (1) the nationwide recognition of the REHS/RS credential, (2) the continual update of the REHS/RS examination and study guide based on an ongoing assessment of the environmental health field, and (3) the tracking of an individual's continuing education by NEHA.
- Certified food safety professional (CFSP): NEHA has created a credential especially for food safety professionals. The CFSP is designed for individuals within the public and private sectors whose primary responsibility is the protection and safety of food. The exam for this prestigious credential integrates food microbiology, Hazard Analysis and Critical Control Point principles, and regulatory requirements into questions that test problem-solving skills and knowledge.
- Certified environmental health technician (CEHT): The CEHT is for individuals who are interested in field-intensive environmental health activities (e.g., testing, sampling, and inspections) and who are required to provide information on safe environmental health practices and to eliminate environmental health hazards.
- Registered environmental technician (RET): NEHA's RET is a baseline credential for entry-level hazardous materials professionals. The credential is an excellent way for recent, 2-year graduates (associate degrees) or career-changing professionals to demonstrate competency in the core requirements of hazardous materials handling and management.
- Registered hazardous substances professional (RHSP): The RHSP provides technically qualified professionals with national recognition for proven expertise in hazardous materials and toxic substances management.
- Registered hazardous substances specialist (RHSS): The RHSS credential is for individuals who follow protocols for field-intensive hazardous materials activities (e.g., testing, sampling, and handling) and who ensure personal, public, and site safety.
- BCSP offers the Certified Safety Professional CSP credential.

TABLE 9-5 Environmental Health Competency Expectations for Graduates of MPH Degree Programs

1. Describe the direct and indirect human, ecological, and safety effects of major environmental and occupational agents.
2. Describe genetic, physiologic, and psychomotor factors that affect susceptibility to adverse health outcomes following exposure to environmental hazards.
3. Describe federal and state regulatory programs, guidelines, and authorities that control environmental health issues.
4. Specify current environmental risk assessment methods
5. Specify approaches for assessing, preventing, and controlling environmental hazards that pose risks to human health and safety.
6. Explain the general mechanisms of toxicity in eliciting a toxic response to various environmental exposures.
7. Discuss various risk management and risk communication approaches in relation to issues of environmental justice and equity.
8. Develop a testable model of environmental injury.

Reproduced from the Association of Schools of Public Health (ASPH) MPH Core Competency Development Process, Version 2.3. Washington, DC: ASPH, 2006. Available at http://www.asph.org. Accessed June 15, 2014.

- American Board of Industrial Hygiene offers the Certified Industrial Hygienist (CIH) and Certified Associate Industrial Hygienist (CAIH) credentials.
- Council on Certification of Health, Environmental, and Safety Technologists offers the Occupational Health and Safety Technologist certification, which has requirements that are less stringent than for CSP, CIH, or CAIH credentials. This remains a voluntary credential, although many employers encourage or require certification.

In addition to NEHA, the web site of the American Academy of Environmental Engineers (www.aaees.net) is another useful resource for environmental engineers. The Environmental Health Section of the American Public Health Association's web site (www.apha.org) is another good source of information for environmental health. Schools and graduate programs of public health are among the institutions that offer graduate degrees in environmental and occupational health. The Association of Schools of Public Health (www.aspph.org) has identified a panel of core environmental health competencies appropriate for all students receiving the master's of public health (MPH) degree. These competencies provide a useful baseline for professional practice and summarize what an MPH graduate should be able to do (**Table 9-5**).

CONCLUSION

Careers in environmental and occupational health cover a wide range of duties and roles at a variety of levels. Career development opportunities in this area of public health practice are plentiful. A mix of education and experience prepares environmental health workers for increasing responsibility in public-sector agencies as well as the private sector. The field already well down the path toward competency-based credentials and certifications. Ongoing education and training are especially relevant concerns for this occupational category. Demand for these positions is steady, and prospects will likely increase over the next few decades, except within the public sector.

REFERENCES

1. Bureau of Labor Statistics, U.S. Department of Labor. Databases and tables. www.bls.gov/data/. Accessed June 15, 2014.
2. Health Resources and Services Administration (HRSA), Bureau of Health Professions, National Center for Health Workforce Information and Analysis and Center for Health Policy, Columbia School of Nursing. *Public Health Workforce Enumeration 2000*. Washington, DC: HRSA; 2000.
3. National Association of County and City Health Officials. *2013 National Profile of Local Health Departments*. Washington, DC: NACCHO; 2014.
4. Association of State and Territorial Health Officials. *Profile of State Health, Volume Three, 2012*. Washington, DC: ASTHO; 2014.

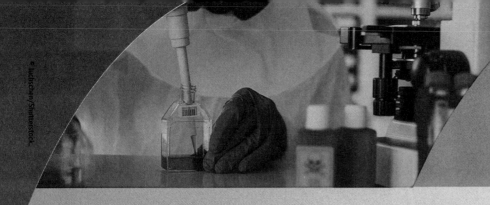

CHAPTER **10**

Public Health Nursing

LEARNING OBJECTIVES

Given the need for nurses in the public health system, describe key features of occupations and careers in public health nursing and how these contribute to carrying out public health's core functions and essential services. Key aspects of this competency expectation include being able to

- Describe several different occupational titles in this category
- Identify specific essential public health services that are critical for positions in this category
- Describe important and essential duties for several job titles in this category
- Identify minimum qualifications and describe general workplace considerations, salary expectations, and career prospects for positions in this category

The title public health nurse designates a nursing professional with educational preparation in public health and nursing science with a primary focus on population-level outcomes. The primary aim of public health nursing is to promote health and prevent disease for entire population groups. This may include assisting and providing care to individual members of the population. It also includes the identification of individuals who may not request care but who have health problems that put themselves and others in the community at risk, such as those with infectious diseases.

The focus of public health nursing is not on providing direct care to individuals in community settings. Public health nurses support the provision of direct care through a process of evaluation and assessment of the needs of individuals in the context of their population group. Public health nurses work with other providers of care to plan, develop, and support systems and programs in the community to prevent problems and provide access to care.

As defined by the Public Health Nursing section of the American Public Health Association (APHA), public health nursing is the practice of promoting and protecting the health of populations using knowledge from nursing, social, and public health sciences. Public health nursing practice is a systematic process by which

- The health and healthcare needs of a population are assessed in order to identify subpopulations, families, and individuals who would benefit from health promotion or who are at risk of illness, injury, disability, or premature death.
- A plan for intervention is developed with the community to meet identified needs that takes into account available resources, the range of activities that contribute to health, and the prevention of illness, injury, disability, and premature death.
- The plan is implemented effectively, efficiently, and equitably.
- Evaluations are conducted to determine the extent to which the interventions have an impact on the health status of individuals and the population.
- The results of the process are used to influence and direct the delivery of care, deployment of health resources, and the development of local, regional, state, and national health policy and research to promote health and prevent disease.

Table 10-1 illustrates an average day in the life of a public health nurse.

TABLE 10-1   A Typical Day for a Public Health Nurse

7:30 a.m.	Breakfast meeting with visiting nursing agency to discuss interagency coordination
8:30 a.m.	Consult with clinic staff on issues requiring follow-up, such as missed appointments
9:00 a.m.	Visit home of family missing recent appointments
10:15 a.m.	Back in office for meeting to update director of nursing
10:45 a.m.	Meeting with communicable disease control and epidemiology staff regarding community concerns over West Nile Virus threat
11:45 a.m.	Informal lunch meeting with community college faculty and students to promote interest in public health nursing careers
1:00 p.m.	Back in office to discuss referrals from clinic and communicable disease staff
1:30 p.m.	Visit patient receiving directly supervised therapy for tuberculosis; identify need for job training assistance and assist with referral
3:00 p.m.	Back in office, assist clinic staff with back-to-school physicals and immunizations
4:30 p.m.	Time to complete paperwork and follow-up phone calls for today's activities
5:15 p.m.	Review and plan tomorrow's schedule
7:00 p.m.	Attend community meeting regarding West Nile Virus concerns to assist epidemiology and environmental health staff

OCCUPATIONAL CLASSIFICATION

There is no standard occupational category specific to public health nurses. There is a more generic standard occupational category registered nurse that encompasses professional nursing positions in any healthcare or health services organization. This standard occupational category is one of the administrative occupations within the white collar grouping of occupations.

Public health nurses plan, develop, implement, and evaluate nursing and public health interventions for individuals, families, and populations at risk of illness or disability. This category covers all positions identified at the registered nurse (RN) level, unless specified as performing work defined under some other professional occupational category (such as epidemiologist or occupational health and safety specialist) and includes graduates of diploma and associate degree programs with the RN license. Common job titles for public health nurses include community health nurse, nurse consultant, school nurse, public health nurse, occupational health nurse, home health nurse, and RN case manager. Public health nurses holding administrative positions have titles such as supervising nurse, nursing coordinator, program director, and director of nursing. Public health nurses who provide clinical services often function with titles such as staff nurse, nurse clinician, or nurse practitioner. Licensed practical (or vocational) nurses (LPNs/LVNs) and nursing assistants are considered as technical rather than professional workers in this classification.

OUTSIDE-THE-BOOK THINKING 10-1

© Alfred Bondarenko/Shutterstock.

What will be the most important new or expanded roles for public health nursing in the 21st century?

There were 2.7 million RNs and 705,000 LPNs/LVNs employed in the United States in 2013. Only 13% of RNs (300,000) work in community or public health settings. Bureau of Labor Statistics (BLS) data indicated that in 2013, 193,000 nurses (145,000 RNs and 48,000 LPNs) worked for federal, state, and local governmental agencies.[1] *Public*

Health Workforce Enumeration 2000 data identified 64,000 public health nurses and an estimated 15,000–20,000 LPNs/LVNs working for governmental public health organizations, with another 8,000 RNs working for voluntary-sector agencies in the year 2000.[2] Surveys in 2012 and 2013 identified nearly 40,000 RNs and more than 3,000 LPNs/LVNs working in state and local public health agencies.[3,4] Data from these various sources are used throughout this chapter.

PUBLIC HEALTH PRACTICE PROFILE

Nurses have long been the professional core of the public health workforce. Nurses provide both clinical and community health services in a wide variety of public and private organizations. Services are provided within maternal and child health programs, communicable disease prevention and control, immunization, and school health programs, to name just a few. Many nurses trained in public health take on supervisory and management roles and serve as chief administrator or as part of the senior management team for many local public health agencies. Nurses also serve as program coordinators and consultants for state and federal health agencies. Their broad expertise and professional credibility assists in advocacy and coalition-building activities and in the evaluation of programs within the community. Public health nurses are also active in community health planning and community health improvement initiatives across the United States. Nurses are directly involved in a wide variety of health promotion and disease and injury prevention efforts. Their skills are critical to achieving community health objectives and broader public health goals through performing one or more of the essential public health services. As a result, public health nurses are involved in a wider array of public health purposes and essential public health services than most other public health occupational categories. It is somewhat misleading to highlight only a few public health purposes and essential public health services that are most closely associated with public health nursing. Virtually all fit within the scope of their professional expertise. For the sake of consistency with other public health occupations and titles addressed in this book, three public health purposes and five essential public health services are identified for public health nurses in **Table 10-2**.

TABLE 10-2   Public Health Practice Profile for Public Health Nurses

Public Health Nurses Make a Difference by:
Public Health Purposes
✓ Preventing epidemics and the spread of disease
Protecting against environmental hazards
Preventing injuries
✓ Promoting and encouraging healthy behaviors
Responding to disasters and assisting communities in recovery
✓ Ensuring the quality and accessibility of health services
Essential Public Health Services
✓ Monitoring health status to identify community health problem
Diagnosing and investigating health problems and health hazards in the community
✓ Informing, educating, and empowering people about health issues
Mobilizing community partnerships to identify and solve health problems
Developing policies and plans that support individual and community health efforts
Enforcing laws and regulations that protect health and ensure safety
✓ Linking people with needed personal health services and ensuring the provision of health care when otherwise unavailable
Ensuring a competent public health and personal healthcare workforce
✓ Evaluating effectiveness, accessibility, and quality of personal and population-based health services
✓ Researching new insights and innovative solutions to health problems

IMPORTANT AND ESSENTIAL DUTIES

Nursing positions within public health organizations have many different titles. In some organizations, all RNs are covered by one series usually termed public health nurse. In other organizations, RNs performing clinical duties may be distinguished from those performing community and public health nursing duties. Some organizations employ nurse practitioners to provide primary medical care. In addition to RNs, some public health organizations employ LPNs or LVNs to provide supportive nursing services for clinical care programs. The focus in this chapter will be on three nursing positions: entry-level public health nurse, senior-level public health nurse, and LVN.

> ## OUTSIDE-THE-BOOK THINKING 10-2
>
> © Alfred Bondarenko/Shutterstock.
>
> What are the most important contributions to improving the health of the public that public health nurses make today?

Public Health Nurse (Entry Level)

Under direction, entry-level public health nurses provide public health nursing services, including health education, the promotion of health awareness, and the prevention and control of diseases. This is the entry and first working level in the public health nurse class series. Incumbents must have requisite public health nursing certification but have limited public health nursing work experience. As experience is gained, incumbents learn to perform the full scope of public health nursing duties. Entry-level public health nurses are distinguished from midlevel public health nurses who independently perform a larger scope of public health nursing duties and activities. Midlevel public health nurses perform a larger range of duties and activities on a more independent basis and are distinguished from senior public health nurses in that senior public health nurses perform more complex, specialized assignments, as well as provide lead direction, work coordination, and training for other professional nursing and support staff. Entry-level and midlevel public health nurses generally report to a senior public health nurse or the director of nursing services. Entry-level positions do not supervise other staff.

Important and essential duties for entry-level public health nursing positions may include

- Participate in planning, organizing, and providing public health nursing services, health instruction, counseling, and guidance for individuals, families, and groups regarding disease control, health awareness, health maintenance, and rehabilitation in a clinic setting
- Identify and interact with local care providers in the coordination of health care
- Provide referrals to other community-based health and social services
- Teach and demonstrate health practices to individuals and groups
- Instruct clients in immunization procedures, family planning, and sexually transmitted disease prevention and follow-up
- Identify individual and family problems that are detrimental to good health
- Make home visits to assess a patient's progress and intervene accordingly
- Work with families to alleviate health problems and promote good health habits
- Refer and coordinate the care of individuals and families with other public and private agencies
- Identify special health needs for assigned cases, recommending and implementing services to meet those needs
- Assist individuals and families with implementing physician recommendations
- Participate in planning, directing, and performing epidemiologic investigations in homes, schools, workplaces, the community, and public health clinics
- Prepare appropriate records and case documentation, arranging follow-up services based on findings
- Confer with physicians, nursing staff, and other staff regarding public health programs, patient reports, evaluations, medical tests, and related items
- Participate in multidisciplinary teams for the purpose of creating a plan of service for at-risk families
- Participate and collaborate with community groups to identify public health needs, develop needed public health services, and improve existing public health services
- Prepare reports and maintain records
- Compile statistical information for appraisal and planning purposes

Public Health Nurse (Senior Level)

Under direction, senior public health nurses provide lead direction and work coordination for other professional nursing and support staff. Senior public health nurses plan and conduct a variety of public health nursing clinics and services and provide complex, specialized, and general nursing, health education, and health consulting services, including the prevention and control of diseases and the promotion of health awareness. This is the advanced level and lead class in the public health nurse series. Incumbents provide the more complex public health nursing services in a specialized public health program, as well as provide lead direction and coordination for other professional nursing staff. This class is distinguished from the midlevel public health nurse by assignment of a higher level of public health program responsibilities and the performance of lead responsibilities for other professional nursing staff. Senior public health nurses report to the director of nursing services and, in turn, provide lead direction and work coordination for entry-level and midlevel public health nurses.

Important and essential duties for senior-level public health nurses may include

- Investigate outbreaks of communicable diseases
- Plan and implement programs for the prevention and control of communicable disease, including tuberculosis, sexually transmitted diseases, and acquired immune deficiency syndrome
- Develop procedures to control the spread of communicable diseases and identify people needing public health services
- Provide interpretations of public health laws and regulations for others
- Assess individuals and families, using health histories, observations of physical condition, and a variety of evaluative methods to identify health problems, health deficiencies, and health service needs
- Identify psychosocial, cultural background, and environmental factors that may hinder the use of or access to healthcare services
- Assist with determining funding needs for specific programs, and monitor budget expenditures within those programs
- Plan and coordinate services for special programs such as family planning, or perinatal, maternal, child, or adolescent programs
- Perform public health nursing activities to promote perinatal, child, and adolescent health
- Provide local case management and coordination within specific programs
- Participate in programs to enhance schoolchildren's health
- Work with community groups to identify needs, develop and facilitate a variety of health services, and improve existing programs
- Refer individuals and families to appropriate agencies and clinics for health services
- Participate in programs to enhance community health services and education
- Attend conferences and workshops related to community health issues
- Assist with the preparation of program and service policies and procedures
- Supervise paraprofessional staff and volunteers
- Prepare reports and maintain records
- Compile and analyze statistical information for appraisal and planning purposes
- Provide lead direction, training, and work coordination for other professional nurses

Licensed Vocational/Practical Nurse

Under general supervision, LPNs/LVNs perform a variety of health-related activities in the provision of basic nursing care, including administering immunizations and vaccinations, hearing and vision screening, basic skin and blood tests, and blood pressure monitoring. LPN/LVNs assist with a variety of activities related to implementation of various agency health programs. Workers in this title do not have the necessary education, experience, or license requirements to qualify as either an RN or a public health nurse. Workers perform a variety of clinical and basic nursing duties consistent with their license and experience. LPN/LVNs report to a midlevel or senior-level public health nurse or to the director of nursing. These positions do not carry supervisory responsibility.

Important and essential duties for LPN/LVN positions may include:

- Perform, read, and evaluate skin, hearing, vision, and blood tests
- Perform and evaluate blood pressure readings
- Provide health education sessions
- Administer immunizations and vaccinations
- Participate in healthcare clinics, coordinating activities as assigned
- Maintain a current inventory of clinic supplies
- Operate a mobile health van

- Evaluate medical records and determine the need for immunization or vaccination
- Prepare patients for physical examinations
- Weigh and measure patients
- Assist with examinations
- Refer clients to other healthcare providers
- Prepare specimens for mailing
- Provide basic health information and instruction to individuals and families
- Answer health-related questions from the public
- Sterilize equipment
- Maintain safety requirements in a clinical setting
- Triage requests for information

MINIMUM QUALIFICATIONS

Nurses working in public health come from a wide variety of backgrounds and academic preparation. The number of RNs produced by 4-year baccalaureate programs is steadily increasing, but there are many RNs from diploma programs in the public health workforce as well. Many nursing schools offer master's-level preparation in community health nursing, school health, and other public health specializations. As described later in this chapter, there is a highly respected, competency-based credential that is offered for community health nurses. Nonetheless, many of those working as nurses in public health settings, including those holding public health nursing titles, do not qualify for this credential due to not having attained the necessary academic credentials.

Typical Minimum Qualifications for Entry-Level Public Health Nurse

Knowledge, Skills, and Abilities

The typical entry-level public health nurse generally has knowledge of:

- Principles, methods, practices, and current trends of general and public health nursing and preventive medicine
- Community aspects of public nursing including community resources and demography
- Federal, state, and local laws and regulations governing communicable disease, public health, and disabling conditions
- Environmental, sociological, and psychological problems related to public health nursing programs
- Child growth and development
- Causes, means of transmission, and methods of control of communicable disease

- Methods of promoting child and maternal health and public health programs
- Principles of health education

A typical entry-level public health nurse has the skills and ability to:

- Learn to organize and carry out public health nursing activities in an assigned program
- Collect, analyze, and interpret technical, statistical, and health data
- Analyze and evaluate health problems of individuals and families, and take appropriate action
- Provide instruction in the prevention of diseases
- Develop and maintain health records, and prepare clear and concise reports
- Communicate effectively orally and in writing
- Interact tactfully and courteously with the public, community organizations, and other staff when explaining public health issues and providing public health services
- Establish and maintain cooperative working relationships
- Effectively represent the agency and nursing division in contacts with public, other staff, and other governmental agencies

Experience and Education

Any combination of training and experience that provides the required knowledge and abilities will qualify an individual for this position. A typical way to obtain the required knowledge and abilities is to complete a bachelor degree and have adequate work experience to meet existing state certification requirements. These often call for 1 year of previous public health nursing experience comparable to an entry-level public health nurse with the hiring organization. Special requirements include possession of a valid state license as an RN. A state-issued certificate as a public health nurse and possession of a valid state driver's license may also be required by some agencies.

Typical Minimum Qualifications for Senior-Level Public Health Nurse

Knowledge, Skills, and Abilities

In addition to those required for entry-level public health nurses, senior-level public health nurses generally have knowledge of:

- Unique psychosocial and cultural issues encountered in a rural health program

- Principles of health education
- Program planning, evaluations, and development principles
- Principles of lead direction, program and work coordination, and training
- Community health assessment principles, strategies, and tools

A senior-level public health nurse generally has the skills and ability to:

- Plan, organize, and carry out public health nursing activities and services for an assigned service area or program
- Develop and maintain effective working relationships with clients, staff, community groups, and other government organizations
- Collect, analyze, and interpret technical, statistical, and health data
- Analyze and evaluate health problems of individuals and families, and take appropriate action
- Provide work direction and coordination for other staff
- Provide instruction in the prevention and control of diseases
- Communicate effectively in writing and orally
- Develop and maintain health records and prepare clear and concise reports

Experience and Education

Any combination of training and experience that provides the required knowledge and abilities will qualify an individual for this position. A typical way to obtain the required knowledge and abilities is to complete sufficient education and experience to meet state certification requirements. This may require 1 year of public health nursing experience comparable to a midlevel public health nurse. In addition, special requirements may include possession of a valid state license as an RN, state certification as a public health nurse, and a valid state driver's license.

Typical Minimum Qualifications for Licensed Practical/Vocational Nurses

Knowledge, Skills, and Abilities

An LPN/LVN generally has knowledge of:

- Principles, methods, and procedures of general nursing
- Causes, means of transmission, and methods of controlling communicable diseases

- Basic medical terminology
- Principles and procedures of medical record keeping
- Health problems and requirements of infants, children, adolescents, and the elderly
- State laws relating to reporting child abuse and neglect

An LPN/LVN generally has the skills and ability to:

- Operate a variety of standard medical testing equipment
- Communicate effectively in writing and orally
- Follow oral and written instructions
- Provide responsible nursing care and services
- Maintain confidentiality of material
- Interview patients and families to gather medical history
- Perform skin tests and interpret results
- Prepare medical forms and records
- Work responsibly with physicians and other members of the healthcare team
- Effectively represent the agency in contacts with the public, community organizations, and other government agencies
- Establish and maintain cooperative working relationships with patients and others

Experience and Education

Any combination of training and experience that provides the required knowledge and abilities will qualify an individual for this position. A typical way to obtain the required knowledge and abilities is through 1 year of vocational nursing experience and completion of nursing studies and curriculum sufficient to obtain requisite state licenses. In addition, special requirements may include possession of a valid state license as an LVN and a valid state driver's license.

WORKPLACE CONSIDERATIONS

Public health nurses have long been one of the most important, and most numerous, categories within the professional public health workforce. Public health nurses are especially prominent in local public health agencies, where they are involved in a wide range of disease prevention, health promotion, and health service programs. They are also found in state and federal health agencies, although not as frequently today as in past decades. Public health nurses play key roles in maternal and child health services, Women, Infants, and

Children programs, immunization and communicable disease control programs, and in the clinical operations of local public health agencies. Their professional background also makes them effective links with other community health organizations and agencies, especially local hospitals and schools. Public health nurses need to know medical terminology and how to perform various medical screening tests and basic nursing procedures.

Work is performed in clinics and healthcare offices, at work sites, and in home environments with occasional exposure to communicable diseases and blood borne pathogens as well as saliva, urine, and feces. Nurses are expected to understand and follow recommended practices and precautions for prevention of disease transmission. Ongoing contact with other staff and the public is part of the daily routine for public health nurses. Public health nurses may need to travel to various locations within the community, including to remote or unsafe areas in all weather conditions in order to perform their duties. Personal safety is enhanced through safety training, use of cell phones and identification badges, and not traveling alone to neighborhoods with high crime rates.

Typical physical requirements for nurses at all levels include the ability to sit and stand for extended periods, normal manual dexterity and eye-hand coordination, the ability to lift and move objects weighing up to 50 pounds, hearing and vision corrected to normal range, verbal communication skills, and the ability to properly use medical and office equipment, including computer, telephone, calculator, copiers, and fax machines.

OUTSIDE-THE-BOOK THINKING 10-3

© Alfred Bondarenko/Shutterstock.

What features make public health nursing a career worth pursuing?

POSITIONS, SALARIES, AND CAREER PROSPECTS

In 2013, there were 2,662,000 RNs employed in the United States, with 145,000 working for federal, state, and local governmental agencies. In addition, there were 705,000 employed LPNs/LVNs, of whom 48,000 worked in government agencies. **Table 10-3** identifies the number of total workers and the number employed by government for the standard occupational categories considered in this chapter. Projections for the year 2022 are also provided. The numbers of both RNs and LPNs/LVNs has been increasing in recent years, a trend that is expected to continue well into the future. For these two nursing categories, job growth has been somewhat less for government employment than outside government.

The overall number of positions for RNs is expected to grow to 3,200,000 by the year 2022, but with no increase in the number employed by government agencies. LPN/LVN positions are projected to increase to 921,000 during

TABLE 10-3 Number of Workers in 2013 and Projected for 2022 for All Industries and Government and Number of Positions to Be Filled 2012–2022 for All Industries

Occupational Category	Workers in All Industries			Workers in Government	
	2013	Projected 2022	2012–2022 Positions To Be Filled	2013	Projected 2022
Registered Nurses	2,661,890	3,238,400	1,052,600	145,110	148,700
Licensed Vocational and Licensed Practical Nurses	705,200	921,300	363,100	47,800	49,900
Nursing Assistants	1,427,880	1,792,000	593,600	60,460	63,900
Home Health Aides	806,710	1,299,300	590,700	14,890	16,500
Nurse Practitioners	113,370	147,300	58,500	2,850	3,100

Data from Bureau of Labor Statistics, U.S. Department of Labor. Selected Occupational Projections Data. Available at www.bls.gov/data/. Accessed June 15, 2014.

TABLE 10-4 Number and Salary Profile for Federal and State/Local Workers for Selected Occupations, 2013

Occupational Category	2013 Government Workers			
	Federal Workers	State / Local Workers	Median Annual Salary	25th–75th Percentile Salary Range
Registered Nurses	69,810	75,350	$69,010	$56,500–$84,170
Licensed Vocational and Licensed Practical Nurses	17,480	30,310	$42,750	$36,730–$48,200
Nursing Assistants	12,740	47,720	$30,708	$24,460–$35,770
Home Health Aides	–	14,890	$22,570	$17,970–$31,550
Nurse Practitioners	10	2,840	$83,610	$72,780–$98,030

Notes: Federal: excludes postal service; State/Local: excludes hospitals and education

Data from Bureau of Labor Statistics, U.S. Department of Labor. Employment and Wages from Occupational Employment Statistics (OES) Survey. Available at www.bls.gov/data/. Accessed June 15, 2014.

that period with only a modest increase (to 50,000) for the number employed by government agencies. Based on the growth in the number of positions and the need to fill other positions because of job changes and retirement, more than 1 million RN positions and 363,000 LPN/LVN positions will be filled between 2012 and 2022. Only a small percentage of these positions will be filled in the government sector. Public health nurses often move up into unit and agency leadership positions and higher salaries. It is not uncommon for the director of a small- or medium-sized public health agency to be an experienced public health nurse. Nonetheless, the ever expanding nongovernmental health sector of the U.S. economy will offer the vast majority of RN positions over the next decade. Job growth for RNs in the government sector will lag behind the growth rate for RN positions in the overall economy.

Salaries differ considerably between the RN and LPN/LVN categories and even within the RN category itself, based on academic degrees, credentialing, experience, and the market conditions related to the shortage of nurses in any given area. The median salary for RNs employed by government agencies in 2013 was $69,000, with the middle 50% earning between $56,000 and $84,000 (**Table 10-4**). Average salaries for RNs working in governmental agencies were similar to those for nurses working in the private and voluntary sectors. Entry-level salaries were in the $44,000–$52,000 range.

The median salary for LPNs/LVNs employed by government agencies in 2013 was $43,000, with the middle 50% earning between $36,000 and $48,000. Entry-level salaries were in the $30,000–$34,000 range.

Nurses remain in short supply throughout the health sector, making the recruitment and retention of public health nurses a continuing issue for potential employers, both public and private. Public sector agencies, such as local and state health departments as well as community and national not-for-profit organizations, often are not able to match salary and benefit levels available through private employers (such as hospitals, clinics, and health plans). Competition with private-sector employers has increased nursing salaries to some extent and in some locations. Public health agencies generally are not able to match the salaries and benefits (including signing bonuses) available within the acute care and primary care sectors.

As the largest professional category employed by public health agencies, and because of the growing shortage of RNs, there are many opportunities for all levels of nurses within the public health workforce. Working hours and conditions for nurses working in public health agencies can be attractive, and many nurses appreciate the importance and impact of working in public health. Still, public health nurses are the number one worker category identified as needed now and in the future for public health agencies. *Public Health Workforce Enumeration 2000* data identified 50,000 public health nurses in 2000, nearly all of whom worked in state and local public health agencies.

The number of undergraduate and graduate students entering nursing training programs has been increasing steadily in recent years. As noted earlier, the demand for public health nurses is also increasing, and even faster than the supply.

OUTSIDE-THE-BOOK THINKING 10-4

© Alfred Bondarenko/Shutterstock.

In which organizations and geographic regions will the need for public health nursing expand most rapidly in the next two decades?

ADDITIONAL INFORMATION

There are many good sources of information on public health nursing. Several sources of information are available on educational programs for these occupations as well as for continuing education and leadership development for public health nurses.

The Public Health Nursing section of the APHA web site (www.apha.org) is a great source of information on public health nursing. The Public Health Nursing section has a long history and currently has many members, making it one of APHA's largest and most active sections.

Schools of public health are among the institutions offering master's and doctoral degrees in public health for nurses. The Association of Schools and Programs of Public Health web site (www.aspph.org) provides information on accredited schools and programs of public health and on the characteristics of public health students and degree concentrations.

State licensing boards (which license RNs), schools of nursing, the American Nurses Association (ANA), and its many state affiliates are also rich sources for additional information on public health nurses. The American Nursing Credentialing Center (ANCC) is the credentialing arm of the ANA (http://www.nursecredentialing.org/Certification.aspx) and awards a registered nurse, board certified certification. ANCC certifies community health nurses who meet all the following requirements:

- Active RN license in the United States
- Two full years of public health nursing practice in the United States
- Bachelor or higher degree in nursing
- Two thousand or more hours of clinical practice within the past 3 years (can include nursing administration, education, client care, and research)
- Thirty contact hours of continuing education within the past 3 years

The Quad Council of Public Health Nursing Organizations is an alliance of the four national nursing organizations that address public health nursing issues. Its members are the Association of Community Health Nurse Educators, the ANA's Congress on Nursing Practice and Economics, the APHA's Public Health Nursing Section, and the Association of State and Territorial Directors of Nursing. The Quad Council was founded in the early 1980s to address priorities for public health nursing education, practice, leadership, and research, and to serve as a unified voice for public health nursing. Public health nursing competencies are an ongoing priority for the Quad Council.

The current Quad Council public health nursing competency framework is designed to be consistent with other competency principles and frameworks of its partner organizations. The framework complements the definition of Public Health Nursing adopted by the APHA's Public Health Nursing Section, the ANA's Scope and Standards of Public Health Nursing Practice, and the Public Health Practitioner Competencies established by the Council on Linkages between Academia and Public Health Practice.[5-7]

Practice competencies for public health nurses were revised by the Quad Council in 2011, in part to promote consistency with the domains and three tiers of public health practitioner competencies established by the Council on Linkages between Academia and Public Health Practice. Eight competency domains address:

- Analytic and assessment skills
- Policy development and program planning skills
- Communication skills
- Cultural competency skills
- Community dimensions of practice skills
- Public health science skills
- Financial planning and management skills
- Leadership and systems thinking skills[7,8]

Similar to the approach taken by the Council on Linkages between Academic and Public Health Practice, the Quad Council also established three tiers of competencies for public health nurses.

- Tier 1 Core Competencies apply to generalist public health nurses who carry out day-to-day functions in state and local public health organizations, including clinical, home visiting and population-based services, and who are not in management positions. Responsibilities of the PHN may include working directly with at-risk populations, carrying out health promotion programs at all levels of prevention, basic data collection and analysis, field work, program planning, outreach activities, programmatic support, and other organizational tasks. Although the Council on Linkages competencies and the Quad Council competencies are primarily focused at the population level, public health nurses must often apply these skills and competencies in the care of individuals, families, or groups. Therefore, Tier 1 competencies reflect this practice.

- Tier 2 Core Competencies apply to PHNs with an array of program implementation, management and/or supervisory responsibilities, including responsibility for clinical services, home visiting, community-based and population-focused programs. For example, responsibilities may include implementation and oversight of personal, clinical, family focused, and population-based health services; program and budget development; establishing and managing community relations; establishing timelines and work plans, and presenting recommendations on policy issues.
- Tier 3 Core Competencies apply to PHNs at an executive/senior, management level and leadership levels in public health organizations. In general, these competencies apply to PHNs who are responsible for oversight and administration of programs or operation of an organization, including setting the vision and strategy for an organization and its key structural units, e.g., a public health nursing division. Tier 3 professionals generally are placed at a higher level of positional authority within the agency/organization, and they bring similar or higher level knowledge, advanced education and experience than their Tier 2 counterparts.[5,8]

In developing their competencies, the Quad Council determined that the generalist level would reflect preparation at the bachelor level. Although recognizing that in many states much of the public health nursing workforce does not have a bachelor degree, the Quad Council believes that those nurses may require job descriptions that reflect a different level of practice or may require extensive orientation and education to achieve the competencies identified. Further, the specialist-level competencies described in this document reflect preparation at the master's level in community/public health nursing or public health. Again, while recognizing that there may be other public health nurses who are promoted or appointed to managerial or consultant positions that require specialist competencies,

a master's degree prepares public health nurses for the specialist-level competencies identified in this document. At both levels, it is expected that on-the-job training and continuing education for nurses hired for these positions who have less than a bachelor or master's degree (as appropriate to the level) will ensure that these competencies are attained.

The Quad Council based its competency framework on several relevant assumptions. Public health nurses must first possess the competencies common to all nurses with bachelor degrees and then demonstrate additional competencies specific to their roles in public health. The progression from awareness to knowledge to proficiency is a continuum, and there are no discrete boundaries between those levels of competence. Both levels reflect competencies for a reasonably prudent public health nurse who has experience in the role (i.e., not a novice and not in a specialized or limited focus role). Defined competencies are intended to reflect the standard for public health nursing practice, not necessarily what is occurring in practice today. Importantly, in any practice setting, the job descriptions may reflect components from each level, depending on the agency's structure, size, leadership, and services.

CONCLUSION

Public health nurses remain the largest category of health professionals in the public health workforce. They are active in community as well as clinical services and at all levels of public health organizations, including serving as public health managers and administrators. Although there are 2.7 million nurses in the United States, only a small fraction work for governmental public health organizations, and relatively few of those have formal training in public health. The national nursing shortage, particularly acute for nursing positions in hospitals and long-term care facilities, also limits the ability of public health organizations to attract and retain qualified nurses. Recruitment and retention initiatives for public health nurses are now receiving widespread attention within the public health community, a testimony to the continuing importance of public health nurses if public health goals and objectives are to be achieved.

REFERENCES

1. Bureau of Labor Statistics, U.S. Department of Labor. Databases and tables. www.bls.gov/data/. Accessed June 15, 2014.
2. Health Resources and Services Administration (HRSA), Bureau of Health Professions, National Center for Health Workforce Information and Analysis and Center for Health Policy, Columbia School of Nursing. *Public Health Workforce Enumeration 2000*. Washington, DC: HRSA; 2000.

3. National Association of County and City Health Officials. *2013 National Profile of Local Health Departments*. Washington, DC: NAC-CHO; 2014.

4. Association of State and Territorial Health Officials. *Profile of State Health, Volume Three, 2012*. Washington, DC: ASTHO; 2014.

5. Quad Council Competency Workgroup. Competencies for Public Health Nurses, Summer 2011. Available at http://www.resourcenter.net/images/ACHNE/Files/QuadCouncilCompetenciesForPublic-HealthNurses_Summer2011.pdf.. Accessed June 18, 2014.

6. American Nurses Association. Scope and Standards of Public Health Nursing Practice.

7. Council on Linkages between Academia and Public Health Practice. Core Competencies for Public Health Professionals. Available at http://www.phf.org/resourcestools/documents/core_public_health_competencies_iii.pdf. Accessed June 19, 2014.

8. Swider SM, Krothe J, Reyes D and Cravetz M. The Quad Council practice competencies for public health nursing. *Public Health Nursing*, 2013; *30*: 519–536. doi: 10.1111/phn.12090.

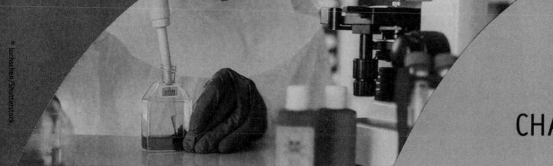
© luchschen/Shutterstock.

CHAPTER **11**

Epidemiology and Disease Control

Epidemiology is often called the mother science of public health practice. Epidemiologists investigate and describe the determinants and distribution of disease, disability, and other health outcomes and help develop the means for their prevention and control. Epidemiology works hand in hand with biostatistics and field investigations to provide information and insights into factors that contribute to health and disease in a population. John Snow's methods of examining cholera outbreaks in 1854 demonstrated the usefulness of epidemiologic methods even when little was known about the microorganism causing these outbreaks. Epidemiology and biostatistics are essential tools for research and evaluation into causative factors as well as into the effectiveness of clinical and community interventions.

Recent concerns over bioterrorism threats and events have raised awareness of the important role played by epidemiologists and related occupations. One of the major objectives of increased funding for bioterrorism preparedness and response is to rapidly increase the number of epidemiologists working in state and local public health agencies. **Table 11-1** provides a snapshot of an average day in the life of an epidemiologist.

OCCUPATIONAL CLASSIFICATION

Two standard occupational categories used for public health workers (epidemiologist and statistician) are addressed in this chapter. Epidemiologist is a standard occupational category that is commonly found in public health organizations. Biostatisticians are a subset of statisticians. Both categories are professional white-collar categories. Another important and related occupational category, disease investigators, is not included among the standard occupational titles but will also be described in this chapter, because their work complements that of epidemiologists and biostatisticians.

- The role of epidemiologist encompasses positions that investigate, describe, and analyze the distribution and determinants of disease, disability, and other health outcomes, and develop the means for their prevention and control. Epidemiologists also describe and analyze the efficacy of programs and interventions. This category includes individuals specifically trained as epidemiologists as well as those trained in another discipline (such as medicine, nursing, or environmental health) working as epidemiologists under such job titles as nurse epidemiologist. Bureau of Labor Statistics (BLS) data indicate that in 2013 there

TABLE 11-1   A Typical Day for an Epidemiologist

7:30 a.m.	Phone discussion from home with state epidemiologist regarding current status of West Nile Virus and follow-up on last week's foodborne illness outbreak involving local fast-food establishment
8:30 a.m.	Meeting with public health student completing internship project analyzing childhood asthma morbidity
9:00 a.m.	Staff meeting to review priorities for week
10:15 a.m.	Meet with agency director, health education, and planning staff regarding completion of community health assessment
10:45 a.m.	Meet with communicable disease control and public health nursing staff regarding community concerns over West Nile Virus threat
11:45 a.m.	Interview candidates for vacant entry-level epidemiologist position
12:15 p.m.	Lunch at desk while catching up with e-mail and phone messages
1:00 p.m.	Grand Rounds presentation at community hospital on nosocomial infections
2:30 p.m.	Office time to respond to e-mail and phone messages
3:00 p.m.	Conference call with epidemiologists and environmental health staff of neighboring jurisdictions and state health department regarding current status of West Nile Virus
4:00 p.m.	Review information suggested by staff for tonight's community meeting on West Nile Virus
4:30 p.m.	Brief agency director on West Nile Virus
5:15 p.m.	Complete final report on last week's foodborne illness outbreak involving local fast-food establishment
7:00 p.m.	Represent agency at community meeting regarding West Nile Virus concerns

were 5,300 epidemiologists in the United States, with state and local governments employing 2,800 of these workers.[1] The *Public Health Workforce Enumeration 2000* study identified 1,400 epidemiologists working in federal, state, and local governmental public health agencies in 2000.[2] The combined results of surveys conducted in 2012 and 2013 identified nearly 4,500 epidemiologists working in state and local public health agencies.[3,4] These findings likely reflect a combination of disease investigators and actual epidemiologists. Data from these various sources are used throughout this chapter. Hospitals, scientific research and development companies, and educational institutions are also important sources of employment for epidemiologists. A 2004 survey conducted by the Council of State and Territorial Epidemiologists (CSTE) identified 2,600 epidemiologists working in state and local public health agencies, although it is likely that this number also included some disease investigator positions.[5]

- The role of infection control/disease investigator includes positions that assist in identifying and locating individuals or groups at risk of specified

health problems and incorporating those people into appropriate health promotion and disease prevention programs. This category includes public health investigators or sexually transmitted infection investigators without reference to educational preparation. Disease investigators may be undercounted if individuals with specific professional preparation (such as nursing, environmental health, or laboratory science) are primarily performing investigations but are employed under another professional title. Because this title is not one of the standard occupational categories tracked by the Bureau of Labor Statistics, it is not clear how many disease investigator positions exist. The *Public Health Workforce Enumeration 2000* report identified 1,200 infection control and disease investigator positions in governmental public health agencies.[2] It is likely that there is some overlap between these positions and those designated as epidemiologists or general program specialists.

- Biostatisticians apply statistical reasoning and methods in addressing, analyzing, and solving problems in public health; health care; and biomedical, clinical, and population-based research. The precise number of biostatisticians is not known. BLS data indicates that there were 25,000 statisticians in the United States in 2013, with 6,400 working for governmental agencies.[1] The federal government alone employed over 4,300 statisticians. The *Public Health Workforce Enumeration 2000* study identified 1,800 biostatisticians in governmental public health agencies in 2000, the majority working for federal and state agencies.[2]

OUTSIDE-THE-BOOK THINKING 11-1

© Alfred Bondarenko/Shutterstock.

What will be the most important new or expanded roles for epidemiologists and biostatisticians in the 21st century?

PUBLIC HEALTH PRACTICE PROFILE

Epidemiologists, biostatisticians, and disease investigators primarily address public health responsibilities for preventing disease and injury and protecting against environmental hazards. These occupational groups may also be involved in emergency preparedness and response and, not infrequently, with assessing the impact and quality of health services within a community.

OUTSIDE-THE-BOOK THINKING 11-2

© Alfred Bondarenko/Shutterstock.

What are the most important contributions to improving the health of the public that epidemiologists and biostatisticians make today?

Among the 10 essential public health services, epidemiologists and related occupations are especially important for four: monitoring health status, diagnosing and investigating health events and threats in the community, assessing the impact and quality of services, and researching innovative solutions to health problems. **Table 11-2** summarizes public health purposes and essential public health services at the

TABLE 11-2   Public Health Practice Profile for Epidemiology and Disease Control

Epidemiology and Disease Control Professionals Make a Difference by:
Public Health Purposes
✓ Preventing epidemics and the spread of disease
✓ Protecting against environmental hazards
✓ Preventing injuries
Promoting and encouraging healthy behaviors
Responding to disasters and assisting communities in recovery
Ensuring the quality and accessibility of health services
Essential Public Health Services
✓ Monitoring health status to identify community health problems
✓ Diagnosing and investigating health problems and health hazards in the community
Informing, educating, and empowering people about health issues
Mobilizing community partnerships to identify and solve health problems
Developing policies and plans that support individual and community health efforts
Enforcing laws and regulations that protect health and ensure safety
Linking people with needed personal health services and ensuring the provision of health care when otherwise unavailable
Ensuring a competent public health and personal healthcare workforce
✓ Evaluating effectiveness, accessibility, and quality of personal and population-based health services
✓ Researching new insights and innovative solutions to health problems

core of positions for epidemiologists and disease control professionals.

IMPORTANT AND ESSENTIAL DUTIES

There are many job titles and positions in the public health workforce that investigate and analyze health problems and risks. The focus in this chapter will be on four positions: communicable disease investigator, entry-level epidemiologist, senior-level epidemiologist, and biostatistician. Each of these positions and a representative panel of their important and essential duties are described in this section.

Communicable Disease Investigator

This position investigates confirmed or suspected cases of communicable diseases to ensure patient treatment and follow-up. Duties are often characterized by the responsibility to implement key aspects of a communicable disease control program. This position performs communicable disease investigative work, bringing to treatment those patients with positive laboratory tests and providing information on sexually transmitted and other communicable diseases. Communicable disease investigator titles may include higher level titles responsible for supervising the work of communicable disease investigators and providing the more difficult and sensitive pretest and posttest counseling to patients and families. Entry-level and midlevel communicable disease investigators exercise no supervision over other workers.

Operational duties related to identifying and obtaining treatment for carriers of communicable diseases include identifying target populations, conducting epidemiologic investigations, testing patients, and making referrals for social or community services. This position administers tuberculin skin tests, obtains laboratory samples, and performs epidemiologic investigations. Many personnel systems have several levels for disease investigators.

Important and essential duties of a communicable disease investigator include

- Interviews clients and contacts; performs risk assessment and counseling; performs disease testing; performs partner counseling and referral service to contacts of infected persons; counsels patients diagnosed as having a communicable disease regarding the disease process (such as the sequence of symptoms), appropriate medications, complications, and prevention so that they will be encouraged to be treated and give names, addresses, and phone numbers of contacts who have been exposed when this is appropriate
- Provides referrals to service providers
- Provides transportation for infected clients and their partners to get appropriate medical care
- Manages cases to closure including successful treatment or failure to comply
- Locates contacts by phone or field visits and informs contacts of infected persons of possible exposure to a sexually transmitted or other communicable disease; maintains confidentiality of information
- Reviews information (such as epidemiologic reports) from other jurisdictions regarding persons exposed to sexually transmitted and other communicable disease; initiates and provides such information for use by other agencies; consults with medical providers regarding a specific client's diagnosis, treatment plan, infection history, and location; consults with laboratory microbiologist regarding complex test results
- Attends meetings and inservice training on identification, testing, and treatment protocols for sexually transmitted and other communicable diseases; may serve as an agency resource or act on behalf of the program coordinator in that person's absence in an assigned program area
- Maintains professional knowledge in applicable areas and keeps abreast of changes in job-related rules, statutes, laws, and new business trends; makes recommendations for the implementation of changes; reads and interprets professional literature; attends training programs, workshops, and seminars as appropriate
- Identifies, contacts, and recruits high-risk patients for participation in communicable disease education and prevention programs
- Provides health education to community organizations, schools, and groups about risky lifestyles and contracting communicable diseases
- Maintains epidemiologic control record of patients, contacts, and suspects
- Maintains a central record file on communicable diseases
- Maintains records of locations where high risk activity occurs
- Participates as member of a multidisciplinary team on disease surveillance and investigations with epidemiologists, biostatisticians, healthcare professionals, environmental health practitioners, health information specialists, and staff of regulated industries (such as restaurants, hospitals, and nursing homes)
- Maintains cooperative relationships with officials of the armed forces, state department of public health, and local police departments

Epidemiologist (Entry Level)

This position performs epidemiologic investigations of human morbidity and mortality; compiles, maintains, and analyzes health data and reports; identifies causative agents resulting in adverse health conditions and proposes corrective actions; and provides public health information and consultative services. This is the entry-level professional epidemiologist performing duties under the direct supervision of a higher level epidemiologist.

Entry-level epidemiologists work in the investigation, analysis, prevention, and control of injuries or communicable, chronic, or environmentally induced diseases. An entry-level epidemiologist is responsible for conducting ongoing epidemiologic studies in order to investigate, identify, and analyze incidence, prevalence, trends, and causes of injuries or communicable, chronic, or environmentally induced diseases. An entry-level epidemiologist is also responsible for assisting with the development of intervention strategies, policies, and procedures and the evaluation of new and existing prevention and control programs based on epidemiologic findings. Work involves communicating with healthcare providers; social service agencies; schools; federal, state, and local officials; the media; and others concerning disease and injury investigation, prevention, and control. This position may supervise subordinate staff, such as communicable disease investigators. Work is subject to general review and direction by a higher level epidemiologist, program administrator, or other designated superior; however, an entry-level epidemiologist works with considerable independence within established policies and procedures.

Important and essential duties of an entry-level epidemiologist include

- Assists in the design of or conducts epidemiologic studies of disease or injury occurrence, including evaluation of behavioral and clinical interventions
- Reviews and evaluates disease or injury reporting and surveillance systems and advises program administrators of important incidence or prevalence changes within reporting areas
- Conducts or assists in investigations of disease clusters using epidemiologic methods, including gathering information and biologic specimens
- Conducts field interviews of case subjects, potential case and control subjects, government officials, and others to ascertain disease incidence and prevalence
- Maintains contact with community physicians, hospital staff, and other healthcare professionals to encourage proper reporting of injuries and communicable, chronic, or environmentally induced diseases and conditions
- Participates as member of a multidisciplinary team on disease surveillance and investigations with disease investigators, biostatisticians, healthcare professionals, environmental health practitioners, health

information specialists, and staff of regulated industries (such as restaurants, hospitals, and nursing homes)

- Communicates with healthcare providers; social service agencies; schools; federal, state, and local officials; the media; and others concerning disease and injury investigation, prevention, and control
- Conducts epidemiologic investigations, surveys, and special studies relating to public health, including assessment of risk behaviors or continuing risk of exposure to specific agents
- Conducts evaluations of control measures related to communicable, chronic, or environmentally induced diseases or injuries
- Prepares investigation reports, statistical analyses, and summaries on completed epidemiologic studies and evaluations
- Participates in preparing grant applications, research reports, and other public health documents

Epidemiologist (Senior Level)

This position coordinates, conducts, analyzes, interprets, and reports the findings from public health surveillance systems and advanced epidemiologic studies that identify the causes of morbidity and mortality; designs and coordinates appropriate preventive health measures based upon investigative results; and determines which specific public health issues require further epidemiologic studies. Medical epidemiologists (such as physicians, veterinarians, dentists, and nurses) provide professional medical consultation in the performance of these duties. This is the highest level position in the series. Incumbents at this level independently propose and direct epidemiologic investigations or act as the principal investigator on local, state, or federal health research grants. Positions at this level may supervise or lead lower-level epidemiologists or other research staff.

Important and essential duties of senior-level epidemiologists include

- Conducts case control, cohort, or cross-sectional studies to identify the incidence, prevalence, or causes of human morbidity or mortality; prepares formal written reports of findings, including a description of the methods used, the findings, and the interpretation of the findings
- Conducts disease outbreak investigations to identify causative agents and environmental conditions resulting in disease outbreaks

- Performs statistical analyses of health data, such as analysis of variance, trend analysis, multiple logistic regression, survival analysis, and so on
- Trains interviewers and clerical staff in project-specific tasks as necessary
- Obtains, as necessary, approval from human subject review boards to conduct investigations or research
- Interacts during the course of investigations with health providers or other persons performing clinical or health research
- Collects surveillance information of reportable human morbidity and mortality as required by state law
- Compiles, maintains, and analyzes health data and reports using statistical methods
- Identifies corrective actions to environmental conditions resulting in adverse health conditions
- Independently proposes and supervises epidemiologic investigations of human morbidity or mortality
- Participates as member of a multidisciplinary team on disease surveillance and investigations with disease investigators, biostatisticians, healthcare professionals, environmental health practitioners, health information specialists, and staff of regulated industries (such as restaurants, hospitals, and nursing homes)
- Collaborates with a broad spectrum of public health constituents and participants including federal, state, and local public health officials, as well as government officials, private individuals, and senior researchers in academic settings
- Communicates health risks to public officials, the media, and the public
- Coordinates local, state, and federal health research programs
- Serves as principal investigator on local, state, and federal health research grants
- Supervises the work of lower level epidemiologists

Biostatistician

This position conducts statistical analyses of morbidity and mortality data, quality assurance, clinical data, surveillance and other data, and serves as a resource for epidemiology and other agency staff.

Important and essential duties of a biostatistician include

- Provides usable reports to epidemiology, program, and clinical staff
- Advises and assists epidemiology staff with research design, statistical design, and statistical analysis of quantitative research projects and databases

- Designs research protocols
- Provides direction on sample size and distribution
- Directs appropriate measures for proper data handling and cleaning
- Analyzes statistical databases, such as birth, death, or disease records, for proper organization and treatment of data
- Suggests revisions based on statistical and research implications
- Writes research design and statistical portions of proposals and papers
- Works closely with epidemiologists to appropriately frame information for reports or papers
- Cultivates sources of population-based data and information available from other public and private agencies
- Participates as member of a multidisciplinary team on disease surveillance and investigations with epidemiologists, disease investigators, healthcare professionals, environmental health practitioners, health information specialists, and staff of regulated industries (such as restaurants, hospitals, and nursing homes)
- Assists with outbreak investigations, when needed; in unusual instances, such as a bioterrorism event or disease outbreak, the biostatistician may need to assist with interviewing victims, analyzing data, arranging sample collection, and so on, as directed by the agency leadership team

MINIMUM QUALIFICATIONS

Epidemiologists come from a variety of professional and experiential backgrounds. Among positions in state health agencies, 10% are physicians, another 16% have some other doctoral degree, 45% have a master's degree, 24% have a bachelor degree, and 5% have less than a bachelor degree.[3]

Epidemiologists and communicable disease investigators work together in investigations of disease patterns and outbreaks. Epidemiologists often have graduate degrees, and some possess other professional credentials. Biostatistics is a specialized field in which master's and doctoral degrees are common. Communicable disease investigators may or may not have education and training equivalent to a bachelor degree. Typical minimum qualifications for communicable disease investigators, entry-level and midlevel epidemiologists, and biostatisticians are detailed below.

Typical Minimum Qualifications for Communicable Disease Investigator

Knowledge, Skills, and Abilities

A typical communicable disease investigator generally has knowledge of:

- Transmission, diagnosis, and treatment of sexually transmitted and other communicable disease
- Symptoms of sexually transmitted and other communicable diseases
- Methods and techniques used to conduct disease investigations
- Methods of infection control
- Laws and legal issues related to the control of communicable diseases
- Diagnostic and therapeutic problems involved in the control of communicable diseases
- Basic medical terminology, clinical practices, and medical procedures
- Principles and practices of customer service
- Available community and social service agencies
- Diverse cultural practices and customs
- Personal computers and related software

A typical communicable disease investigator generally has the skills and ability to:

- Understand, interpret, and apply laws, regulations, policies, and procedures relating to communicable disease reporting
- Interview tactfully and effectively, and work cooperatively with other agencies involved in the control of sexually transmitted and other communicable diseases
- Deal firmly and fairly with clients of various socio-economic backgrounds and temperaments
- Maintain accurate records and document actions
- Make referrals to local and regional providers of social, medical, and other specialized services
- Maintain confidentiality of information; recognize and respect limits of authority and responsibility
- Conduct interviews of a highly personal nature
- Exercise initiative and tact in tracing contacts and bringing them in to seek treatment
- Gain the confidence of many varied personalities
- Communicate and work effectively with coworkers, supervisors, and the general public sufficient to exchange or convey information and to receive work direction
- Communicate effectively both orally and in writing

- Understand program objectives in relation to departmental goals and procedures
- Establish and maintain effective working relationships with officials, the general public, and personnel from other government agencies
- Operate personal computers, including spreadsheet database, word processing, presentation, and other related software

Experience and Education

Any combination of training and experience that provides the required knowledge and abilities will qualify an individual for this position. A typical way to obtain the required knowledge and experience is through 1 year of experience in a clinical or other healthcare setting requiring contact with the general public, and at least an associate degree or trade school diploma, preferably as a medical assistant or a closely related field with college-level course work in psychology, health education, or social work. Another path to these qualifications is through an associate degree in allied health or a related field and 2 years of experience providing emergency medical treatment as an emergency medical technician, medical technician, military corpsman, or related experience; or an equivalent interchange of related education and experience sufficient to successfully perform the essential duties of the job. Still another path is through graduation from an accredited college with a degree in biologic or behavioral sciences or a related field and 1 year of professional experience in public health, hospital services, or a related field. Qualifying experiences may substitute for the required education on a year-for-year basis.

Special requirements often necessary for this position include a valid driver's license, ability to travel independently, bilingual skills, and the ability to work in an environment that may include exposure to communicable diseases. Disease investigators may be required to work outside normal business hours and sign a statement agreeing to comply with state laws and regulations relating to child abuse reporting.

Typical Minimum Qualifications for Entry-Level Epidemiologists

Knowledge, Skills, and Abilities

A typical entry-level epidemiologist generally has knowledge of:

- Modern epidemiologic principles and practices, including the symptoms, causes, means of transmission, and methods of control of communicable and chronic diseases

- Microbiology and pathophysiology
- Basic medical terminology
- Modern research procedures including biostatistical methodology
- Computers and programming in database management and statistical software
- Community organizations and resources related to the field of public health and epidemiology
- Epidemiologic techniques, methods, and surveillance systems, particularly those related to communicable, chronic, or environmentally induced diseases or injury control
- Current research and analytical methods related to public health and epidemiology
- Scientific methods and the pathobiology of disease or injury occurrence
- Nature and objectives of statewide public health programs addressing individual and community health problems
- Organization and operation of federal, state, and local governmental agencies relating to public health

A typical entry-level epidemiologist generally has the skills and ability to:

- Apply laws, rules, and regulations to problems of disease control
- Communicate clearly and concisely orally and in writing on both technical and nontechnical levels
- Prepare grant proposals and budgets
- Implement and evaluate program activities relating to the prevention and control of injuries and communicable, chronic, or environmentally induced diseases
- Analyze and interpret epidemiologic data
- Assess a disease outbreak situation and make appropriate decisions
- Prepare or assist in preparing scientific articles, making presentations to professional groups, and clearly communicating the findings of epidemiologic studies
- Establish and maintain effective working relationships with other employees, healthcare providers, social service agencies, schools, the media, the public, and federal, state, and local officials

Experience and Education

Any combination of training and experience that provides the required knowledge and abilities will qualify an individual for this position. A typical pathway to obtain the required knowledge and experience is through a master's degree in epidemiology or a master's degree in public health (MPH) with specialization in epidemiology and 1 year of experience in epidemiology research and analysis. Another path is through 1 year of professional experience in chronic disease, communicable disease, human nutrition, injury control, environmental epidemiology, or infection control, which includes disease or injury investigation and risk assessment, and a master's degree from an accredited college or university in nursing, nutrition/dietetics, healthcare administration, biostatistics, sociology, psychology, anthropology, or a biological, physical, or environmental science. Another pathway is through 2 years of professional experience above the entry level in chronic disease, communicable disease, human nutrition, injury control, environmental epidemiology, or infection control, which includes disease or injury investigation and risk assessment, such as a position as a research analyst, program specialist, environmental specialist, nutritionist, community health nurse, or health educator.

Typical Minimum Qualifications for Senior-Level Epidemiologists

Knowledge, Skills, and Abilities

In addition to the knowledge and abilities required for the entry-level epidemiologist just listed, this position requires knowledge of disease control methods, recent developments in the field of epidemiology, and basic management skills. It also requires the skill and ability to supervise and lead lower-level staff and develop grant proposals.

Experience and Education

Any combination of training and experience that provides the required knowledge and abilities will qualify an individual for this position. A typical pathway to obtain the required knowledge and experience is through a doctoral degree in epidemiology or biostatistics and 2 years of experience in epidemiology research and analysis. Another path is through a doctoral degree in a health science field, with a master's degree in epidemiology or an MPH with specialization in epidemiology and 2 years of experience in epidemiology research and analysis. A third pathway is through a master's degree in epidemiology, or an MPH with specialization in epidemiology and 6 years of experience in epidemiology research and analysis. Yet another pathway is through a medical degree with a master's degree in epidemiology or an MPH with specialization in epidemiology and 2 years of experience in epidemiology research and analysis. It is possible that completion of related training or experience such as with the Centers for Disease Control and Prevention (CDC) or the National Institutes of Health could substitute for the

MPH degree. When a medical doctor is selected, a license to practice medicine in the state is necessary.

Biostatistician

Knowledge, Skills, and Abilities

A typical biostatistician generally has knowledge of:

- Biostatistics and statistics with basic knowledge of medicine and epidemiology, including research designs, probability, distributions, rates, proportions, odds, categorical variable analyses, regression, logistic regression, survival analysis, sample size calculations, and power analysis essentials
- Modern, high-level database management and statistical languages such as SAS and SPSS (and possibly S-Plus, StatXact and SigmaPlot), in addition to Microsoft Office software including Excel and Access
- Both parametric and nonparametric statistics
- Sample survey design and analysis including the survey software SUDAAN, FoxPro, Dbase, Oracle, SQL, Visual Basic languages, and database formats

A typical biostatistician generally has the skills and ability to:

- Effectively interact with multidisciplinary teams and outside investigators
- Develop novel approaches for new situations and exhibit the leadership skills needed for successful implementation
- Prioritize conflicting tasks in a fast-paced environment with minimal supervision
- Communicate easily and successfully, both orally and in writing, remain calm under pressure, work as part of a team, and meet deadlines while paying meticulous attention to detail
- Relate well with others and be flexible in unpredictable, ever changing work environments

Experience and Education

Any combination of training and experience that provides the required knowledge and abilities will qualify an individual for this position. A typical way to obtain the required knowledge and experience is through a master's degree in biostatistics, epidemiology, or a related field and 4 years of experience in research analysis and database management, either as part of an educational process or as paid employment. Experience should be in a science, social science, or community-based research setting and involve extensive use of statistical methodologies.

WORKPLACE CONSIDERATIONS

Physical requirements for positions in this occupational category are similar to those for many other public health occupations. Most epidemiologist, biostatistician, and communicable disease investigator positions call for workers to be able to sit for extended periods and to frequently stand and walk short distances. Normal manual dexterity and eye-hand coordination and hearing and vision corrected to within the normal range are also important considerations. Normally, public health professionals must be able to communicate verbally and be able to use office equipment including computers, telephones, calculators, copiers, and fax machines. Although much of the work is performed in an office environment, frequent or continuous contact with staff and the public is also necessary. In some situations, a valid driver's license may be required.

Physical abilities necessary for most public health occupations include the ability to exert light physical effort in sedentary to light work, which may involve some lifting, carrying, pushing, and pulling of objects and materials of light weight (5–10 pounds). Tasks may involve extended periods of time at a keyboard or workstation. When epidemiologists and communicable disease investigators work outside the office, they must have the ability to work under conditions in which exposure to communicable disease risks and environmental factors poses a risk of moderate injury or illness.

> ## OUTSIDE-THE-BOOK THINKING 11-3
>
> © Alfred Bondarenko/Shutterstock.
>
> What features make epidemiology and biostatistics a career worth pursuing?

POSITIONS, SALARIES, AND CAREER PROSPECTS

In 2013, there were 5,300 epidemiologists and 25,000 statisticians employed in the United States, with 2,800 epidemiologists and 6,400 statisticians working for federal, state, and local governmental agencies. **Table 11-3** identifies the number of total workers and the number employed by government for the two standard occupational categories considered in this chapter. Projections for the year 2022 are also provided. The numbers of both epidemiologists and statisticians have been increasing in recent years, a trend that

TABLE 11-3 Number of Workers in 2013 and Projected for 2022 for All Industries and Government and Number of Positions to Be Filled 2012–2022 for All Industries

Occupational Category	Workers in All Industries			Workers in Government	
	2013	Projected 2022	2012–2022 Positions To Be Filled	2013	Projected 2022
Epidemiologists	5,350	5,700	1,600	2,790	2,800
Statisticians	24,950	34,900	16,100	6,430	7,800

Data from Bureau of Labor Statistics, U.S. Department of Labor. Selected Occupational Projections Data. Available at www.bls.gov/data/. Accessed June 15, 2014.

is expected to continue well into the future. For these two occupational categories, job growth has been somewhat less for government employment than outside government.

The total number of positions for epidemiologists is expected to grow to 5,700 by the year 2022 with about 2,800 employed by government agencies. Statistician positions are projected to increase to 35,000 during that period with only a modest increase (to 7,800) for the number employed by government agencies. Based on the growth in the number of positions and the need to fill other positions because of job changes and retirement, more than 1,600 epidemiologist positions and 16,100 statistician positions will be filled between 2012 and 2022. Job growth in the government sector, notably, will lag behind the growth rate for epidemiologist and statistician positions in the overall economy.

Salaries differ considerably between the epidemiologists and statisticians. The median salary for epidemiologists employed by government agencies in 2013 was $61,000, with the middle 50% earning between $50,000 and $75,000 (**Table 11-4**). Average salaries for epidemiologists working in governmental agencies were notably lower than those for epidemiologists working in the private and voluntary sectors. Entry-level salaries were in the $40,000–$48,000 range. Many midsize and small local health departments do not employ an epidemiologist. Larger local health departments and state

health agencies often have several. Larger governmental public health agencies can offer salaries that are somewhat competitive with those in the private and voluntary sectors. Epidemiologists with professional credentials, especially physicians, dentists, veterinarians, and nurses, may be able to attract salaries in the six-figure range.

A 2004 CSTE survey found the highest ratios of epidemiologists to population on the East and West Coasts (1 per 100,000). The South and the Midwest lag behind, with 0.7 and 0.8 epidemiologists per 100,000 population, respectively.

The median salary for statisticians employed by government agencies in 2013 was $82,000, with the middle 50% earning between $56,000 and $105,000. Entry-level salaries were in the $39,000–$52,000 range. Salary information for biostatisticians is not very straightforward, because biostatisticians are lumped with other types of statisticians in employment and wage surveys. Mean salaries for statisticians working for federal agencies are notably higher than those for statisticians working in state and local agencies.

Based on information from current job postings, salaries for communicable disease investigators fall in the $35,000–$55,000 range.

According to surveys of state and territorial health agencies, epidemiologic capacity needs to be increased by 50%.[5] Recent increases in epidemiologists have largely benefited

TABLE 11-4 Number and Salary Profile for Federal and State/Local Workers for Selected Occupations, 2013

Occupational Category	2013 Government Workers			
	Federal Workers	State / Local Workers	Median Annual Salary	25th–75th Percentile Salary Range
Epidemiologists	–	2,790	$61,290	$49,850–$75,120
Statisticians	4,320	2,110	$82,370	$56,730–$105,220

Notes: Federal: excludes postal service; State/Local: excludes hospitals and education

Data from Bureau of Labor Statistics, U.S. Department of Labor. Employment and Wages from Occupational Employment Statistics (OES) Survey. Available at www.bls.gov/data/. Accessed June 15, 2014.

bioterrorism preparedness and response efforts, often at the expense of communicable disease, chronic disease, injury, and environmental epidemiologic capacity. As a result, there is consensus that additional epidemiologists are needed, especially infectious disease, chronic disease, and terrorism-related epidemiologists. The Bureau of Labor Statistics also identifies epidemiologists as an occupation that will grow more rapidly than the average for all occupations over the next 10 years.

OUTSIDE-THE-BOOK THINKING 11-4

© Alfred Bondarenko/Shutterstock.

In which organizations and geographic regions will the need for epidemiologists and biostatisticians expand most rapidly in the next two decades?

ADDITIONAL INFORMATION

There are many good sources of information on epidemiologists, disease investigators, and biostatisticians. Several sources are available for information on educational programs for these occupations as well as for continuing education and leadership development for practitioners.

The CSTE Web site (www.cste.org) and the CDC Epidemiologic Intelligence Service (EIS) Web site (www.cdc.gov/eis/) head the list of useful information sources. CSTE has more than 1,000 members working in state and local public health agencies. The EIS is an elite unit of CDC that provides technical assistance and human resources to state and local governments during unusual or large outbreaks.

Schools of public health are among the institutions offering graduate degrees in health administration. The Association of Schools and Programs of Public Health (www.aspph.org) has identified a battery of core epidemiology and biostatistics competencies appropriate for all students receiving the MPH degree. These competencies provide a useful baseline for professional practice and summarize what an MPH graduate should be able to do (see **Table 11-5**).

The epidemiology section and statistics section of the American Public Health Association's (APHA) Web site (www.apha.org) are also good sources of information for epidemiologists and biostatisticians. The epidemiology section has a long history and currently has 3,000 members, making it one of APHA's largest and most active sections.

TABLE 11-5 Epidemiology and Biostatistics Competency Expectations for Graduates of MPH Degree Programs

1. Identify key sources of data for epidemiologic purposes.
2. Identify the principles and limitations of public health screening programs.
3. Describe a public health problem in terms of magnitude, population affected, time, and place.
4. Explain the importance of epidemiology for informing scientific, ethical, economic, and political discussion of health issues.
5. Comprehend basic ethical and legal principles pertaining to the collection, maintenance, use, and dissemination of epidemiologic data.
6. Apply the basic terminology and definitions of epidemiology.
7. Calculate basic epidemiology measures.
8. Communicate epidemiologic information to lay and professional audiences.
9. Draw appropriate inferences from epidemiologic data.
10. Evaluate the strengths and limitations of epidemiologic reports.
11. Describe the role biostatistics serves in the discipline of public health.
12. Describe basic concepts of probability, random variation, and commonly used statistical probability distributions.
13. Describe preferred methodological alternatives to commonly used statistical methods when assumptions are not met.
14. Distinguish among the different measurement scales and the implications for selection of statistical methods to be used based on these distinctions.
15. Apply descriptive techniques commonly used to summarize public health data.
16. Apply common statistical methods for inference.
17. Apply descriptive and inferential methodologies according to the type of study design for answering a particular research question.
18. Apply basic informatics techniques with vital statistics and public health records in the description of public health characteristics and in public health research and evaluation.
19. Interpret results of statistical analyses found in public health studies.
20. Develop written and oral presentations based on statistical analyses for both public health professionals and educated lay audiences.

Reproduced from the Association of Schools of Public Health (ASPH). MPH Core Competency Development Process, Version 2.3. Washington, DC: ASPH: 2006. Available at http://www.asph.org. Accessed June 15, 2014.

Additional sources of relevant information include the American College of Preventive Medicine (www.acpm.org), the American College of Epidemiology (www.ace-pidemiology.org), the American Epidemiology Society (www.americanepidemiologicalsociety.org), the Association for Professionals in Infection Control and Epidemiology (www.apic.org), the International Epidemiological Association (www.ieaweb.org), and the Society for Epidemiologic Research (www.epiresearch.org).

CONCLUSION

Epidemiology is one of the virtual operating systems for public health practice, and epidemiologists are in great demand. Although recent events have emphasized bioterrorism threats and events, epidemiologists, biostatisticians, and disease investigators work across the entire spectrum of diseases, conditions, and health risks. Due to a variety of highly visible developments and events, such as the anthrax letters in 2001, epidemiologists and other disease investigators have been spotlighted and interest in these careers has grown. Because disease investigators acquire practical skills in the field, they often seek to complement their experience with additional education and training, establishing a practical career ladder. Current and future public threats will serve to ensure that epidemiologists, biostatisticians, and disease investigators remain vital components of the public health workforce.

REFERENCES

1. Bureau of Labor Statistics, U.S. Department of Labor. Databases and tables. Available at www.bls.gov/data/. Accessed June 15, 2014.
2. Health Resources and Services Administration, Bureau of Health Professions, National Center for Health Workforce Information and Analysis and Center for Health Policy, Columbia School of Nursing. *Public Health Workforce Enumeration 2000*. Washington, DC: HRSA; 2000.
3. National Association of County and City Health Officials. *2013 National Profile of Local Health Departments*. Washington, DC: NAC-CHO; 2014.
4. Association of State and Territorial Health Officials. *State Health Profile, Volume Three, 2012*. Washington, DC: ASTHO; 2014.
5. Council of State and Territorial Epidemiologists. 2004 National Assessment of Epidemiologic Capacity: Findings and Recommendations. Washington, DC: CSTE; 2004. Available at www.cste.org. Accessed March 20, 2014.

CHAPTER **12**

Public Health Education and Information

LEARNING OBJECTIVES

Given the need for public health educators, public information specialists, and community health workers in the public health system, describe key features of occupations and careers in public health education and information and how these contribute to carrying out public health's core functions and essential services. Key aspects of this competency expectation include being able to

- Describe several different occupational titles in this category
- Identify specific essential public health services that are critical for positions in this category
- Describe important and essential duties for several job titles in this category
- Identify minimum qualifications and describe general workplace considerations, salary expectations, and career prospects for positions in this category

Public health education has been one of the fastest growing public health professions. Public health educators play important roles in a variety of public health programs and in community relations in general. Chronic disease prevention programs, injury prevention and control activities, and community health planning and community health improvement initiatives all rely heavily on the expertise of health educators. At the state and local level, about one half of the public health educators are professionally certified. **Table 12-1** provides a snapshot of an average day in the life of a public health educator.

Health education is closely linked with two other occupations increasingly found in public health agencies—public information specialists and community health workers.

Recent concerns over bioterrorism threats and events have raised awareness as to the importance of risk communication and public information skills within the public health workforce. This has prompted public health agencies to employ individuals with public relations and public information skills. At the same time, public health agencies have been utilizing community health workers for outreach and community engagement activities. Together these three occupations comprise one of the few growth areas within the public health workforce.

OCCUPATIONAL CLASSIFICATION

Three standard occupational categories for public health workers are addressed in this chapter—health educators, public relations specialists, and community health workers.

A health educator is a white collar, professional category encompassing positions that promote, maintain, and improve individual and community health by assisting individuals and communities to adopt healthy behaviors. Health educators collect and analyze data to identify community needs prior to planning, implementing, monitoring, and evaluating programs designed to encourage healthy lifestyles, policies, and environments. Health educators serve as resources to individuals, other professionals, and the community, and may administer fiscal resources for health education programs. Data from the Bureau of Labor Statistics (BLS) indicate that in 2013 there were 57,000 health educators working in the United States.[1] Federal, state, and local governmental agencies are among the largest employers

TABLE 12-1   A Typical Day for a Public Health Educator

7:30 a.m.	Breakfast meeting with steering committee of community health coalition for community health improvement plan
8:30 a.m.	Office time for phone messages and e-mail
9:00 a.m.	Staff meeting to review priorities for week
10:15 a.m.	Meeting with agency director, epidemiology, and planning staff on community health assessment
10:45 a.m.	Set up conference room for satellite downlink program
11:00 a.m.	Satellite downlink program on establishing a medical reserve corps unit, followed by staff discussion
12:15 p.m.	Lunch at desk revising presentation slides for staff orientation
1:00 p.m.	Staff orientation presentation on "What Is Public Health, and Where Do I Fit In?"
2:00 p.m.	Review draft for agency press release if West Nile Virus outbreak occurs
3:00 p.m.	Conference call meeting with technical program committee for state public health association annual meeting
4:00 p.m.	Review information to be distributed at tonight's community meeting on West Nile Virus threat
4:30 p.m.	Review and analyze participant evaluations from today's orientation program for new employees; revise presentation materials for next month's orientation
5:15 p.m.	Prepare remarks for tonight's community meeting
7:00 p.m.	Represent agency at community meeting regarding West Nile Virus concerns

of health educators; these agencies employ 13,000 health educators. *Public Health Workforce Enumeration 2000* data identified 3,500 public health educator positions in governmental public health agencies in the year 2000.[2] Aggregated data from surveys conducted in 2012 and 2013 identified more than 7,500 health educators working in state and local public health agencies.[3,4] Data from these various sources are used throughout this chapter.

Public information specialist is a position title comparable to the standard occupational classification public relations specialist, which includes positions that engage in promoting or creating goodwill for individuals, groups, or organizations by writing or selecting material and releasing it through various communications media. Public relations and media specialists present public health issues to the media and the public, often serving as spokespersons for public health agencies. These positions may prepare and arrange displays and make speeches and other presentations. There were nearly 21,000 public relations and public information positions in federal, state, and local governmental agencies in 2013. The *Public Health Workforce Enumeration 2000* study identified 900 public information positions in governmental public health agencies.[2] More recent surveys of state and local public health agencies identified nearly 900 public information specialists.[3,4]

OUTSIDE-THE-BOOK THINKING 12-1

© Alfred Bondarenko/Shutterstock.

What will be the most important new or expanded roles for health educators, public information specialists, and community health workers in the 21st century?

Community health workers may perform a variety of duties including assisting individuals and communities to adopt healthy behaviors, conducting outreach for medical personnel or health organizations to implement programs in the community that promote, maintain, and improve individual and community health, providing information on available resources, providing social support and informal counseling, advocating for individuals and community health needs, and providing services such as first aid and blood pressure screening. Community health workers may collect data to help identify community health needs. There were 46,000 community health workers in 2013, with 8,000 working for public sector agencies. The *Public Health Enumeration 2000*

TABLE 12-2 Public Health Practice Profile for Public Health Education and Information Professionals

Public Health Education and Information Professionals Make a Difference by:
Public Health Purposes
✓ Preventing epidemics and the spread of disease
Protecting against environmental hazards
✓ Preventing injuries
✓ Promoting and encouraging healthy behaviors
Responding to disasters and assisting communities in recovery
Ensuring the quality and accessibility of health services
Essential Public Health Services
Monitoring health status to identify community health problems
Diagnosing and investigating health problems and health hazards in the community
✓ Informing, educating, and empowering people about health issues
✓ Mobilizing community partnerships to identify and solve health problems
✓ Developing policies and plans that support individual and community health efforts
Enforcing laws and regulations that protect health and ensure safety
✓ Linking people with needed personal health services and ensuring the provision of healthcare when otherwise unavailable
✓ Ensuring a competent public health and personal healthcare workforce
Evaluating effectiveness, accessibility, and quality of personal and population-based health services
Researching new insights and innovative solutions to health problems

study did not specifically identify community health workers, but NACCHO's 2013 survey of LHDs reported an estimated 6,700 working in LHDs nationally.[3]

PUBLIC HEALTH PRACTICE PROFILE

Health education and information occupations are primarily involved with addressing public health responsibilities for promoting healthy behaviors and preventing disease and injury. These occupational categories may also be involved in emergency preparedness and response and sometimes in assessing the impact and quality of health services within a community.

OUTSIDE-THE-BOOK THINKING 12-2

© Alfred Bondarenko/Shutterstock.

What are the most important contributions to improving the health of the public that health educators, public information specialists, and community health workers make today?

Among the 10 essential public health services, public health education and information workers are especially important for four—informing and educating the public, mobilizing community partnerships, developing policies and plans that support community health improvement, and ensuring a competent workforce. Community health workers also play an especially important role in linking individuals and communities to needed services. **Table 12-2** summarizes public health purposes and essential public health services at the core of positions for public health education and information occupations.

IMPORTANT AND ESSENTIAL DUTIES

There are several job titles and positions in the public health workforce that specialize in public health education and information services. The focus in this chapter will be on three professional positions: (1) entry-level public health educator, (2) senior-level public health educator, and (3) public information specialist/coordinator. Each of these positions and a representative panel of their important and essential duties are described in the following section. Community health workers, a technical occupation, will be addressed in relevant sections later in this chapter.

Public Health Educator (Entry Level)

This position encompasses entry-level professional work in the development and coordination of public health education and health promotion activities. Public health educators assist in the formulation of the health education plan and in the development and implementation of health promotion programs. Work includes providing technical assistance and training to local health professionals, schools, community organizations, government agencies, businesses, and individuals. Supervision is received from a higher level health educator or other designated administrative superior; however, the employee is expected to work with considerable independence within established policies and procedural guidelines.

Essential and important duties for an entry-level public health educator include

- Assists in the development and implementation of health education, behavioral risk reduction, and health promotion programs for schools, work sites, communities, and individuals; provides healthy intervention strategies that meet specified and measurable objectives
- Collects, analyzes, and disseminates information regarding major health problems, behavioral risk factors, and health attitudes and knowledge using epidemiologic procedures; assists in the formulation of disease prevention and health promotion strategies
- Develops various educational materials, such as brochures, exhibits, videotapes, and slides; employs mass media, group process, and counseling techniques in health education, health promotion, and behavioral risk reduction program activities
- Assists in development of training programs and works with others to plan and implement health promotion programs, policies, and legislation
- Maintains knowledge and skills in health education and health promotion research through review of professional literature, participation in conferences, and continuing education
- Provides assistance in the submission of applications for health education, behavioral risk reduction, and health promotion program funds; monitors existing programs for compliance with federal and state regulations

Public Health Educator (Senior Level)

Under direction, this position plans, develops, supervises, evaluates, and monitors specific health education programs for the agency. Senior-level public health educators are distinguished from lower-level public health educators by their responsibility for the preparation, administration, and evaluation of specific public health education programs, grant contracts, and budgets. In addition, a senior public health educator supervises staff assigned to specific programs. This position is distinguished from the health education program manager in that the latter manages the overall agency public health education program, but this position is responsible for the preparation, administration, and evaluation of the public health education efforts of specific programs.

Essential and important duties of senior-level public health educators include

- Plans, implements, and evaluates specific public health education programs
- Assesses and identifies community needs for educational services in specific program areas
- Plans, organizes, designs, develops, and evaluates public health education activities; carries out or directs others to carry out public health education activities, including educational presentations and workshops
- Assists in the development and adaptation of data collection instruments and designs for assessment and evaluation activities
- Develops educational literature and flyers and provides information to the community
- Selects, trains, directs, evaluates, and handles disciplinary problems of subordinate staff
- Seeks funding sources for specific public health education programs
- Prepares grant proposals
- Develops memoranda of understanding and budgets
- Negotiates and monitors contracts with funding agencies and other subcontractors
- Develops and maintains contact with state and local public health agencies, community organizations, and the media
- Serves as the community leader of public health education efforts for specific programs
- Inputs, accesses, and analyzes data in a computer database

Public Information Specialist/Coordinator

This position is a midlevel informational and public relations professional for a public health organization. Public information specialists prepare and disseminate informational materials to support and promote the programs and services of their agency. Work includes composing and editing copy for press releases, articles, bulletins, newsletters, pamphlets, and other publications. Work may involve interpreting and communicating agency programs to employees, special interest groups, and the general public. Supervision is received from an administrative superior who reviews work in progress and upon completion.

Public health information coordinators perform more advanced duties in the coordination of informational and public relations activities in an agency or specialized program and serve as assistants to a public information administrator, or perform a comparable level of work. Work involves collecting, preparing, and disseminating informational material to support and promote agency programs and services, including composing and editing text and producing graphic and photographic illustrations for publication or distribution to the news media and other groups. Work includes interpreting and communicating agency programs to employees, special interest groups, and the general public. Supervision may be exercised over professional, technical, or clerical staff. General supervision is received from a public information administrator or other administrative superior; consequently, the employee is expected to work with considerable independence and technical skill in the area of communication and public relations.

Essential and important duties of public information specialists/coordinators include

- Gathers, compiles, and verifies information; composes and edits copy for newsletters, brochures, web pages, and other publications
- Prepares news releases to inform and educate the public concerning agency programs and services
- Composes or edits articles for internal agency news bulletins; edits articles or correspondence for staff members
- Develops spot announcements and scripts for radio and television
- Answers requests for literature and information; maintains files of photographs, clippings, and agency publications
- Meets with agency officials and attends staff meetings for the purpose of discussing activities and securing newsworthy information
- Researches available material to assist in the preparation of speeches for agency officials
- Operates still and video cameras
- Creates illustrations and does layout work
- Assists with agency-sponsored and interagency public relations activities and special events

- Coordinates informational and public relations activities in a specialized program, serves as an assistant to a public information administrator, or performs work of comparable level and scope
- Provides assistance to higher level management on matters pertaining to public relations and informational policy
- Develops and maintains working relationships with media representatives and public, private, labor, business, and civic organizations to ensure the effective dissemination of informational material
- Estimates costs, develops specifications, and makes recommendations on securing and accepting bids for printing; maintains contact with printing contractors to ensure quality control; reviews and corrects printers' galley proofs
- Arranges public appearances and media engagements for agency officials; prepares or edits the material to be presented
- Makes presentations and serves as a spokesperson for assigned agency programs to special interest groups, employee groups, and the general public
- Informs management of public reaction to programs, suggests strategies for future communications, and makes recommendations for modified or new programs
- Coordinates special events and develops materials, displays, and programs to promote agency services, missions, and goals and to enhance consistency and accuracy in those efforts
- Provides training to improve the techniques of supervisory and professional staff in furthering public understanding of the services offered by the agency
- Supervises, trains, and evaluates subordinate staff

MINIMUM QUALIFICATIONS

Public health educators and public information staff work in professional positions often supported by administrative support and clerical positions. There are generally several steps in the health educator and public information series that allow for advancement and career development. Comparable positions exist in local public health agencies of all sizes, making career advancement from a small to larger employer not uncommon for these workers.

Public health training programs in schools of public health and other academic institutions produce health educators and other communications specialists. The vast majority of current workers in these titles, however, do not have a public health degree. This allows for variability in the types of experience and training that agencies require when filling these positions. As with virtually all public health positions, both experience and education are important considerations for hiring and promotion. Experience and education both contribute to necessary knowledge, skills, and abilities required for workers in this field. Typical minimum qualifications for entry-level and senior-level health educators and public information specialists/coordinators are detailed in this section.

Typical Minimum Qualifications for Entry-Level Public Health Educator

Knowledge, Skills, and Abilities

A typical entry-level public health educator generally has knowledge of:

- Current principles, practices, and processes employed in the health education and health promotion component of a public health program
- Principles, techniques, and application of behavioral epidemiology as related to health education and health promotion
- The psychological, social, economic, and cultural determinants of behavior and methods to promote healthy lifestyles
- Educational methods and techniques of developing and presenting health education to individuals and groups
- Community organization principles and resources, and community health needs
- Current trends and developments in public health, medical sciences, and health care
- Research methods as applied to health education and health promotion

A typical entry-level public health educator has the skills and ability to:

- Assist in the planning, development, implementation, and evaluation of effective health education and health promotion programs for various populations
- Perform statistical computations
- Explain complex medical information to civic and community groups and to public officials, and present ideas effectively
- Establish and maintain effective working relationships with other employees, community groups, and the public

Experience and Education

Any combination of training and experience that provides the required knowledge and abilities will qualify an individual for this position. A typical way to obtain such knowledge and abilities is through graduation from an accredited 4-year college or university with a bachelor degree with major specialization in health education or health promotion, or a master's degree in health education, health promotion, or public health with specialization in health education.

Typical Minimum Qualifications for Senior-Level Public Health Educator

Knowledge, Skills, and Abilities

A typical senior-level public health educator generally has knowledge of:

- The principles of public health education, including program planning and evaluation
- Public health education methods and materials, including teaching methods and curriculum design
- Assessment techniques to identify community health problems in specific program areas
- Existing methods of intervention and control and the health education needs of various target groups
- Principles and practices of community organization for enhancing public health
- The philosophy, concepts, and principles of public health
- The functions and services of local community health agencies and community organizations
- Publicity and media practices and procedures
- Grant proposal writing and budgeting techniques
- Principles and practices of staff supervision and training

A typical senior-level public health educator has the skills and ability to:

- Plan, organize, implement, and evaluate public health education services
- Design, effectively use, and evaluate public health education methods and materials
- Provide public health education consultation, and develop cooperative relationships with a wide range of individuals and representatives of organizations and the news media
- Prepare and present a variety of clear and concise written and oral reports
- Develop and nurture funding sources

- Analyze and prepare grant proposals, contracts, and related budgets
- Negotiate and monitor contracts
- Originate, prepare, and distribute informational and publicity materials
- Plan, assign, direct, and evaluate the work of staff
- Interpret legislation regulations, administrative policies, and procedures
- Input, access, and analyze data in a computer database

Experience and Education

Any combination of training and experience that provides the required knowledge and abilities will qualify an individual for this position. A typical way to obtain such knowledge and abilities is through 2 years of experience in public health education, promotion, or a related field that provides the knowledge and abilities previously identified. Some agencies may require a master's degree in health education from an accredited college and a valid driver's license.

Typical Minimum Qualifications for Public Information Specialist/Coordinator

Knowledge, Skills, and Abilities

A typical public information specialist/coordinator generally has knowledge of:

- Journalism, photography, film/video production, graphic arts, publication, and printing
- News media operation and its proper utilization for dissemination of information
- Principles and methods of establishing and maintaining good public relations
- Community resources and organizations
- Commercial art methods and the general principles of layout and design
- Marketing and advertising practices and techniques
- Journalistic principles and practices, including techniques of planning, composing, and editing informational materials
- Use of methods and techniques of disseminating information to the public
- Public relations techniques and procedures
- Agency organizational structure, including programs, administrative rules and regulations, and staff
- Operation of still and video cameras and developing, processing, and editing the film or video

A typical public information specialist/coordinator generally has the skills and ability to:

- Compose and produce a variety of informational materials
- Use a variety of desktop publishing software packages and Web formatting languages
- Establish and maintain working relationships with media representatives, agency officials, other employees, and the general public
- Communicate with special interest groups, employee groups, and the general public
- Produce graphic art, photographs, and other materials
- Interpret and explain agency policies, laws, and operations
- Stimulate public interest and gain support for agency programs
- Compose and produce a variety of informational materials for release to the media or other publications
- Conduct research to find pertinent and newsworthy information
- Advise and train agency staff in public relations methods and techniques

Experience and Education

Any combination of experience and training that results in the acquisition of the knowledge and skills described above will qualify an individual for this position. A typical way to acquire these qualifications is through graduation from an accredited 4-year college or university with specialization in journalism, communications, English, public relations, advertising, marketing, or closely related areas. Professional experience in the areas of journalism, advertising, marketing, film/video production, or public relations and information may be substituted on a year-for-year basis for the required education. For a public information coordinator, requirements may include 1 year as public information specialist or 2 years of professional experience in public relations, advertising, or journalism; and graduation from an accredited 4-year college or university with specialization in journalism, communications, English, public relations, advertising, marketing, or closely related areas. Professional experience in the areas of journalism, advertising, marketing, film/video production, or public relations and information may be substituted on a year-for-year basis for the stated education. Graduate work in the educational areas previously listed may be substituted on a year-for-year basis for 1 or more years of the stated experience.

WORKPLACE CONSIDERATIONS

In 2013, state and local governmental agencies employed approximately 13,000 health educators and 8,000 community health workers, and there is every indication that even greater numbers will be employed by these agencies over the next decade.

Physical requirements for positions in this occupational category are similar to those for other professional public health positions. Most health educator, public information, and community health worker positions call for workers to be able to sit for extended periods and to frequently stand and walk short distances. Normal manual dexterity and eye-hand coordination and hearing and vision corrected to within the normal range are also important considerations. Normally, public health educators and public information staff will be able to communicate verbally and be able to use office equipment including computers, telephones, calculators, copiers, and fax machines. Although much of the work is performed in an office environment, frequent or continuous contact with staff and the public is also necessary. In many situations, people filling these positions may be required to possess a valid driver's license.

OUTSIDE-THE-BOOK THINKING 12-3

© Alfred Bondarenko/Shutterstock.

What features make health education and public information careers worth pursuing?

POSITIONS, SALARIES, AND CAREER PROSPECTS

In 2013, there were 57,000 health educators, 203,000 public relations/public information specialists, and 46,000 community health workers employed in the United States, with 13,600 health educators, 20,700 public information specialists, and 8,000 community health workers working for federal, state, and local governmental agencies. **Table 12-3** identifies the number of total workers and the number employed by government for the three standard occupational categories considered in this chapter. Projections for the year 2022 are also provided. The numbers of health educators, public information specialists, and community health workers have been increasing in recent years, a trend that is expected to continue well into the future. For these occupational categories, job growth has been somewhat less for government employment than for outside government. This trend in all likelihood will continue.

The total number of positions for health educators is expected to grow to 70,000 by the year 2022 with 14,000 employed by government agencies. Community health workers are forecast to grow to 51,000 with 8,500 employed by government agencies. Public information specialist positions are projected to increase to 257,000 during that period with only a modest increase (to 21,500) for the number employed by government agencies. Based on the growth in the number of positions and the need to fill other positions because of job changes and retirement, nearly 276,000 health educator positions, 21,000 community health worker positions, and 59,000 public relations/public information specialist positions will be filled between 2012 and 2022. Only about one fourth of these positions will be filled in the government sector. Job growth in the government sector will lag well behind the growth rate for health educator, community health worker, and public relations specialist positions in the overall economy.

TABLE 12-3   Number of Workers in 2013 and Projected for 2022 for All Industries and Government and Number of Positions to Be Filled 2012–2022 for All Industries

Occupational Category	Workers in All Industries			Workers in Government	
	2013	Projected 2022	2012–2022 Positions To Be Filled	2013	Projected 2022
Health Educators	56,720	70,100	26,600	12,550	13,700
Public Relations Specialists	202,530	256,500	58,800	20,670	21,500
Community Health Workers	45,800	50,700	20,800	7,880	8,500

Data from Bureau of Labor Statistics, U.S. Department of Labor. Selected Occupational Projections Data. Available at www.bls.gov/data/. Accessed June 15, 2014.

TABLE 12-4   Number and Salary Profile for Federal and State/Local Workers for Selected Occupations, 2013

Occupational Category	2013 Government Workers			
	Federal Workers	State / Local Workers	Median Annual Salary	25th–75th Percentile Salary Range
Health Educators	3,030	9,520	$52,270	$40,360–$78,000
Public Relations Specialists	5,040	15,630	$59,630	$44,290–$77,990
Community Health Workers	–	7,880	$37,360	$29,480–$48,020

Notes: Federal: excludes postal service; State/Local: excludes hospitals and education

Data from Bureau of Labor Statistics, U.S. Department of Labor. Employment and Wages from Occupational Employment Statistics (OES) Survey. Available at www.bls.gov/data/. Accessed June 15, 2014.

The median salary for health educators employed by government agencies in 2013 was $52,000, with the middle 50% earning between $40,000 and $78,000 (**Table 12-4**). Average salaries for health educators working in governmental agencies were higher than those for health educators working in the private and voluntary sectors. Entry-level salaries were also higher for government employment ($31,000–$37,000) than for all industries ($26,000–$33,000). Many small local health departments do not employ health educators. Larger local health departments and state health agencies often have several.

The median salary in 2013 for community health workers employed by government was $37,000 with the middle 50% earning between $29,000 and $48,000.

The median salary in 2013 for public information specialists employed by government agencies was $60,000, with the middle 50% earning between $44,000 and $78,000. Entry-level salaries were in the $33,000–$40,000 range. Salary information for public relations/public information specialists for all industries is difficult to interpret because the duties outside government vary considerably.

As is the case with several other public health occupations, health educators and public information specialists can advance from entry-level to midlevel to senior-level positions in their specialty. But in view of their strong communication and information skills, these workers may be used by agencies for both program-specific work (i.e., as program staff for an assigned program) and at the agency level to deal with community and other public interactions. For example, health educators play a major role in organizing and coordinating community health planning efforts that lead to community health needs assessments, community health report cards, and ultimately to community health improvement initiatives. Because community health improvement efforts have become a central role of local and state public health agencies, and as they continue to grow over the next decade, the need for health educators will continue to grow in comparison with other public health occupations. This greater emphasis on community planning and partnerships, as well as the need for more effective risk communication capabilities for bioterrorism and other threats, also increases the need and demand for public information specialists and coordinators.

Community health workers are considered technical or paraprofessional staff and there is no formal career ladder to positions such as health educators. A career ladder, however, is possible in some situations. It is likely that several elements of the Affordable Care Act, including the need for patient navigators, community liaisons, and program outreach workers, will foster the growth and professionalization of this occupational category.

Public health education, an increasingly recognized and important occupational category within the public health workforce, has developed a credential for highly skilled health educators. Certified health education specialists (CHES) illustrate the movement toward credentialing as a means of increasing the professional stature of an occupation. Many public health workers currently providing health education services, however, do not qualify to sit for the CHES exam because they have not completed a degree program in health education at the bachelor or master's level. For either group, however, ongoing continuing education initiatives will be important to strengthen the corps of workers providing health education services to the public.

OUTSIDE-THE-BOOK THINKING 12-4

© Alfred Bondarenko/Shutterstock.

In which organizations and geographic regions will the need for health educators, public information specialists, and community health workers expand most rapidly in the next two decades?

ADDITIONAL INFORMATION

There are many good sources of information on health education and public information as careers. Several sources are available for information on educational programs for health education as well as for continuing education and leadership development for practicing health educators seeking a professional credential.

Schools of public health are among the institutions offering graduate degrees in health administration. The Association of Schools and Programs of Public Health (www.aspph.org) has identified a battery of behavioral science competencies appropriate for all students receiving the master's of public health (MPH) degree. These competencies provide a useful baseline for professional practice and summarize what an MPH graduate should be able to do (**Table 12-5**).

Additional sources of information on health education include the web sites of several other organizations, including the Directors of Health Promotion and Education (www.dhpe.org), the American College Health Association (www.acha.org), the American School Health Association (www.ashaweb.org), the Association of State and Territorial Directors of Health Promotion and Public Health Education (www.astdhpphe.org), and the Coalition of National Health Education Organizations (www.cnheo.org). The coalition, for example, has as its primary mission the mobilization of the resources of the health education profession in order to expand and improve health education, regardless of the setting.

The American Public Health Association Web site (www.apha.org) has several sections active in health education issues, including the public health education and health promotion section and the school health education section. Yet another useful resource for health education and information is the *Healthy People 2020* web site.

Central to making health education a profession are the efforts of the Society of Public Health Educators and the National Commission for Health Education Credentialing (www.nchec.org) with its competency-based credentialing program for professional health educators (CHES). CHES competencies focus on: assessing needs, assets and capacity for health education; planning, implementing, managing, and evaluating health education interventions; and communicating, advocating, and serving as a resource for health education.[5]

TABLE 12-5   Social and Behavioral Science Competency Expectations for Graduates of MPH Degree Programs

1. Identify basic theories, concepts, and models from a range of social and behavioral disciplines that are used in public health research and practice.
2. Identify the causes of social and behavioral factors that affect the health of individuals and populations.
3. Identify individual, organizational, and community concerns, assets, resources, and deficits for social and behavioral science interventions.
4. Identify critical stakeholders for the planning, implementation, and evaluation of public health programs, policies, and interventions.
5. Describe steps and procedures for the planning, implementing, and evaluating of public health programs, policies, and interventions.
6. Describe the role of social and community factors in both the onset and solution of public health problems.
7. Describe the merits of social and behavioral science interventions and policies.
8. Apply evidence-based approaches in the development and evaluation of social and behavioral science interventions.
9. Apply ethical principles to public health program planning, implementation, and evaluation.
10. Specify multiple targets and levels of intervention for social and behavioral science programs and/or policies.

Reproduced from the Association of Schools of Public Health (ASPH). MPH Core Competency Development Process, version 2.3. Washington, DC: ASPH: 2006. Available at http://www.asph.org. Accessed June 15, 2014.

CONCLUSION

In an age of communications and information technology and community engagement, it is no wonder that public health educators, public information professionals, and community health workers play key roles in public health practice. Public health agencies are increasingly adding staff with these capabilities and utilizing existing staff across programs to address community-wide concerns and issues. Public health educators have led the way in establishing a credential that is based on relevant practice competencies and respected in practice settings. It is expected that opportunities will continue to grow for public health educators, public information specialists, and community health workers over the next decade.

REFERENCES

1. Bureau of Labor Statistics, U.S. Department of Labor. Databases and tables. www.bls.gov/data/. Accessed June 15, 2014.
2. Health Resources and Services Administration, Bureau of Health Professions, National Center for Health Workforce Information and Analysis and Center for Health Policy, Columbia School of Nursing. *Public Health Workforce Enumeration 2000.* Washington, DC: HRSA; 2000.
3. National Association of County and City Health Officials. *2013 National Profile of Local Health Departments.* Washington, DC: NACCHO; 2014.
4. Association of State and Territorial Health Officials. *State Health Profile, Volume Three, 2012.* Washington, DC: ASTHO; 2014.
5. National Commission for Health Education Credentialing, Inc. (NCHEC), *Society for Public Health Education (SOPHE), American Association for Health Education (AAHE). (2010a). A competency-based framework for health education specialists, 2010.* Whitehall, PA: NCHEC; 2010.

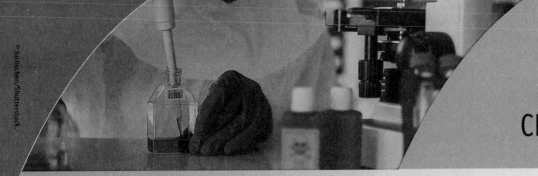

CHAPTER **13**

Additional Public Health Professional and Technical Occupations

This chapter is organized a bit differently from the other chapters focusing on public health professional and technical occupations. This chapter highlights selected professional and technical public health occupations within the public health workforce, as well as several commonly used position titles that do not fit neatly into one of the standard occupational classifications (SOCs) established by the United States Bureau of Labor Statistics (BLS) These professional occupational categories, their related technical occupational categories, and several commonly used position titles are addressed individually in this chapter, except for those that are closely related in practice settings. To a large degree, the career links are not as clear for these occupations as for those addressed in earlier chapters.

Many SOCs carry out professional roles or perform technical duties in support of professionals. Within the public health workforce, these include a variety of professional occupations, including nutritionists and dietitians,

healthcare social workers, mental health and substance abuse social workers, substance abuse and behavioral disorder counselors, medical and clinical laboratory technologists, physicians, veterinarians, pharmacists, optometrists, oral health professionals, and administrative judges/hearing officers—just to name a few. A variety of technical occupations support the efforts of these professional categories. Home health aides, nursing assistants, emergency medical technicians, and laboratory technicians represent a few of the technical occupations in the public health workforce. This chapter provides information and data for 20 such SOCs.

Nutritionists and dietitians work in a variety of settings for governmental public health agencies, voluntary organizations, and healthcare providers. Public health social workers often have positions in maternal and child health programs or in mental health services offered by public agencies. Mental health substance abuse social workers and substance abuse and behavioral disorder counselors work with psychologists and other mental health providers in programs that offer mental health services.

Not all public health agencies have laboratories, but those that provide public health and clinical laboratory services employ medical and clinical laboratory technologists and technicians. Those labs also employ public health laboratory scientists with special expertise in microbiology, chemistry, and physics.

Physicians were once one of the largest and most active professional occupational categories in the public health workforce. Today, however, they represent only a small percentage of the public health workforce. Veterinarians now play key roles in animal control and communicable disease control programs, and pharmacists and emergency medical technicians are increasingly involved in clinical and emergency preparedness and response roles. Oral health professionals, including dentists and dental hygienists, coordinate oral health programs within public health agencies as well as provide clinical dental services. Administrative law judges/hearing officers are important personnel in a variety of administrative and regulatory processes of governmental public health agencies. Together, these varied occupational categories, and several not yet identified, demonstrate the multidisciplinary and interdisciplinary nature of modern public health practice.

In addition to these 20 occupations, there are several important positions within public health organizations that don't fall neatly into one of the existing BLS SOCs, or may actually fall into several. Public health program specialists/coordinators, policy analysts, and public health information specialists are prime examples. This chapter will also discuss these positions, although BLS data on numbers, salary distribution, and forecasted job openings are not available. When possible, information and data from other sources is included.

This chapter examines this veritable army of public health professional and supporting technical occupations that make up key subsets of the overall public health workforce. Data from several sources are used throughout this chapter, including the Bureau of Labor Statistics (BLS), the *Public Health Workforce Enumeration 2000* study, and the most recent survey of local health departments (LHDs) and state health agencies (SHAs) conducted by the National Association of County and City Health Officials (NACCHO) and the Association of State and Territorial Health Officials.[1-4]

The professional and technical occupations addressed in this chapter are presented in alphabetical order except for a few occupational groupings that share similar functions and duties. There is no attempt to treat each occupation equally in terms of functions, skills, qualifications, and data. Greater attention and detail are devoted to those that have the greatest overall impact or that play unique roles in public health practice. **Table 13-1** offers a general public health practice profile for each of these groupings or separate occupational categories, pointing out the prime public health purposes and essential public health services addressed by each. **Table 13-2** summarizes BLS data on the number of jobs in all industries and government for each SOC in 2013 and projected for 2022, as well as the number of job openings

TABLE 13-1   Public Health Practice Profile for Selected Public Health Professional and Technical Occupations

Selected Public Health Professional Occupations								
Make a Difference by:								
	Nutr	BH	Lab	Docs	Oral	Law	Prog	Pol
Public Health Purposes								
Preventing epidemics and the spread of disease	✓		✓	✓	✓	✓		✓
Protecting against environmental hazards			✓			✓	✓	✓
Preventing injuries							✓	
Promoting and encouraging healthy behaviors	✓	✓		✓	✓		✓	
Responding to disasters and assisting communities in recovery		✓						
Assuring the quality and accessibility of health services	✓	✓	✓	✓	✓	✓		✓
Essential Public Health Services								
Monitoring health status to identify community health problems	✓		✓	✓	✓		✓	
Diagnosing and investigating health problems and health hazards in the community			✓	✓			✓	
Informing, educating, and empowering people about health issues	✓	✓			✓			✓
Mobilizing community partnerships to identify and solve health problems		✓						✓
Developing policies and plans that support individual and community health efforts		✓				✓	✓	✓
Enforcing laws and regulations that protect health and ensure safety			✓			✓	✓	
Linking people with needed personal health services and assuring the provision of health care when otherwise unavailable	✓	✓		✓	✓			

TABLE 13-1   Public Health Practice Profile for Selected Public Health Professional and Technical Occupations (*continued*)

Selected Public Health Professional Occupations								
Make a Difference by:								
	Nutr	**BH**	**Lab**	**Docs**	**Oral**	**Law**	**Prog**	**Pol**
Essential Public Health Services								
Assuring a competent public health and personal healthcare workforce						✓		
Evaluating effectiveness, accessibility, and quality of personal and population-based health services	✓	✓	✓	✓	✓	✓	✓	✓
Researching new insights and innovative solutions to health problems	✓		✓	✓		✓		✓

Notes: Nutr: nutritionists and dietitians; BH: behavioral health professionals; Lab: public health laboratory workers; Docs: physicians, veterinarians, optometrists, pharmacists; Oral: oral health professionals; Law: administrative judges and hearing officers: Spec; public health program specialists/coordinators; Pol: policy analysts.

TABLE 13-2   Number of Workers in 2013 and Projected for 2022 for All Industries and Government and Number of Positions to Be Filled 2012–2022 for All Industries

	Workers in All Industries			Workers in Government	
Occupational Category	**2013**	**Projected 2022**	**2012–2022 Positions To Be Filled**	**2013**	**Projected 2022**
Animal Control Workers	13,590	15,700	4,500	12,310	13,600
Audiologists	11,550	17,300	7,000	140	200
Administrative Law Judges, Adjudicators, and Hearing Officers	14,270	14,700	2,400	14,260	14,700
Dental Hygienists	192,330	256,900	113,500	1,670	1,700
Dentists (General)	96,000	146,400	51,200	1,880	2,100
Dietitians and Nutritionists	59,530	81,600	22,100	8,720	9,400
Emergency Medical Technicians and Paramedics	237,660	294,400	120,600	70,310	75,700
Healthcare Social Workers	141,830	185,500	70,200	15,370	16,800
Home Health Aides	806,710	1,299,300	590,700	14,890	16,500
Medical and Clinical Laboratory Technicians	157,080	209,400	90,200	5,090	5,400
Medical and Clinical Laboratory Technologists	162,630	187,100	65,800	6,860	6,500
Mental Health Counselors	115,580	165,100	64,000	10,410	12,200
Mental Health and Substance Abuse Social Workers	110,010	140,200	50,200	16,290	17,500
Microbiologists	19,880	21,600	7,100	4,620	4,700
Optometrists	32,040	41,200	17,700	530	500
Pharmacists	287,420	327,800	109,800	9,080	9,600
Physician Assistants	88,110	120,000	48,900	3,150	3,200
Physicians (General and Family Practitioners)	120,860	142,100	49,200	2,890	3,700
Substance Abuse and Behavioral Disorder Counselors	83,120	117,700	47,200	9,000	10,600
Veterinarians	59,230	78,700	31,000	2,130	2,300

Note: Comparable data for public health program specialists, public health policy analysts, and public health information specialists not available.

Data from Bureau of Labor Statistics, U.S. Department of Labor. Selected Occupational Projections Data. Available at www.bls.gov/data/. Accessed June 15, 2014.

TABLE 13-3   Number and Salary Profile for Federal and State/Local Workers for Selected Occupations, 2013

Occupational Category	2013 Government Workers			
	Federal Workers	State/Local Workers	Median Annual Salary	25th–75th Percentile Salary Range
Animal Control Workers	–	12,310	$32,240	$25,570–$40,560
Audiologists	–	140	$63,710	$52,130–$74,280
Administrative Law Judges, Adjudicators, and Hearing Officers	3,890	10,360	$87,190	$58,420–$115,450
Dental Hygienists	650	1,030	$54,190	$48,240–$62,170
Dentists (General)	–	1,880	$121,840	$105,260–$151,310
Dietitians and Nutritionists	2,000	6,720	$53,670	$41,210–$67,950
Emergency Medical Technicians and Paramedics	–	70,310	$35,320	$26,130–$49,920
Healthcare Social Workers	–	15,370	$50,230	$40,340–$60,620
Home Health Aides	–	14,890	$22,570	$17,970–$31,550
Medical and Clinical Laboratory Technicians	3,340	1,750	$40,300	$34,090–$46,830
Medical and Clinical Laboratory Technologists	5,150	1,720	$61,680	$53,740–$68,880
Mental Health Counselors	–	10,410	$49,060	$39,260–$61,050
Mental Health and Substance Abuse Social Workers	–	16,290	$46,380	$36,180–$58,430
Microbiologists	2,490	2,130	$75,680	$55,180–$100,920
Optometrists	430	90	$82,120	$34,000–$92,560
Pharmacists	6,820	2,250	$110,490	$97,980–118,530
Physician Assistants	2,410	740	$88,190	$78,530–$94,420
Physicians (General/Family Practice and General Internists)	–	2,890	$149,420	$117,040–$184,010
Substance Abuse and Behavioral Disorder Counselors	–	9,010	$44,480	$35,510–$54,770
Veterinarians	1,330	790	$85,150	$75,830–$95,290

Notes: Federal: excludes postal service; State/Local: excludes hospitals and education. Comparable data for public health program specialists, public health policy analysts, and public health information specialists not available.

Data from Bureau of Labor Statistics, U.S. Department of Labor. Employment and Wages from Occupational Employment Statistics (OES) Survey. Available at www.bls.gov/data/. Accessed June 15, 2014.

anticipated between 2012 and 2022 due to job growth and turnover. **Table 13-3** offers additional detail for these SOCs on the number of workers for each level of government as well as salary data for workers employed by government.

OUTSIDE-THE-BOOK THINKING 13-1

© Alfred Bondarenko/Shutterstock.

Which of the occupations covered in this chapter is likely to play important new or expanded roles in the public health system of the 21st century?

ADMINISTRATIVE LAW JUDGES AND HEARING OFFICERS

Administrative law judges, adjudicators, and hearing officers conduct hearings to recommend or make decisions on claims concerning government programs or other government-related matters. Duties often include determining liability, sanctions, or penalties, or recommending the acceptance or rejection of claims or settlements.

Administrative judges and hearing officers provide legal advice to public health agencies, provide legal representation of public health officials in courts and administrative law proceedings, and preside over administrative law hearings of various kinds. The *Public Health Workforce Enumeration 2000* study identified 900 administrative judges/hearing officers working in federal, state, and local public health agencies. There were 14,000 administrative judges/hearing officers in the United States in 2013. Virtually all worked for government agencies. The median salary in 2013 was $87,000 with the middle 50% earning between $58,000 and $116,000. Job growth is expected to be very slow with only about 2,400 positions to be filled through increased demand and job turnover over the next decade. Jobs in the public sector, however, are not expected to increase.

ANIMAL CONTROL WORKERS

Animal control workers handle animals for the purpose of investigations of mistreatment, or control of abandoned, dangerous, or unattended animals. Animal control programs are sometimes operated by local health departments, but in many communities these programs are located in other agencies of local government. BLS data document nearly 14,000 animal control workers with about 90% working for local governments. Only 1,200 of these positions were in LHDs.[3] The median salary for public sector animal control workers in 2013 was $32,000, with the middle 50% earning between $25,000 and $41,000. Job growth is expected to be modest with about 4,500 positions to be filled through increased demand and job turnover over the next decade. Jobs in the public sector, however, are not expected to increase.

AUDIOLOGISTS

Audiologists assess and treat persons with hearing and related disorders. Duties may include fitting hearing aids, providing auditory training, and performing research related to hearing problems. Of the nearly 12,000 audiologists employed in the United States in 2013, only 140 worked for government agencies. The median salary for these public sector audiologists in 2013 was $64,000, with the middle 50% earning between $52,000 and $75,000. This occupation is expected to grow substantially with 7,000 positions to be filled through increased demand and job turnover over the next decade. Positions will likely increase in government agencies.

BEHAVIORAL, SOCIAL, SUBSTANCE ABUSE, AND MENTAL HEALTH PROFESSIONALS

Public health social workers, mental health and substance abuse social workers, and mental health, substance abuse and behavioral disorder counselors promote and encourage healthy behaviors and often participate in responses to disasters and public health emergencies. These professionals diagnose and investigate health problems; inform, educate, and empower people about issues; mobilize community partnerships; and link people with needed personal health

services. Throughout the first decade of the 20th century, public health organizations increasingly employed a variety of behavioral and mental health workers, including mental health and substance abuse social workers, substance abuse and behavioral disorder counselors, and psychologists and other mental health providers. This trend was interrupted by the national recession of 2008/2009, which forced many public health organizations to cut or reduce programs that provide personal health services. This aggregate category examines 4 SOCs: healthcare social workers, mental health and substance abuse social workers, mental health counselors, substance abuse and behavioral disorder counselors. More than 50,000 workers in these SOCs are employed by government agencies, although fewer than 10,000 work in local and state public health agencies.[3,4]

Healthcare social workers provide individuals, families, and groups with the psychosocial support needed to cope with chronic, acute, or terminal illnesses. Services include advising family care givers, providing patient education and counseling, and making referrals for other services. Healthcare social workers may also provide care and case management or interventions designed to promote health, prevent disease, and address barriers to access to health care. In 2013, there were 142,000 healthcare social workers in the United States, with 15,000 working for government agencies, virtually all at the state and local levels. The median salary for healthcare social workers employed by government agencies in 2013 was $50,000 with the middle 50% earning between $40,000 and $61,000. Growth prospects for this occupation are strong, with 70,000 positions expected to be filled through increased demand and job turnover over the next decade. Job growth will be especially strong for positions outside the public sector.

Mental health and substance abuse social workers assess and treat individuals with mental, emotional, or substance abuse problems, including abuse of alcohol, tobacco, and/or other drugs. Activities may include individual and group therapy, crisis intervention, case management, client advocacy, prevention, and education. There were 110,000 mental health and substance abuse social workers in the United States in 2013, with 16,000 employed by state and local governmental agencies. The median salary for public sector mental health and substance abuse social workers in 2013 was $46,000 with the middle 50% earning between $36,000 and $59,000. Job growth for this occupation is expected to be moderate through 2022, with 50,000 positions to be filled due to increased demand and job turnover over the next decade. Job growth will be slower for government employment.

Mental health counselors counsel with emphasis on prevention, work with individuals and groups to promote optimum mental and emotional health, and help individuals deal with issues associated with addictions and substance abuse, stress management, self-esteem, family, parenting, marital problems, and aging. There were 116,000 mental health counselors in the United States in 2013, with 10,400 working for public sector agencies. The median salary for public sector mental health counselors in 2013 was $49,000 with the middle 50% earning between $39,000 and $62,000. Job growth for this occupation is expected to be strong through 2022, with 64,000 positions to be filled through increased demand and job turnover. Jobs will increase but a lower rate for government agencies.

Substance abuse and behavioral disorder counselors counsel and advise individuals with alcohol, tobacco, drug, or other problems, such as gambling and eating disorders. Duties may include counseling individuals, families, or groups or engaging in prevention programs. There were 83,000 substance abuse and behavioral disorder counselors in the United States in 2013, with 9,000 working for public sector agencies. The median salary for public sector substance abuse and behavioral disorder counselors in 2013 was $44,500 with the middle 50% earning between $35,000 and $55,000. Job growth for this occupation is expected to be strong through 2022, with 47,000 positions to be filled through increased demand and job turnover. Jobs will increase but at a lower rate for government employment.

DENTAL/ORAL HEALTH PROFESSIONALS

Oral health professionals examine, diagnose, and treat diseases, injuries, and malformations of teeth and gums. General dentists treat diseases of nerve, pulp, and other dental tissues affecting oral hygiene and retention of teeth, fit dental appliances, and provide preventive care. Dental hygienists clean teeth and examine oral areas, head, and neck for signs of oral disease. Many dental hygienists also educate patients on oral hygiene, take and develop x-rays, or apply fluoride or sealants. In public health settings, oral health professionals also plan, develop, implement, and evaluate oral health programs to promote and maintain optimum oral health of the public. The *Public Health Workforce Enumeration 2000* study identified 3,100 dental workers (both dentists and hygienists) in federal, state, and local public health agencies. More recent surveys in 2012 and 2013 indicate a similar number of oral health professionals working in local and state health agencies.[3,4]

There were 96,000 general dentists in the United States in 2013, with only about 2,000 working for public sector agencies. The median salary for public sector general dentists in 2013 was $122,000 with the middle 50% earning between $105,000 and $152,000. Job growth for this occupation is expected to be very strong through 2022, with 51,000 positions to be filled through increased demand and job turnover. Jobs will increase very little for government agencies.

There were 192,000 dental hygienists in the United States in 2013, with only about 2,000 working for public sector agencies. The median salary for public sector dental hygienists in 2013 was $54,000 with the middle 50% earning between $48,000 and $63,000. Similar to that for general dentists, job growth for this occupation is expected to be very strong through 2022, with 113,000 positions to be filled through increased demand and job turnover. Jobs will increase very little for government agencies.

DIETITIANS AND NUTRITIONISTS

Dietitians and nutritionists plan and conduct food service or nutritional programs to assist in the promotion of health and control of disease. Duties may include supervising activities of a department providing quantity food services, counseling individuals, or conducting nutritional research. Dietitians and nutritionists primarily work toward preventing the spread of diseases and conditions related to diet and exercise. These categories monitor health status to identify community health problems; inform, educate, and empower people about health issues; and link people with needed personal health services. They may also be involved in research activities.

Nutritionists and dietitians may supervise the activities of a program or unit providing nutrition or food services, counsel individuals, or conduct nutritional research. Nutritionists, dietitians, and dietetic technicians work in community-oriented programs such as the federally funded WIC program or state and locally funded maternal and child health programs, as well as in clinical settings, such as prenatal and well child clinics.

BLS data indicate that there were 59,500 nutritionists and dietitians employed in the United States in 2013. Most nutritionists and dietitians work for hospitals, long-term care facilities, and community care facilities for the elderly. Only 8,700 nutritionists work for federal, state, and local governmental agencies, primarily public health departments. The *Public Health Workforce Enumeration 2000* study identified 6,700 public health nutritionists in governmental public health agencies in 2000, largely based on information provided by the Association of State and Territorial Public Health Nutrition Directors (ASTPHND).

About the same number were identified in more recent surveys of state and local public health agencies conducted in 2012 and 2013.[3,4]

Within state and local health agencies, most nutritionists work in WIC programs. WIC is short for Supplemental Foods Program for Women, Infants, and Children, which is funded by the U.S. Department of Agriculture. Nutrition positions are also found in regulatory programs for hospitals, nursing homes, day care centers, and other facilities as well as in Child and Adult Care Food Program (food stamps) and state Medicaid and school lunch programs.

Entry-level public health nutritionists plan and conduct nutritional programs that assist in the promotion of health and control of disease. Midlevel and senior-level nutritionists may supervise activities of a program or unit of an agency providing quality food services, counsel individuals, or conduct nutritional research. Many nutritionists and dietitians seek the registered dietitian (RD) credential.

Entry-level professional public health nutritionists are responsible for participating in the implementation of nutrition programs and services. Work involves providing nutrition program services to local health units or health and human services professionals. General supervision is received from an administrative superior, with professional supervision received from a higher-level nutritionist.

Essential and important duties of an entry-level public health nutritionist include

- Carries out program policies and procedures in implementing nutritional components of general or specialized public health programs
- Coordinates nutrition program services with other nutrition or public health programs within an assigned area
- Confers with public health personnel on food and nutrition related to health programs or problems
- Participates in conducting studies and surveys of the relationships of dietary factors to health and disease, including compilation of data and interpretation of results
- Conducts formal training using educational materials and visual aids in the education of students and public health staff, and assists in the evaluation and recommendation for improvement of such materials
- Participates and works with higher-level nutritionists or consultants in inservice training of health personnel
- Prepares reports, records, and other data related to nutritional services

- Assists in monitoring local health units for compliance with federal or state regulations related to nutrition programs or grant projects

Key knowledge, skills, and abilities for entry-level public health nutritionists include

- Working knowledge of the principles and practices of nutrition and food, particularly in relation to health and disease
- Knowledge of current developments in public health nutrition and their application to statewide and/or local nutrition programs
- Knowledge of social, cultural, and economic problems and their impact on public health nutrition
- Knowledge of the general organization and function of public health agencies
- Ability to effectively use educational materials for the nutrition education of individuals and groups
- Ability to gather, interpret, evaluate, and use statistical data
- Ability to present ideas clearly and concisely
- Ability to establish and maintain working relationships with professional and lay groups, other employees, and the general public

Minimum qualifications, in terms of experience and training, for entry-level public health nutrition positions may call for graduation from an accredited 4-year college or university with a bachelor degree, including or supplemented by at least 15 semester hours in foods and nutrition including at least one course in diet therapy and one course in community nutrition or nutrition in life cycle; or completion of an undergraduate curriculum accredited or approved by the American Dietetic Association (ADA). Registration or current eligibility for registration by the Commission on Dietetic Registration (CDR) may be accepted in lieu of other specified qualifications. A registered dietitian is identified by the RD credential.

As noted previously, there were 59,500 nutritionists and dietitians employed in the United States in 2013, with 8,700 working for government agencies at the federal, state, or local level. The median salary for nutritionists and dietitians employed in the governmental sector in 2013 was also $54,000 with the middle 50% earning between $41,000 and $68,000. Entry-level salaries were in the $33,000–$40,000 range. The Bureau of Labor Statistics projects there will be 82,000 positions overall, including 9,400 positions in the governmental sector in the year 2022. Because of job growth, retirements, and other job changes, more than

22,000 positions have been or will be filled between 2012 and 2022, although growth among government agencies will be substantially less.

EMERGENCY MEDICAL TECHNICIANS AND PARAMEDICS

Emergency medical technicians (EMTs) assess injuries, administer emergency medical care, and extricate trapped individuals. Duties often include transporting injured or sick persons to medical facilities. Paramedics are trained to provide more complex and sophisticated medical care under the general supervision of physicians.

There were 238,000 EMTs and paramedics in the United States in 2013, with 70,000 working for public sector agencies. The median salary for public sector EMTs and paramedics in 2013 was $35,000 with the middle 50% earning between $26,000 and $50,000. Job growth for this occupation is expected to be moderate through 2022, with 121,000 positions to be filled through increased demand and job turnover. Jobs will increase but a lower rate for government employment.

LABORATORY WORKERS

Public health laboratories require a variety of professional and technical workers, including public health scientists and laboratory technologists and technicians. Public health scientists are not one of the standard occupational categories tracked by the Bureau of Labor Statistics, although there are several other standard occupational categories that work in this capacity (such as microbiologists and biochemists). Technologists and technicians working in medical and clinical labs, including public health labs, are among the occupations for which national data are compiled. Public health laboratory workers prevent the spread of disease, protect against environmental hazards, and ensure the quality of services. Lab workers diagnose and investigate health problems and disasters, evaluate the effectiveness and quality of services, and research new insights and innovative solutions to health problems. *Public Health Workforce Enumeration 2000* data identified 22,000 public health laboratory workers in governmental public health agencies in the year 2000. Far fewer laboratory workers (6,100) were identified in more recent surveys of state and local public health agencies conducted in 2012 and 2013.[3,4]

Public health laboratory scientists are professionals who plan, design, and implement laboratory procedures to identify and quantify agents in the environment that may be hazardous to human health; biologic agents believed to be involved in the etiology of diseases in animals or humans, such as bacteria, viruses, and parasites; or other physical, chemical, and biologic hazards. Titles include microbiologist, chemist, toxicologist, physicist, and entomologist.

Public health laboratories rely heavily on the work of technologists and technicians in order to perform a variety of chemical, serologic, viral, or bacteriologic analyses of clinical or environmental specimens according to established procedures. Work involves performing complex tests under general supervision, ensuring the accuracy of the tests through quality control procedures, notifying appropriate scientific and supervisory staff when a test system is not functioning, and, in consultation with appropriate authorities, implementing and documenting appropriate remedial and corrective actions. Work may also involve communicating with health professionals in other agencies regarding routine questions concerning specimen requirements and tests offered. Work is performed under general supervision; however, public health laboratory scientists are expected to exercise independent judgment within the framework of established procedures and policies.

Public health laboratory scientists include microbiologists, biochemists, and biophysicists. Microbiologists investigate the growth, structure, development, and other characteristics of microscopic organisms, such as bacteria, algae, or fungi. Biochemists and biophysicists study the chemical composition and physical principles of living cells and organisms, their electrical and mechanical energy, and related phenomena. They may conduct research to further understanding of the complex chemical combinations and reactions involved in metabolism, reproduction, growth, and heredity. Biochemists may also determine the effects of foods, drugs, serums, hormones, and other substances on tissues and vital processes of living organisms.

Essential and important duties of a public health laboratory scientist include

- Performs routine serologic tests for the presence of antibodies or antigens to various disease agents
- Performs a variety of bacteriologic examinations for the presence of disease agents or contaminants in clinical or other specimens, such as feces, urine, sputum, spinal fluid, blood cultures, water specimens, dairy products, foods, and beverages
- Performs microscopic examinations of animal heads for rabies

- Performs microscopic examinations for tissue and intestinal protozoans, helminths, and nematodes
- Performs cultural and microscopic examinations for gonorrhea, and cultural, biochemical, and serologic examinations for various species of bacteria
- Performs analytic chemical analysis on clinical and environmental samples using a variety of methodologies and instrumentation
- Evaluates methods and instruments for determination of blood alcohol content in breath, blood, urine, or saliva; periodically performs quality assurance checks of field units; testifies in court as required
- Performs screening and confirmatory tests to detect inborn errors of metabolism and sickle cell disease
- Performs, records, and reviews quality control results to determine the validity, accuracy, or precision of tests performed and to ascertain the quality of reagents, chemicals, or media used for analysis
- Participates in sample accessioning and record keeping to ensure that all specimens are accounted for, appropriately handled, and properly and completely tested
- Records and reports results in the proper manner for the technical area of analysis; checks reports for accuracy; maintains confidentiality of reports
- Consults with public health personnel, physicians, other laboratory workers, and healthcare professionals regarding the interpretation of results, collection of specimens, and the applicability of tests to particular circumstances

Knowledge, skills, and abilities relevant for public health laboratory scientists include

- Knowledge of the principles and practices of microbiology or analytic chemistry
- Knowledge of accepted analytic techniques
- Knowledge of laboratory methods, materials, techniques, and safety procedures
- Knowledge of the principles, practices, and methods of a public health, medical, or other health-related analytic laboratory
- Knowledge of common laboratory equipment and apparatus, and when appropriate, some knowledge of the operation, maintenance, and repair of specific instruments, such as gas chromatographs, atomic absorption units, fluorescent microscopes, and spectrophotometer readers
- Working knowledge of statistics, the metric system, and mathematics for interpreting data and reporting results

- Ability to perceive colors and, when applicable, eyesight sufficiently strong to permit extended microscopic work
- Ability to perform assigned tasks exactly according to prescribed procedures, to accurately observe and interpret results, and to make reports
- Ability to communicate effectively
- Ability to establish and maintain working relationships with staff members, public health personnel, physicians, other laboratories, and the public
- Ability to effectively organize work

Minimum qualifications for public health laboratory scientists often call for 2 years of professional experience as a chemist, microbiologist, medical technologist, or associate public health laboratory scientist, and graduation from an accredited 4-year college or university with a bachelor degree with major specialization in a biologic or chemical science, or medical technology. In some instances, possession of Clinical Laboratory Improvement Amendments of 1988 certification will substitute for the educational requirements. Graduate education in the above areas may substitute on a year-for-year basis for the stated experience.

Microbiologists investigate the growth, structure, development, and other characteristics of microscopic organisms, such as bacteria, algae, or fungi. This category includes medical microbiologists who study the relationship between organisms and disease or the effects of antibiotics on microorganisms. There were 20,000 microbiologists employed in the United States in 2013, with government agencies employing 4,600. Microbiologists employed by government agencies had a median salary of $76,000 in 2013, with the middle 50% earning between $56,000 and $101,000. Mean salaries for microbiologists working for federal agencies are well above the mean salaries at state and local governmental agencies. Only modest growth is projected for this occupation through 2022, with about 7,100 positions to be filled through increased demand and job turnover. Little if any growth is anticipated for microbiology positions employed by government.

Medical and clinical laboratory technologists perform complex medical laboratory tests for the diagnosis, treatment, and prevention of disease. Duties may include training or supervising staff. Medical and clinical laboratory technicians perform routine medical laboratory tests for the diagnosis, treatment, and prevention of disease, often under the supervision of a medical technologist.

Essential and important duties for a public health laboratory technologist include

- Receives, counts, logs, and labels samples submitted by field staff and individuals for testing
- Prepares samples for analysis by racking, centrifuging, filtering, weighing, and so on, and distributes prepared samples to appropriate testing areas
- Pipettes serum samples onto testing plates and adds antigen or reagents in accordance with standard laboratory procedures; stirs, rocks, shakes, and incubates mixture for specified time; reads test results in accordance with established parameters
- Draws blood and collects urine, stool, sputum, and other samples for analysis as ordered by physicians; performs routine analyses of specimens
- Maintains basic records consistent with assigned responsibilities
- Prepares sample specimen kits and shipping boxes for mailing
- Cleans and maintains sample containers, laboratory equipment, and work areas

Key knowledge, skills, and abilities for public health laboratory technologists include

- Knowledge of basic science terminology, concepts, and principles
- Knowledge of laboratory procedures, techniques, and equipment
- Knowledge of blood-drawing techniques
- Ability to properly operate microscopes, centrifuges, autoclaves, sterilizers, or other laboratory equipment
- Ability to apply proper methods of handling and disposing of chemicals and infectious materials
- Ability to perform assigned tasks according to specific instructions and clearly prescribed procedures
- Ability to read, compare, identify, and record laboratory data accurately, such as names, numbers, sample descriptions, and so on
- Ability to perform basic mathematics and make accurate measurements
- Ability to make accurate observations and prepare accurate records of laboratory tests
- Ability to work with other employees, laboratory staff, health professionals, and the general public

Minimum qualifications for these positions may call for 1 year of experience in a medical or public health laboratory

performing routine laboratory tests under the direction of a physician or qualified laboratory technician, and possession of a high school diploma or a general educational development certificate. College coursework with specialization in the chemical, physical, or biologic sciences may substitute on a year-for-year basis for deficiencies in the required experience.

Medical and clinical laboratory technologists numbered 163,000 in 2013. The vast majority work for hospitals, nonhospital-based laboratories, physician offices, and universities. Government agencies employed 7,000 lab technologists. There were 157,000 medical and clinical laboratory technicians employed by the same types of organizations as for lab technologists. Government agencies employed only 5,100 of these workers. The *Public Health Workforce Enumeration 2000* report identified 8,000 public health laboratory technicians working in governmental public health agencies. Despite projections that the number of positions for laboratory technologists and technicians will grow substantially (156,000 positions to be filled due to increased demand and job turnover) between 2012 and 2022, relatively few of these new positions will be filled in the government sector.

The median salary for laboratory technologists employed by government agencies in 2013 was $62,000, with the middle 50% earning between $53,000 and $69,000. Public sector laboratory technicians had a median salary of $40,000 in 2013, with the middle 50% earning between $34,000 and $47,000. Salaries for laboratory technicians working for federal, state, and local governmental agencies are similar.

OPTOMETRISTS

Optometrists diagnose, manage, and treat conditions and diseases of the human eye and visual system. Duties include examining eyes and the visual system, diagnosing problems or impairments, prescribing corrective lenses, and providing treatment. Optometrists may prescribe therapeutic drugs to treat specific eye conditions.

There were 32,000 optometrists in the United States in 2013, with only about 500 working for public sector agencies. The median salary for public sector optometrists in 2013 was $82,000 with the middle 50% earning between $34,000 and $93,000. Job growth for this occupation is expected to be very strong through 2022, with 18,000 positions to be filled through increased demand and job turnover. Jobs will increase very little, if at all, for government agencies.

PHARMACISTS

Pharmacists dispense drugs prescribed by physicians and other health practitioners and provide information to patients about medications and their use. Pharmacists may advise physicians and other health practitioners on the selection, dosage, interactions, and side effects of medications.

Public health pharmacists combine pharmacy and public health skills to plan, organize, and perform drug-related activities with a specific public health focus or within a public health setting. Public health pharmacists may work in agency-run pharmacies or serve as the liaison between private pharmacies and the public health agency in regard to standards, procedures, and education. They also dispense drugs prescribed by physicians and other health practitioners and provide information to patients about medications and their use. Pharmacists advise physicians and other health practitioners on the selection, dosage, interactions, and side effects of medications and are increasingly involved in Strategic National Stockpile planning and operations. The *Public Health Workforce Enumeration 2000* report identified 2,300 public health pharmacists working in federal, state, and local public health agencies in the year 2000.

There were 287,000 pharmacists in the United States in 2013, with only about 9,000 working for public sector agencies. The median salary for public sector pharmacists in 2013 was $110,000 with the middle 50% earning between $97,000 and $119,000. Job growth for this occupation is expected to be moderate through 2022, with 110,000 positions to be filled through increased demand and job turnover. Jobs will increase only slightly for government agencies.

PHYSICIAN ASSISTANTS

Physician assistants (PAs) provide healthcare services typically performed by a physician, under the supervision of a physician. PAs may conduct complete physicals, provide treatment, counsel patients and, in some cases, prescribe medication. Most PAs graduate from an accredited educational program for physician assistants.

There were 88,000 PAs in the United States in 2013, with only about 3,000 working for public sector agencies. The median salary for public sector PAs in 2013 was $88,000 with the middle 50% earning between $78,000 and $95,000. Similar to that for general dentists, job growth for this occupation is expected to be strong through 2022, with 49,000 positions to be filled through increased demand and job turnover. Jobs will increase very little, if at all, for government agencies.

PHYSICIANS

Physicians (general and family practitioners) diagnose, treat, and help prevent diseases and injuries that commonly occur in the general population. General and family practice physicians may refer patients to specialists when needed for further diagnosis or treatment.

Public health physicians identify persons or groups at risk of illness or disability, and develop, implement, and evaluate programs or interventions designed to prevent, treat, or ameliorate such risks. Public health physicians may provide direct medical services within the context of such programs and include physicians with doctor of medicine and doctor of osteopathic medicine degrees working as either generalists or specialists. Relatively few active physicians in the United States work in public health settings, and only a small number of those public health physicians have training in public health or preventive medicine. For example, the number of physicians who are board certified in preventive medicine with a specialization in public health actually decreased from 2,300 in 1980 to 1,800 in 2000. Those with specializations in general preventive medicine increased from 800 to 1,700, and those specializing in occupational medicine increased from 2,400 to 3,000 during that same period. The *Public Health Workforce Enumeration 2000* report identified 9,000 public health physicians working in federal, state, and local public health agencies. Surveys of local and state health departments conducted in 2012 and 2013 identified only about 3,200 public health phyisicns.[3,4] Many public health physicians may fall under other non-physician SOCs, such as chief executive officers, medical and health services managers, and epidemiologists, making a precise enumeration of their number impossible.

There were 121,000 generalist physicians (general and family practitioners) in the United States in 2013, with only about 3,000 working for public sector agencies. The median salary for public sector general physicians in 2013 was $149,000 with the middle 50% earning between $117,000 and $184,000. Overall job growth for this occupation is expected to be strong through 2022, with 49,000 positions to be filled through increased demand and job turnover. Jobs will also increase moderately for government employment.

VETERINARIANS

Veterinarians diagnose, treat, or research diseases and injuries of animals. Some veterinarians conduct research and development, inspect livestock, or care for pets and companion animals. Public health veterinarians/animal control specialists identify and assess health risks to humans from animals; they plan, manage, and evaluate programs to reduce these risks. The *Public Health Workforce Enumeration 2000* study identified more than 3,100 veterinarians and animal control specialists working in governmental public health agencies, indicating that professionals other than veterinarians coordinate and manage animal control programs at the local level.

There were 59,000 veterinarians in the United States in 2013, with only about 2,000 working for public sector agencies. The median salary for public sector veterinarians in 2013 was $85,000 with the middle 50% earning between $76,000 and $95,000. Job growth for this occupation is expected to be strong through 2022, with 31,000 positions to be filled through increased demand and job turnover. Jobs will increase very little for government agencies.

OUTSIDE-THE-BOOK THINKING 13-2

© Alfred Bondarenko/Shutterstock.

What features make one or more of these public health occupations a career worth pursuing?

PUBLIC HEALTH PROGRAM SPECIALISTS

Public health program specialists plan, develop, implement, and evaluate programs or interventions designed to identify persons at risk of specified health problems and to prevent, treat, or ameliorate such problems. This includes public health workers reported as public health program specialists without specific designation of a program, as well as those reported as specialists working in a specific program (e.g., maternal and child health, acquired immune deficiency syndrome awareness, immunization, retail food inspection programs). Public health program specialists have a wide range of educational preparation, including many individuals who have preparation in a specific occupational category or profession (e.g., dental health, environmental health, nutrition, and nursing). The *Public Health Workforce Enumeration 2000* report identified 12,000 public health program specialists.

A large number of public health program specialists work in licensing and regulatory programs performing various types of inspections. Many different titles are used, such as licensure, inspection, and regulatory specialist. These positions audit, inspect, and survey programs, institutions,

equipment, products, and personnel, using approved standards for design or performance. This title includes workers who perform regular inspections of a specified class of sites or facilities, such as restaurants, nursing homes, and hospitals whose personnel and materials present constant and predictable threats to the public, without specification of educational preparation. This classification also includes a number of individuals with preparation in environmental health, nursing, and other health fields. The *Public Health Workforce Enumeration 2000* report identified 21,000 licensure/inspection/regulatory specialists working in federal, state, and local public health agencies.

Public health specialists carry responsibility for planning, performing, or supervising technical and professional work involving public health and consumer protection services. This includes performing inspections, surveys, and investigations to identify and eliminate conditions hazardous to life and health, providing consultative services and assistance in assigned areas of responsibility, ensuring corrective actions are taken to eliminate public health or other hazards, and ensuring compliance with applicable statutes and regulations.

The functions within this job family vary by level and from program to program, but may include the following:

- Develops, implements, and manages projects and initiatives for an assigned program or unit
- Develops and implements activities to ensure effective operations and compliance with established standards and/or contracted goals and objectives
- Serves as a team leader on specific projects
- Coordinates program activities that may include fiscal monitoring; grant writing; monitoring of funded programs or agencies to ensure compliance; report preparation and writing; and assisting with developing and distributing communications, brochures, and educational materials
- Coordinates/oversees activities that may include health education; training; development and oversight of requests for proposals and grants; and developing and distributing communications, brochures, and educational materials
- Collaborates and meets with management staff to -determine program requirements, standards, and goals
- Evaluates projects or initiatives to determine effectiveness and to recommend changes and improvements
- Supervises employees; trains and evaluates staff; and reviews the work of subordinates for completeness, accuracy, and content

- Assists in overseeing specialized research and evaluation projects
- Delivers services according to established program protocols
- Conducts inspections, surveys, and investigations of food establishments, lodging facilities, barber shops, public bathing places, schools, day care centers, nursing homes, hospitals, and other regulated facilities to identify public health hazards or environmental conditions that are detrimental to life and health
- Monitors state food supplies and products; provides training and technical assistance; ensures compliance with applicable laws, rules, and regulations; and assists in the implementation of Hazard Analysis Critical Control Point (HACCP) systems in food establishments and in verifying implementation
- Responds to complaints concerning foodborne illnesses, adulterated foods, food tampering, recalls, insect or rodent infestation, or other issues related to food establishments or the sale of food and food products
- Reviews and acts on various epidemiologic reports and complaints, including animal bites, rabies, and disease outbreaks; conducts environmental assessments and other surveys related to lodging, public bathing, and barber services; and performs inspections for lead contamination and other public health hazards or nuisances
- Provides emergency response services for complaints concerning foodborne illnesses, fires in food establishments, accidents involving the transportation of food, incidents concerning food or water contamination, and power outages or natural disasters involving food products; conducts inspections or investigations on an as-needed basis, including on weekends and at night
- Directs the embargo and disposal of food products found unfit for human consumption; conducts evaluations to determine imminent hazards to life or health that warrant the closure of a facility
- Prepares records, reports, and correspondence concerning regulatory actions as needed; conducts follow-up inspections and surveys to ensure corrective actions have been taken and that public health hazards are eliminated; and testifies at hearings and court proceedings concerning regulatory actions as required

The public health specialist series within a personnel system may include three or more levels that are distinguished by the level of complexity of specific job assignments, the extent of responsibility assigned for specific tasks, the level of expertise required for completion of the assigned work, and the responsibility assigned for providing leadership to others.

For public health program specialists working in an inspection or regulatory program, for example, the entry level of the series involves assigned duties and responsibilities in a training status to build skills in conducting inspections and investigations, performing basic professional analysis, and interpreting state and federal laws. Entry-level public health specialists perform tasks involving the evaluation of inspection or survey data and the preparation of technical records and reports, and assist in making recommendations concerning remedial actions to correct public health hazards and provide for consumer protection.

Knowledge, skills, and abilities required at the entry level include knowledge of the causes, impact, and prevention of public health problems in regulated establishments; food microbiology as it applies to preventing foodborne illness; basic epidemiology and chemistry; mathematical concepts, including basic statistical analysis; food processing techniques such as modified atmospheric packaging; and rules and regulations governing food establishments, public bathing places, nursing homes, schools, day care facilities, or other licensed establishments. Abilities required include the ability to conduct inspections and investigations of regulated facilities; identify the causes of foodborne illnesses and related health hazards; analyze and evaluate environmental and sanitary conditions; organize work and work independently; communicate effectively, both orally and in writing; and use computers to organize data and generate reports.

Experience and education requirements at this level consist of a bachelor degree with at least 30 semester hours in a biologic, medical, or physical science; food science or technology; and chemistry, nutrition, engineering, epidemiology, or closely related scientific field.

Midlevel public health specialist positions involve more advanced assigned duties for inspections, surveys, and investigations related to public health services, consumer protection, and the enforcement of applicable state and federal laws in the assigned area of responsibility. Midlevel public health specialists evaluate inspection and survey data, prepare technical records and reports, make recommendations concerning required remedial actions, and provide technical assistance and training as needed to correct public health or consumer protection problems. Some responsibility may also be assigned for providing limited guidance and training to entry-level employees in performing various consumer protection program duties. In addition, midlevel public health specialist positions may involve a clear specialization in a consumer protection or public health discipline and recognition as an expert in the specialty along with a high degree of technical and administrative freedom to plan, develop, organize, and conduct all phases of the work necessary for completion within broad program guidelines.

Knowledge, skills, and abilities required at this middle level include those identified in the entry level plus the ability to make recommendations concerning the implementation of HACCP systems and verify implementation; conduct preoperational inspections to determine compliance with approved plans; assist in planning and presenting education and training programs; plan and conduct field investigations; ensure that corrective action has been completed to eliminate health hazards; analyze and interpret engineering plans and specifications; and assist in developing HACCP plans for the regulated food industry.

Experience and education requirements at this level consist of those identified for entry-level positions plus 2 years professional work experience in public health or consumer protection or a master's degree in a listed field and successful completion of training in conducting food establishment inspections plus 2 additional years of qualifying experience.

Salary scales vary greatly from agency to agency, although entry-level positions may be in the $30,000–$35,000 range, with midlevel positions in the $40,000–$50,000 range. Higher-level public health specialist positions that oversee several program areas or units can expect salaries equivalent to other midlevel managers in these organizations. Job growth for public health specialists is expected to be about average for all positions in the health field.

POLICY ANALYSTS

Public policy is an important public health tool used to promote conditions in which individuals and communities can be healthy. Public health policy analysts analyze needs and plans for the development of public health and other programs, facilities and resources, and/or analyze and evaluate the implications of alternative policies relating to public health and health care for a defined population. Public health analysts determine the questions that such policies will raise, answer those questions, and help shape policies that make our society a better place to live.

Public health policy analysts function under many different titles, including health planners, researchers, and health economists. Health economists conduct research, prepare reports, or formulate plans to aid in the solution of economic problems arising from the production and distribution of goods and services related to public health and health care. Health economists may collect and process economic and statistical data using econometric and sampling techniques.

Public health policy analysts must be able to dissect a problem, analyze and interpret data, and evaluate and create alternative courses of action. They provide information to government officials and the public about which policies will be most effective in meeting society's public health goals.

Public health policy analysts work in national, state, and local governments, nonprofit agencies, "think tanks," consulting firms, community action groups, and direct service organizations. International health and development organizations also employ public health policy analysts. The *Public Health Workforce Enumeration 2000* report identified nearly 6,000 public health policy analysts, planners, researchers, and economists. Because of the wide variation in titles used for this function, it is likely that there are actually many more public health analyst positions in the public health workforce.

Important and essential duties of a public health policy analyst include

- Conducts site visits to assess the operations and costs of state, federal, and local healthcare programs
- Conducts literature reviews
- Performs quantitative analyses with large databases to determine program outcomes or conduct policy simulations
- Writes chapters of analytic reports and proposals for new projects
- Tracks financial progress of projects using computerized spreadsheets, prepares reports for monthly project reviews, and assists with budget revisions and contract proposals

Key knowledge, skills, and abilities for public health policy analyst positions include

- Knowledge of current policy issues in one or more of the following areas: managed care, public health infrastructure, state health policy, healthcare reimbursement issues, mental health/substance abuse, maternal and child health, disability, long-term care, or other relevant areas
- Knowledge of healthcare policy issues related to employer-based coverage, managed care, Medicaid, Medicare, and the uninsured
- Knowledge of how to use data to affect policy and systemic changes

- Ability to establish collaborative working relationships with diverse interest groups and stakeholders
- Excellent writing and verbal skills, particularly in presenting complex information in a clear, comprehensible format

Minimum qualifications for public health policy analyst positions vary greatly but generally require a master's degree in public policy, public health, economics, statistics, or a related field, or equivalent experience in a clinical field, and extensive knowledge of quantitative and qualitative research methods. In some instances, a bachelor degree and a minimum of 5 years of experience, preferably in healthcare advocacy or policy analysis, may be acceptable. Invariably, work experience with state or federal government, a foundation, a policy research organization, or a healthcare program is desirable.

Salaries for public health analysts vary considerably based on education, experience, and specific duties within an organization. With little information available on employment trends for these positions, it is difficult to assess future job prospects, although the number of such positions does not appear to be declining.

PUBLIC HEALTH INFORMATION SPECIALISTS AND ANALYSTS

Public health information systems and data analysts plan, direct, or coordinate activities in areas such as electronic data processing, information systems, systems analysis, and computer programming. They often work with computer specialists who manage the specialized technical aspects of computer operation, applications, operating systems, and hardware. Common titles include computing consultant, applications programmer, computer service technician, data entry technician, data processing specialist, network technician, information technology specialist, and vital records support specialist. Not included are titles that operate computers as part of administrative or professional tasks.

Important and essential duties of a public health information specialist include

- Plans and coordinates the collection, analysis, and dissemination of complex disease and other health data and information
- Performs health risk and community needs appraisals
- Monitors and evaluates programs for effectiveness and quality

- Collaborates with other agencies, organizations, and stakeholders in the identification and monitoring of community health needs
- Exercises independent judgment in analyzing problems, issues, and situations; develops and implements recommendations
- Plans and conducts meetings
- Presents information and represents the agency at public and other meetings
- Complies with legal standards and requirements
- Collects, researches, verifies, enters, updates, analyzes, summarizes, and presents complex disease and other health information and data
- Records information and data accurately following procedures; prepares complete reports on time with supporting conclusions and recommendations, such as the health status report
- Communicates changes and progress and completes projects on time and within budget
- Formulates recommendations anticipating possible ramifications and appropriately communicates significance of findings

Public health information specialist positions require a bachelor degree in public health or a related field and 5 years of progressively responsible experience in public health evaluation or a related health field. A master's degree in public health is preferred. These positions require knowledge of core public health functions; epidemiologic principles and practices, including symptoms, causes, means of transmission, and methods of control of communicable, chronic, and complex disease; principles of disease investigation, control, and prevention; and emergency response principles and practices. These positions also require familiarity with the operation of computers and a variety of office software including word processing, spreadsheet, database, geographical information systems, mapping, statistical, and other applications related to the area of assignment.

The Public Health Workforce Enumeration 2000 study identified 900 health information specialists and 6,000 computer specialists working for governmental public health agencies. Surveys conducted in 2012 and 2013 identified 3,500 health information specialists working in state and local public health agencies.[3,4] Salaries for health information specialists are often in the $40,000–$50,000 range. Health information specialist jobs are projected to be among the fastest growing in the health sector.

OUTSIDE-THE-BOOK THINKING 13-3

© Alfred Bondarenko/Shutterstock.

In which organizations and geographic regions will the public health occupations presented in this chapter expand most rapidly in the next two decades?

ADDITIONAL INFORMATION

Many sources provide additional and more detailed information for the occupational categories addressed in this chapter.

The American Public Health Association (APHA, www.apha.org) has sections that focus on issues important to each of these occupational categories, including food and nutrition; social work; mental health; alcohol, tobacco, and other drugs; medical care; and oral health. APHA also has a laboratory special interest group, veterinary public health special interest group, and public health law forum.

ASTPHND (www.astphnd.org/) provides information on and resources for public health nutrition professionals. Another resource for nutritionists is the ADA (www.eatright.org/Public/), which has 65,000 members and works in concert with the CDR (www.cdrnet.org/). More than 80,000 dietitians and dietetic technicians across the country and the world have taken CDR exams over the past several decades. CDR currently awards four separate and distinct credentials: RD; Dietetic Technician, Registered; Board Certified Specialist in Renal Nutrition; and Board Certified Specialist in Pediatric Nutrition. The commission's certification programs are fully accredited by the National Commission for Certifying Agencies, the accrediting arm of the National Organization for Competency Assurance.

Web sites of the National Association of Social Workers (www.socialworkers.org) and the Council on Social Work Education (www.cswe.org) provide information on accredited social work programs. The Association of Social Work Boards (www.aswb.org) is a good source of information on licensing requirements and testing procedures used for state licensing purposes.

Information on public health laboratory workers is available from the Association for Public Health Laboratories (www.aphl.org) and the National Center for Public Health Laboratory Leadership (http://www.aphl.org/mycareer/

lablead/pages/default.aspx). The American College of Preventive Medicine (www.acpm.org) and American Medical Association (www.amaassn.org/) Web sites provide information on public health physicians.

The Community Health Planning and Policy Development section of the American Public Health Association (APHA) Web site (www.apha.org) provides useful information for public health policy analysts. Similarly, the American Health Information Management Association (AHIMA, www.ahima.org) is the premier association of health information management professionals, with 50,000 members committed to advancing the health information management profession. AHIMA focuses on advocacy, education, certification, and lifelong learning and works through the Commission on Accreditation for Health Informatics and Information Management Education (CAHIM) to accredit degree-granting programs in health informatics and information management. CAHIM establishes quality standards for the educational preparation of future health information management professionals.

CONCLUSION

Professionals comprise the major share of the public health workforce, although public health professionals are quite diverse in terms of their professional background and experience. Nutritionists are valuable resources for public health agencies and the communities they serve, although most nutritionist positions work within the massive federally funded WIC program. More local public health agencies than state public health agencies provide social, mental, and behavioral health services, because these programs may be funded by and relate to state agencies other than the state health agency in many states. Public health laboratory expertise is essential for disease and threat detection, and one of the major impacts of increased federal spending for terrorism preparedness is resulting in upgraded lab capabilities for state and local public health agencies. Recruiting and retaining the many levels of laboratory professionals and technicians necessary for lab operations has emerged as an important priority for public health as well as national security concerns. Physicians once dominated the field of public health. Today they represent one of many important professions within the public health workforce, standing beside veterinarians, pharmacists, and dental health workers. The regulatory and administrative processes within governmental public health agencies now require a level of legal expertise beyond that called for in the past. These many and varied professional categories provide public health with the multidisciplinary and interdisciplinary muscle needed to battle modern public health threats and issues. Public health organizations use many different titles for public health program staff. Indeed, most public health workers function within a defined program or program-related unit such as environmental health, maternal and child health, Supplemental Food Program for Women, Infants, and Children, or immunization program.

Program specialists work on all aspects of program planning, implementation, and evaluation in concert with professionals, technicians, and administrative support personnel. Because the programs in which they work often have specific goals and objectives, program specialists are at risk of operating in an isolated environment. This contributes to the critique that programs operate as silos within an agency, often unrelated to the operation of the many other silos housed within that same agency. Because of their generalist skills, program specialists may move from one program to another as a means of career and salary advancement. Their crosscutting, core, generalist public health practice skills are generally acquired through work experiences rather than academic preparation. The size and impact of this corps of public health program specialists argue that development and enhancement of these crosscutting competencies should be a central strategy of public health workforce development efforts.

REFERENCES

1. Bureau of Labor Statistics, U.S. Department of Labor. Databases and tables. www.bls.gov/data/. Accessed June 15, 2014.
2. Health Resources and Services Administration, Bureau of Health Professions, National Center for Health Workforce Information and Analysis and Center for Health Policy, Columbia School of Nursing. *Public Health Workforce Enumeration 2000*. Washington, DC: HRSA; 2000.
3. National Association of County and City Health Officials. *2013 National Profile of Local Health Departments*. Washington, DC: NACCHO; 2014.
4. Association of State and Territorial Health Officials. *State Health Profile, Volume Three, 2012*. Washington, DC: ASTHO; 2014.

CHAPTER **14**

Public Health Practice: Future Challenges

This text approaches what public health is and how it works from a unified conceptual framework. Key dimensions of the public health system are examined, including its purpose, functions, capacity, processes, and outcomes. Although it is a simple framework, many of the concepts addressed are anything but simple. As a result, much has been left unsaid, and many important issues and problems facing the public health system have been addressed only in passing. This may serve to whet the appetite of those eager to move beyond the basics and ready to tackle emerging and more complex issues in greater depth. The basic concepts included in this text seek to facilitate that process and encourage outside-the-book thinking. Delving into these other issues without the benefit of a broad understanding of the field and how it works, however, can be hazardous in any field of endeavor. For public health workers, continuously fighting off alligators remains the major deterrent to draining the swamp in order to avert the alligator threat in the first place.

The public health achievements of the 20th century demonstrate that the problems facing public health have

changed over the past century and argue that we can expect them to continue to change throughout the current century. In retrospect, many past problems appear as though they should have been relatively easy to solve in comparison with those on the public health agenda at the beginning of the 21st century; however, we often forget that last century's problems appeared to be quite formidable to public health advocates 100 years ago. Although formidable, they were eventually deemed unacceptable, initiating the chain of events that resulted in an impressive catalog of accomplishments ranging from infectious disease threats to oral health.

Each public health achievement provides valuable lessons and insights into the obstacles to achieving even further gains that lie ahead. Challenges reside at many levels, especially at the level of preparedness for unforeseen and previously unanticipated threats to the public's health. Melding the expectations for addressing ongoing health problems in the community with those for preparing and responding to new threats leads us to the three key questions addressed in this chapter:

1. What are the lessons learned from the threats and challenges faced by public health in 20th century America?
2. What are the limitations and challenges facing public health in the 21st century?
3. How can these limitations and challenges be overcome?

LESSONS FROM A CENTURY OF PROGRESS IN PUBLIC HEALTH

The remarkable achievements of the 20th century did not completely eradicate the public health problems faced in

FIGURE 14-1 Past and Projected Female and Male Expectancy at Birth, United States, 1900–2050

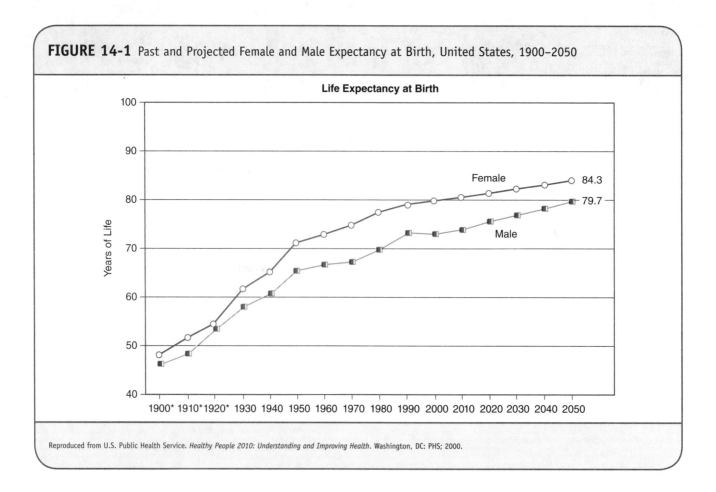

Reproduced from U.S. Public Health Service. *Healthy People 2010: Understanding and Improving Health*. Washington, DC: PHS; 2000.

1900. Many of these continue to threaten the health of Americans and impede progress toward realizing the life span projections presented in **Figure 14-1**. New faces for old enemies have appeared in the form of challenges and obstacles to be overcome in the early decades of the 21st century. Infectious diseases, tobacco, maternal and infant mortality, environmental and occupational health, food safety, cardiovascular disease, injuries, and oral health remain high on the list of leading threats to the public's health. Each presents special challenges.

Infectious Diseases

The continuing battle against infectious diseases will be fought on several fronts because of the emergence of new infectious diseases and the reemergence of old enemies, often in drug-resistant forms. For example, infections caused by Escherichia coli O157:H7 have emerged as a frequent and frightening risk to the public. Initially identified as the cause of hemorrhagic conditions in the early 1980s, this pathogen was increasingly associated with foodborne illness outbreaks in the 1990s, including a major outbreak in the Pacific

Northwest related to E. coli-contaminated hamburgers distributed through a national fast food chain.[1] The source of the E. coli was cattle. Other outbreaks of this pathogen involved swimmers in lake water contaminated by bathers infected with the organism (**Figure 14-2**). Because many of the illnesses are minor and both medical and public health practitioners fail to perform the tests necessary to diagnose E. coli infections properly, current surveillance efforts greatly underreport the extent of this condition.

Multidrug-resistant pathogens represent another emerging infectious disease problem for the public health system. The widespread and, at times, indiscriminate use of antibiotics in agricultural and healthcare settings produces strains of bacteria that are resistant to these drugs. Antimicrobial agents have been increasingly deployed throughout the second half of the 20th century. Slowly, over this period, the consequences of these miracle drugs have been experienced in our communities, as well as our health facilities. The emergence of drug-resistant strains has reduced the effectiveness of treatment for several common infections, including tuberculosis, gonorrhea, pneumococcal infections,

FIGURE 14-2 Emergence of a Public Health Threat: The Escherichia coli 0157: H7 Time Line

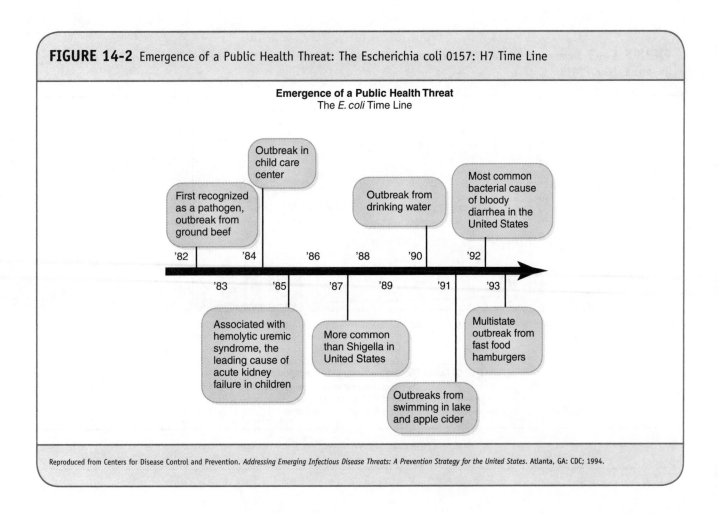

Reproduced from Centers for Disease Control and Prevention. *Addressing Emerging Infectious Disease Threats: A Prevention Strategy for the United States.* Atlanta, GA: CDC; 1994.

and hospital-acquired staphylococcal and enterococcal infections. For tuberculosis, drug resistance and demographic trends, including immigration policies, played substantial roles in this disease's resurgence in the early 1990s. The changing demographics of tuberculosis infections are illustrated in **Figure 14-3**.

Pathogens, both old and new, have devised ingenious ways of adapting to and thwarting the weapons used to control them. Many factors in society, the environment, and global interconnectedness continue to increase the risk of emergence and spread of infectious diseases. An outbreak of monkeypox virus affecting several states in the United States in 2003 demonstrates how unusual diseases in remote parts of the world can affect Americans virtually overnight (**Figure 14-4**). In 2014, Middle East Respiratory Syndrome (MERS) made its first appearance in the United States, again illustrating this threat.

The potential for global outbreaks and massive pandemics is now on the public health radar screen. An outbreak of severe acute respiratory syndrome hit more than two dozen countries in North America, South America, Europe, and Asia in 2003 before it was contained, but not before taking nearly 800 lives. The possibility of a global pandemic of influenza virus looms as even more frightening because it is impossible to predict when the next influenza pandemic will occur or how severe it will be. Wherever and whenever a pandemic starts, everyone everywhere in the world is at risk. Countries might, through measures such as border closures and travel restrictions, delay arrival of the virus, but cannot stop it.

Health professionals remain concerned that the continued spread of a highly pathogenic avian H5N1 virus across eastern Asia and other countries represents a significant threat to human health. The H5N1 virus has raised concerns about a potential human pandemic because:

- It is especially virulent.
- It is being spread by migratory birds.
- It can be transmitted from birds to mammals and in some limited circumstances to humans.
- Like other influenza viruses, it continues to evolve.

FIGURE 14-3 Number and Rate of Tuberculosis Cases Among U.S.-Born and Foreign-Born Persons, by Year Reported, 2000–2013

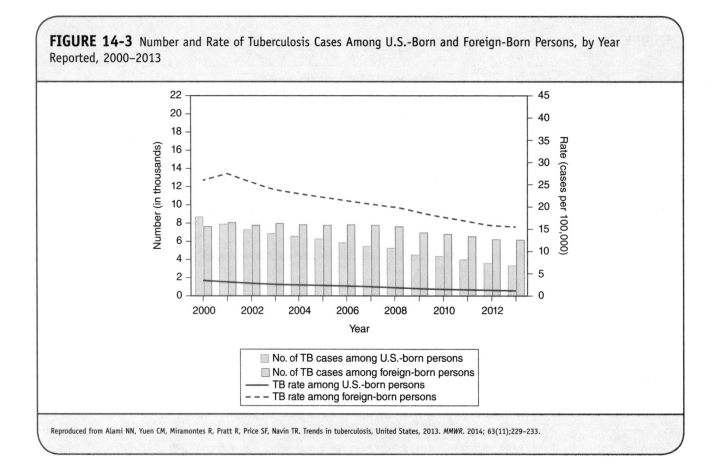

Reproduced from Alami NN, Yuen CM, Miramontes R, Pratt R, Price SF, Navin TR. Trends in tuberculosis, United States, 2013. *MMWR*. 2014; 63(11);229–233.

Since 2003, a growing number of human H5N1 cases have been reported in Asia, Africa, and Europe. More than half of the people infected with the H5N1 virus have died. Most of these cases are all believed to have been caused by exposure to infected poultry. There has been no sustained human-to-human transmission of the disease, but the concern is that H5N1 will evolve into a virus capable of human-to-human transmission.

A massive epidemic of Ebola virus disease, a rare and deadly disease previously known as Ebola hemorrhagic fever, led to an unprecedented international response in 2014 after the case count in West Africa (Guinea, Liberia, Nigeria, Sierra Leone) surpassed 10,000 with case fatality rates in the 70% range (see **Figure 14-5** and **Table 14-1**). This explosion of cases occurred after decades of smaller, intermittent outbreaks affecting a dozen countries in Africa. The importation of travel-related cases to the United States and elsewhere outside West Africa in late 2014, leading to cases among several health care workers, further demonstrated the global risks associated with uncontrolled local outbreaks and the

importance of vigilance and preparedness in dealing with unfamiliar pathogens.

Heightened concerns over the risk of acts of bioterrorism add a new twist to the threats posed by infectious diseases. As noted in our examination of public health emergency preparedness and response, these concerns have raised expectations for public health to serve both national security and personal safety roles.

The influence of infectious diseases in the development of chronic diseases such as diabetes, heart disease, and some cancers further argues that infectious diseases will continue as important health risks in the new century. To battle infectious diseases, the development and deployment of new methods, both in laboratory and epidemiologic sciences, are needed to better understand the interactions among environmental factors as contributors to the emergence and reemergence of infectious disease processes. Also, despite the successes realized in the development and use of vaccines over the past century, substantial gaps persist in the infrastructure of the vaccine delivery system,

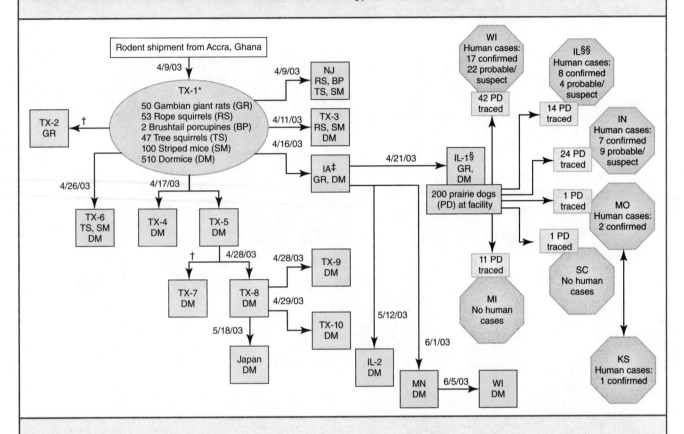

FIGURE 14-4 Movement of Imported African Rodents to Animal Distributors and Distribution of Prairie Dogs from an Animal Distributor Associated with Human Cases of Monkeypox, 11 States, 2003

Notes:

Illinois (IL), Indiana (IN), Iowa (IA), Kansas (KS), Michigan (MI), Minnesota (MN), Missouri (MO), New Jersey (NJ), South Carolina (SC), Texas (TX), and Wisconsin (WI). Japan is included among sites having received rodents implicated in the outbreak.

† Date of shipment unknown.
* Identified as distributor C in MMWR 2003;52:561–564.
§ Identified as distributor B in MMWR 2003;52:561–564.
‡ Identified as distributor D in MMWR 2003;52:561–564.
§§ Includes two persons who were employees at IL-1.

Reproduced from Centers for Disease Control and Prevention. Update: multi-state outbreak of monkeypox—Illinois, Indiana, Kansas, Missouri, Ohio, and Wisconsin, 2003. *MMWR.* 2003;52(27):642–646.

including the roles played by parents, providers, information technology, and biotech and pharmaceutical companies. Improving the coordination of these elements holds the promise of reducing the toll from infectious diseases in the 21st century.

Tobacco Use

The potential gains to be realized from further reduction of tobacco usage are also apparent. Despite the overall decline in tobacco use among adults over the second half of the 20th century, an alarmingly high prevalence of tobacco use among teens persists, and rates among adults are no longer declining, as they did prior to 1980. These trends suggest that concerns over risks related to exposure to environmental tobacco smoke will continue for many years to come. Disparities in tobacco use by race and ethnicity, together with the growth of demographic groups with high use rates, add yet another dimension to the war against tobacco. New approaches and new products will raise new issues of safety, whereas the increase in tobacco use across the globe will transport old and new challenges around the world.

FIGURE 14-5 Cases of Ebola Virus Disease in Africa, 1976-2014

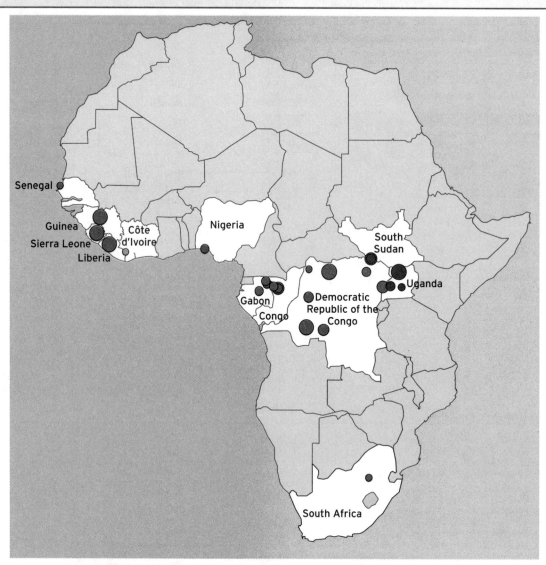

EBOLAVIRUS OUTBREAKS BY SPECIES AND SIZE, 1976-2014

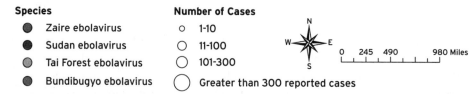

Species	Number of Cases
● Zaire ebolavirus	○ 1-10
● Sudan ebolavirus	○ 11-100
● Tai Forest ebolavirus	○ 101-300
● Bundibugyo ebolavirus	○ Greater than 300 reported cases

Source: Reproduced from Centers for Disease Control and Prevention. Ebola Virus Distribution Map. Available at http://www.cdc.gov/vhf/ebola/outbreaks/history/distribution-map.html. Accessed November 4, 2014.

TABLE 14-1   Ebola Virus Disease – Known Cases and Outbreaks in Reverse Chronological Order, Various Countries, 1976-2014 (through 11/3/2014)

Country	Cases	Deaths	Species	Year
Dem. Rep. of Congo	66	49	*Zaire ebolavirus*	2014
Multiple countries	13540	4941	*Zaire ebolavirus*	2014
Uganda	6*	3*	*Sudan ebolavirus*	2012
Dem. Rep. of Congo	36*	13*	*Bundibugyo ebolavirus*	2012
Uganda	11*	4*	*Sudan ebolavirus*	2012
Uganda	1	1	*Sudan ebolavirus*	2011
Dem. Rep. of Congo	32	15	*Zaire ebolavirus*	2008
Uganda	149	37	*Bundibugyo ebolavirus*	2007
Dem. Rep. of Congo	264	187	*Zaire ebolavirus*	2007
South Sudan	17	7	*Zaire ebolavirus*	2004
Republic of Congo	35	29	*Zaire ebolavirus*	2003
Republic of Congo	143	128	*Zaire ebolavirus*	2002
Republic of Congo	57	43	*Zaire ebolavirus*	2001
Gabon	65	53	*Zaire ebolavirus*	2001
Uganda	425	224	*Zaire ebolavirus*	2000
South Africa	2	1	*Zaire ebolavirus*	1996
Gabon	60	45	*Zaire ebolavirus*	1996
Gabon	37	21	*Zaire ebolavirus*	1996
Dem. Rep. of Congo	315	250	*Zaire ebolavirus*	1995
Côte d'Ivoire (Ivory Coast)	1	0	*Taï Forest ebolavirus*	1994
Gabon	52	31	*Zaire ebolavirus*	1994
South Sudan	34	22	*Sudan ebolavirus*	1979
Dem. Rep. of Congo	1	1	*Zaire ebolavirus*	1977
South Sudan	284	151	*Sudan ebolavirus*	1976
Dem. Rep. of Congo	318	280	*Zaire ebolavirus*	1976

Notes: *Numbers reflect laboratory confirmed cases only. 2014 Democratic Republic of Congo outbreak not related to 2014 outbreak involving multiple countries; Multiple countries in 2014 include Liberia, Sierra Leone, Nigeria, Guinea, United States, Senegal and Spain as of November 4, 2014.

Source: Data from Centers for Disease Control and Prevention. Available at http://www.cdc.gov/vhf/ebola/outbreaks/history/chronology.html. Accessed November 4, 2014

Maternal and Child Health

Even as maternal and child health outcomes have improved dramatically, there has been little change in the prime determinants of perinatal outcomes—the rate of low birth weight and preterm deliveries. This situation must be addressed to even partially replicate the gains realized in the 20th century. Another important risk factor moving in the wrong direction is the rate of unintended pregnancies. Together, these challenges call for improved understanding of the biologic,

social, cultural, economic, psychological, and environmental factors that influence maternal and infant health outcomes and in the effectiveness of intervention strategies designed to address these causative factors.

Motor Vehicle Injuries

The impressive gains realized in reducing motor vehicle injuries have uncovered gaps in our understanding of comprehensive prevention. Challenges include expanding surveillance to monitor nonfatal injuries, detect new problems, and set priorities. Greater research into emerging and priority problems, as well as intervention effectiveness, is also needed, as are more effective collaborations and interagency partnerships. Injuries to pedestrians from vehicles other than automobiles will also challenge public health in the 21st century. The effects of age, alcohol use, seat belt use, and interventions targeting these risks will require greater attention for progress to continue in the battle against motor vehicle injuries.

Cardiovascular Disease

An aging population less threatened by infectious disease and injury will place even more people at risk of ill health related to cardiovascular diseases. Greater attention to research to understand the various social, psychological, environmental, physiologic, and genetic determinants of cardiovascular diseases is needed in the new century. Reducing disparities that exist in terms of burden of disease, prevalence of risk factors, and ability to reach high-risk populations represents another mega challenge. Identifying new and emerging risk factors and their relationships, including genetic and infectious disease factors, will be necessary in both developed and developing parts of the world.

Food Safety

Our understanding of food safety and nutrition made great strides in the 1900s, but both old and new risks will need to be addressed in the new century. Iron and folate deficiencies continue, and many of the advantages related to breastfeeding remain unrealized. The emergence of obesity, often in the midst of food deserts, as an increasingly prevalent condition throughout the population is one of the most startling developments of the late 20th century. Persistent challenges include applying new information about nutrition, dietary patterns, and behavior that promote health and reduce the risk of chronic diseases.

Oral Health

One of the most overlooked achievements of public health in the 20th century was the dramatic decline in dental caries due to fluoridation of drinking water supplies. Ironically, these advances in oral health have contributed to the perception that dental caries are no longer a significant public health problem and that fluoridation is no longer needed. These battles are likely to be fought in political, rather than scientific, arenas, presenting a substantial challenge to public health in the 21st century.

Workplace Safety

Workplaces are now safer than ever before, yet challenges remain on this front, as well. Improved surveillance of work-related injuries and illnesses and better methods of conducting field investigations in high-risk occupations and industries remain formidable challenges. Applying new methods of risk assessment to improve assessment of injury exposures and intervention outcomes, as well as improved research into intervention effectiveness, surveillance methods, and organization of work represent additional challenges for public health practice in the 21st century.

Unfinished Agenda

It is clear that much remains to be done. The national Healthy People process articulates this unfinished agenda by identifying important targets and leading indicators of health status for the United States.[2] These health problems persist on the public health agenda, which has now expanded to include new issues related to alcohol and substance abuse, mental health, violence, and risky sexual behaviors. These are now categorized as important public health problems and have taken their rightful place on the public health agenda. Progress toward these leading health indicators documents the challenges that lie ahead. The public health challenges of the 21st century appear daunting, but those of the preceding century must have seemed even more so.

Applying the lessons learned from the recent century of progress in public health to both new and persisting health threats will be necessary to increase the span of healthy life and eliminate the huge disparities in health outcomes that are the overarching goals of the year 2020 national health objectives. The public health challenges of both centuries call for the application of sound science in an environment that supports social justice in health. This remains the most formidable challenge facing public health practice in the 21st century.

OUTSIDE-THE-BOOK THINKING 14-1

© Alfred Bondarenko/Shutterstock.

What was the most important achievement of public health in the 20th century? Why?

What will likely be the most important achievement of public health in the 21st century? Why?

LIMITATIONS OF 21ST-CENTURY PUBLIC HEALTH

Despite the remarkable achievements of the 20th century, there is much for public health to do in the early decades of the new century. Continued progress is by no means assured because of a new constellation of problems and important limitations of conventional public health efforts. Global environmental threats, the disruption of vital ecosystems, global population overload, persistent and widening social injustice and health inequalities, and lack of access to effective care add to the list of health problems left over from the 20th century.[3] Consider, for example, the implications of the link between social position and health, and a nation growing more and more diverse, with a disproportionate burden of poverty falling on children, minorities, and one-parent families. Further gains in health status may be less related to science than to social policies. For some public health professionals, the limitations of conventional public health are difficult to accept because, in large part, they represent the supporting pillars of the public health enterprise. This reluctance to critically self-assess makes future progress less certain. It is useful to examine these limitations in terms of their relationship to the two major forces shaping public health responses—science and social values.

Among the limitations affecting the science of public health is an undue emphasis on reductionist thinking that seeks molecular-level explanations for social and structural phenomena. Identification of risk factors has been useful for public health efforts, but the emphasis on individual risk factors often obscures patterns that call for multilevel responses. The persistent identification of the association of social deprivation with many of the important health problems of the last century is a case in point. Approaches for reducing coronary heart disease provide another example. Health interventions targeting a reduction in coronary heart disease frequently focus on risk factors at the physiologic level, such as blood pressure control, cholesterol, and obesity and on lifestyle factors at the individual level, including smoking, nutrition, physical activity, and psychosocial factors. However, there are also environmental influences, such as geographic location, housing conditions, occupational risks, and social structure influences, such as social class, age, gender, and race/ethnicity. In this multilevel view of coronary heart disease, interventions that focus on primary and secondary prevention (those addressing the physiologic and individual levels) need to be supplemented by organization-level and community-level interventions (addressing environmental influences) and healthy public policy (addressing the social structure level).

Another limitation of public health's scientific heritage is the penchant for dichotomous thinking and the failure to view health phenomena as continuous. Using coronary heart disease as an example, dichotomous thinking draws attention to individual and physiologic level factors, whereas viewing this condition as continuous encourages a population-wide view and development of interventions that reduce overall incidence and prevalence by affecting frequency distributions in the entire population. A view of health problems as continuous phenomena suggests that efforts be made throughout the population to move the entire frequency distribution for coronary heart disease "to the left," rather than to reduce disease burden only among those groups most heavily impacted. Here it is apparent that science and social values are not pure and mutually exclusive forces.

Discussion and debate over scientific approaches to public health problems are not, however, purely scientific in nature. At the heart of collective actions are collective values as to whether issues affecting individuals are more important than issues affecting communities of individuals and as to the meaning of health itself. Should public health emphasize the health of individuals or the health of communities? In part, these reflect the different perspectives of health described in other chapters. On one hand is a mechanistic view of health as the absence of disease, promoting health interventions that emphasize curative treatment for afflicted individuals. On the other hand is a more holistic view of health that sees health as a complex equilibrium of forces and factors necessary for optimal functioning of that individual. This latter view emphasizes health maintenance and health promotion, often through broad social policies affecting the entire community. Differences in public health systems among societies are largely described by these differences. Some societies, like the United States, focus on individuals using a largely medical treatment approach. Others are more heavily influenced by collectivism and a holistic view of health. At the core of what can be accomplished under either view, however, are basic values and social philosophies that guide the use of the scientific knowledge available at any point in time. These differences in social values also affect perceptions as to what is expected of government and, as a result, the form and leadership of public health efforts. To a large extent, these forces have hastened the development of community public health practice and career opportunities in public health in the United States, a phenomenon described in previous chapters.

THE FUTURE OF PUBLIC HEALTH IN 1988 AND A QUARTER CENTURY LATER

In many respects, the limitations of modern public health are as apparent as its achievements. Persisting, emerging, reemerging, and newly assigned problems will forever challenge public health as a social enterprise. Success will depend on both the structure and the content of the public health response. A continuous, critical, and comprehensive self-examination of the public health enterprise offers the greatest chance for continued success. A series of such self-examinations began with the 1988 report of Institute of Medicine (IOM), The Future of Public Health.[4] A comprehensive reexamination, The Future of the Public's Health in the 21st Century, was completed in 2002.[5] A companion study of issues related to educating public health professionals was also completed by the IOM in 2002.[6] These examinations outlined the limitations of public health efforts in the 20th century, but cast these failings as lessons, challenges, and opportunities for public health in the 21st century.

The Future of Public Health, 1988

The IOM's landmark report, completed in 1988, found much of value in the nation's public health efforts, but it also identified a long list of problems. The most serious problem of all was that Americans were taking their public health system for granted. The nation had come to believe that epidemics of communicable diseases were a thing of the past and that food and water would forever be free of infectious and toxic agents. Americans assumed that workplaces, restaurants, and homes were safe and that everyone had access to the information and skills needed to lead healthy lives. They also assumed that all of this could occur even while public health agencies were being increasingly called on to provide health services to nearly 50 million Americans who had no health insurance or were underinsured; however, across the nation, states and localities were failing to provide the resources that would allow both the traditional public health and more recent health service roles to be carried out successfully. When future benefits compete with immediate needs, the results are predictable.

These circumstances fostered the image of a public health system in disarray. Within this system, neither the public nor those involved in the work of public health appreciated the scope and content of public health in modern America. There was little consensus as to the specific responsibilities to be expected from the various levels of government and even less interest in securing such consensus.

Previous chapters document that several formulations in the IOM report have been widely embraced by the public

health community. These include statements of the mission, substance, and core functions of public health. The mission has been described simply as ensuring conditions in which people can be healthy. The substance consists largely of organized community efforts to promote health and prevent disease. The IOM report identified an essential role for government in public health in organizing and ensuring that the mission gets addressed. An expanded view of the fundamental functions of governmental public health was articulated in the three core functions of assessment, policy development, and assurance. These represent a more comprehensive view of public health efforts than that conveyed by earlier views that public health primarily furnished services and enforced statutes. The new public health differed in its emphasis on problem identification and resolution as the basis of rational interventions and on working with and through other stakeholders, rather than intervening unilaterally.

Perhaps the most motivating aspect of the IOM report, however, was its characterization of the disarray of public health and the significance of that disarray. The IOM report painted a picture of disjointed efforts in the 1980s to deal with immediate crises, such as the epidemic of human immunodeficiency virus infections and an increasing lack of access to health services and enduring problems with significant social impacts, such as injuries, teen pregnancy, hypertension, depression, and tobacco and drug use. With impending crises on the horizon in the form of toxic substances, mental illness, Alzheimer's disease, and public health capacity, the IOM report found the situation to be grimmer still.

The report found a wide gap between the capacity of the public health system of the 1980s and those of a public health system capable of rising to modern challenges. It charted a course to move ever closer to an optimally functioning system. Several enabling steps were identified:

- Improving the statutory base of public health
- Strengthening the structural and organizational framework
- Improving the capacity for action, including technical, political, management, programmatic, and fiscal competencies of public health professionals
- Strengthening linkages between academia and practice[4]

In the end, the report concluded that working through a multitude of society's institutions, rather than through only traditional public health organizations, is the key to improving the public health system. It is also a daunting task, calling for entering into partnerships with sectors such as education, law enforcement, media, faith, corrections, and business, and fostering change through leadership and influence, rather than through command and control. The barriers to effecting these collaborations are the major obstacles to achieving the aspirations outlined in the Healthy People national health objectives. These barriers come in all sizes and shapes and from many different sources. Some are perceived as external barriers; others appear to be more internal.

The IOM report identified important barriers inhibiting effective public health action:

- Lack of consensus on the content of the public health mission
- Inadequate capacity to carry out the essential public health functions of assessment, policy development, and assurance of services
- Disjointed decision making without necessary data and knowledge
- Inequities in the distribution of services and the benefits of public health
- Limits on effective leadership, including poor interaction among the technical and political aspects of decisions, rapid turnover of leaders, and inadequate relationships with the medical profession
- Organizational fragmentation or submersion
- Problems in relationships among the several levels of government
- Inadequate development of necessary knowledge across the full array of public health needs
- Poor public image of public health, inhibiting necessary support
- Special problems that unduly limit the financial resources available to public health[4]

The Future of Public Health, A Quarter Century Later

The IOM advanced these themes through several other reports published in the 1990s and early years of the new century. A brief status report on progress in implementing the 1988 report's major recommendations was completed in the mid-1990s, and a report promoting community health improvement processes appeared later in the decade. A full scale reexamination of the public health enterprise, titled *The Future of the Public's Health in the 21st Century*, was undertaken after the turn of the century and completed in late 2002. That report focused more extensively on multisectoral partnerships with government than had the 1988 report, which mainly emphasized government's role in achieving public health goals.

The 2002 IOM report restated the unique responsibility that government has for promoting and protecting the health of its people. It noted, however, that four factors argue that government alone should not bear full responsibility for the health of the public:

1. Public resources are limited, and public health spending must compete with other valid causes.
2. Democratic societies expressly limit the powers of government and reserve many activities for private institutions.
3. Determinants affecting health derive from multiple sources and sectors, including many social determinants that cannot be addressed by government alone.
4. There is growing evidence that multisectoral collaborations are more powerful and effective than government acting alone.[5]

In light of these factors, the 2002 IOM report examined both the governmental contributions to the public's health and those from other sectors of American society. Recommendations for the governmental enterprise were complemented by recommendations for healthcare providers, business, media, the faith community, and academia. The report proposed six major areas for action:

1. Adopting a population health approach that considers the multiple determinants of health within an ecological framework
2. Strengthening the governmental public health infrastructure, which forms the backbone of the public health system
3. Building a new generation of intersectoral partnerships that also draw on the perspectives and resources of diverse communities and actively engages them in health actions
4. Developing systems of accountability to ensure the quality and availability of public health services
5. Making evidence the foundation of decision making and the measure of success
6. Enhancing and facilitating communication within the public health system (e.g., among all levels of the governmental public health infrastructure, between public health professionals and community members)[5]

Barriers to future progress are apparent in both major IOM reports. Foremost has been the lack of a social-ecological view of health that attempts to understand good and poor health in terms of the multiple factors that interact with each other at the personal, family, community, and population level. Another set of important barriers affecting public health is the prevailing values of the American public—in particular, those restricting the ability of government to identify and address factors that influence health. Social values determine the extent to which government can regulate human behavior, such as through controlling the production and use of tobacco products or requiring bicycle or motorcycle helmet use. These values also determine whether and to what extent family planning or school-based clinic services are provided in a community and determine the content of school health education curricula. Some of these social values find strange bedfellows. For example, many Americans oppose control of firearms on the basis of principles of self-protection embodied in the U.S. Constitution; gun companies also oppose control, although on the basis of more direct economic considerations.

Economic and resource considerations are common themes, as well. One obvious issue is that most public health activities remain funded from the discretionary budgets of local, state, and federal government. At all levels, discretionary programs have been squeezed by true entitlement programs, such as Medicaid and Medicare, as well as by some governmental responsibilities that have become near entitlements, such as public safety, law enforcement, corrections, and education. The war on terrorism with military campaigns in Iraq and Afghanistan further squeezed the national budget and any chance of significant health or human service initiatives at home. Funding one set of health-related services from governmental discretionary funds while other health services are financed through a competitive marketplace widens the imbalance between treatment and prevention as investment strategies for improved health status. There are powerful economic interests among health sector industries, as well as among industries whose products affect health, such as the tobacco, alcohol, pesticide, and firearms industries. One can only dream that equally powerful lobbies, other than those made up of pharmaceutical companies, might develop for hepatitis or drug-resistant tuberculosis.

All too often, the complex problems and issues of public health, with causes and contributing factors perceived to lie outside its boundaries, lead public health professionals to believe that they should not be held accountable for failure or success; however, many facets of public health practice itself could be further improved. These include relationships with the private sector and medical practice and some internal reengineering of public health processes. Fear and suspicion of the private sector can lead to many missed opportunities. Just as the three most important factors determining real estate values are location, location, and location, it can be argued that the three most important factors for health are

jobs, jobs, and jobs. If this is anywhere near true, suspicions of the private sector need to be put to rest. There is little question that employment is a powerful preventive health intervention, in terms of both individual and community health status. Community development activities that bring new businesses and jobs to a community can affect health status more positively than a public health clinic on every corner. Furthermore, businesses have been major forces behind the growth of managed care systems in the United States. Their partnership with public health interests will be essential to secure new resources or to shift the balance between treatment and prevention strategies. Increased partnerships with medical care interests will also be necessary. Unfortunately, there is widespread ignorance of the medical care sector among public health workers.

Among barriers internal to public health agencies is one that often goes unnoticed—the persistent and widespread use of categorical approaches to the deployment of interventions, which often fragments and isolates individual programs, one from another. In addition to the unnecessary proliferation of information, management, and other administrative processes, each program tends to develop its own assortment of interest and constituency groups, including those involving program staff members, who often work to oppose meaningful consolidation and integration of programs.

Another limiting factor is the generalized inability to prioritize and focus public health efforts, despite the wealth of information as to which factors most affect health at the national, state, and even local levels. Time and time again, tobacco, alcohol, diet, and violence have been shown to lie at the root of most preventable mortality and years of potential life lost. Ideally, resource allocation decisions would be made on the basis of the most important attributable risks, rather than being spread around to address, ineffectively, risks both large and small. With scores of priorities, there are really none, and without clear priorities, accountability is seldom expected. Public health has always operated at the interface of science and politics; political issues and compromises are natural. Still, inconsistencies between stated public health priorities and actual program priorities, as demonstrated through funding, are themselves barriers to public understanding and support for public health work. Comprehensive and systematic approaches must replace current silo strategies.

Other factors that influence public understanding and support for public health relate to the transition from conditions caused by microorganisms to those caused by human behaviors. It is more difficult for the public to appreciate the scientific basis for public health interventions when social, rather than physical sciences, guide strategies. This occurs at a time when government is increasingly portrayed as both incompetent and overly intrusive. Largely because governmental processes are considered by the public to be intensely political, the public view of public health processes, including programs and regulations, is that of highly politicized and partly scientific exercises.

There has been considerable debate as to whether the 1988 IOM report accurately captured the problems and needs of the American public health system. In many respects, the report restated the fundamental values and concepts underlying public health in terms of its emphasis on prevention, professional diversity, collaborative nature, community problem solving, loosely attached constituencies, assurance functions, need to draw other sectors into the solution of public health problems, and lack of an identifiable constituency. Taken together, these features appear to represent disarray; however, the cause of this disarray may not lie with public health but rather with our social and governmental institutions, more generally. Posing solutions that restructure the public health system's components may do little more than rearranging the deck chairs on the Titanic would have done.

It may be necessary to more broadly restructure the tasks and functions of public health to deal with modern public health problems. The larger work of public health is to get the threat protection, disease prevention, and health promotion job done right, rather than to get it done through a traditional structuring of roles and responsibilities. Preventing disease and promoting health must be embraced throughout society and its health institutions, rather than existing in a parallel subsystem. There is no evidence to support the contention that public health activities are best organized through public health agencies of government. Other nations have emphasized social policies that have brought them better overall health outcomes for their populations at much lower cost. It is the mission and the effort that are important and not necessarily the organization from which those efforts are generated.

OUTSIDE-THE-BOOK THINKING 14-2

© Alfred Bondarenko/Shutterstock.

Using an academic grading scale from A to F, how effective is the public health system in the United States? How did you arrive at this rating?

CONCLUSION: THE NEED FOR A MORE EFFECTIVE PUBLIC HEALTH SYSTEM

The perpetual frustration for public health is the gap between what has been achieved and what could have been achieved. The unfulfilled promise of public health should not be viewed as some unfortunate accident but as a direct result of a series of past decisions and actions undertaken quite purposefully. Sadly, they reflect both a history of disregard and the consequences of battles over the legitimacy, scope, professional authority, and political reach of public health.[7] A recent example is the use of tobacco settlement funds.

The various settlements in 1998 with a group of the major tobacco companies will provide $250 billion to the states over a 25-year period. These settlements were initially viewed as a colossal success for public health over one of its most important enemies. Although still in the middle years of this possible quarter-century windfall, state legislative and executive branch leaders have opted to use this money for a variety of purposes, some for health purposes but much for other ends. It was expected that approaches would vary from state to state, with most using some portion of the money to support tobacco cessation and prevention interventions. Early indications, however, are that as little as one third of the settlement funds were earmarked for health programs and that the health share declined rapidly in the face of state budget deficits throughout the first and second decades of the century.

The tobacco company settlement can be viewed as a success story or as part of a full accounting of the massive failure of public health efforts in the battle against tobacco use. Why did it take 3 decades to change public perceptions and values to the point that settlement became inevitable? Without attention to the lessons of this saga and to strengthening the public health system, tobacco will be the first of many health hazards that are inadequately addressed and for which a negotiated settlement will eventually occur. If we look at the tobacco settlement as a signal of the failure of public health and evidence of a weak public health infrastructure, this windfall becomes, at best, a bittersweet victory. Perhaps the tobacco settlement windfall would best be directed toward averting the next tobacco-like settlement. Difficult questions arise, even in otherwise good times!

In any event, the settlement offered the possibility of a sustained increase in public health resources to the tune of about $10 billion annually for 25 years. Considering that only approximately $43 billion was expended for governmental public health activities in 2000, the tobacco funds represented a possible 25% increase. Additional funding to governmental public health agencies for bioterrorism preparedness on top of the tobacco settlement funds provided for a possible doubling of governmental public health activities in the early years of the 21st century. As we have seen, however, this was an illusion that never materialized.

These circumstances and other key issues and challenges facing the future of public health defy simple summarization. This chapter has examined several, including those offered by the achievements and limitations of public health practice in the 20th century and others offered by the IOM reports; other chapters presented many more. Which of these are most important remains a point of contention. It would be useful to have an official list that represents the consensus of policy makers and the public alike; however, because an official list is lacking, several general conclusions as to the critical challenges and obstacles facing the future of public health in the United States are offered here. They summarize some of the important themes of this text in describing why we need more effective public health efforts.

The Easy Problems Have Already Been Solved

Major successes have been achieved through public health efforts over the past 150 years, largely related to massive reductions in infectious diseases but also involving substantial declines in death rates for injuries and several major chronic diseases since about 1960. The list of current problems for public health includes the more difficult chronic diseases, new and emerging conditions, including bioterrorism, and broader social problems with health effects (teen pregnancy and violence are good examples) that have identifiable risk and contributing factors that can be addressed only through collective action. The days of command-and-control approaches to relatively simple infectious risks are behind us. In the past, environmental sanitation and engineering could collaborate with communicable disease control expertise to address important public health problems. The collaborations needed for violence prevention or bioterrorism preparedness require very different skills and relationships.

To a Hammer, the Entire World Looks Like a Nail

Behind the aphorism that to a hammer, the entire world looks like a nail is the perception that common education and work experiences foster common professional perspectives. The danger lies in believing that one's own professional tools are adequate to the task of dealing with all of the problems and needs that are served by the profession. Each profession has its own scientific base and jargon. Problems are given labels or diagnoses, using the profession's specialized language, so that the tools of the profession can be brought to bear on those problems. All too often, however, the problems come to be considered as the domain of that profession, and the potential contributions of other professions and disciplines are underappreciated. Although public health professionals are remarkably diverse in terms of their educational and experiential backgrounds, we can also fall into this trap. When we do, bridges to other partners are not built, and collaborations do not take place. As a result, problems that can be addressed only through collaborative, intersectoral approaches flourish unabated.

A Friend in Need Is a Friend Indeed

Finding the means to build such bridges can be difficult, but some key collaborations appear to be absolutely essential for the work of public health to succeed. Certainly, links between public health and medical care must be improved for both to prosper in a reforming health system. Links with businesses also represent another avenue for mutually successful collaborations. The key is to find major areas of common purpose. For medical care interests, the common denominator is that prevention saves money and rewards those who use it as an investment strategy. For business interests, the bottom line has to be improved, and businesses must accept the premise that improving health status in the community serves their bottom lines through healthier, more productive workers and healthier and wealthier consumers.

You Get What You Pay For

There is good cause to question the current national investment strategy as it relates to health. The excess capacity that has been established in the American health system is becoming increasingly unaffordable, and the results are nothing about which to write home. Still, the competition for additional dollars is intense among the major interests that dominate the health industry, and there is only minimal movement to alter the current balance between treatment and prevention strategies. With less than 5% of all health expenditures supporting public health's core functions and essential services and only about 1% supporting population-based prevention, even small shifts could reap substantial rewards. The argument that resources are limited and that there simply are not adequate resources to meet treatment, as well as prevention purposes, is uniquely American and quite inimical to the public's health. More disconcerting yet are the lost opportunities in securing and using recent tobacco settlement and bioterrorism preparedness funding to shore up a sagging public health infrastructure.

It's Not My Job?

The job description of public health has never been clear. As a result, public health has become quite proficient in delivering specific services, with less attention paid to mobilizing action toward those factors that most seriously affect community health status. Among traditional health-related factors, tobacco, alcohol, and diet are factors responsible for much of modern America's mortality (or lack thereof) and morbidity. Nonetheless, the resources supporting interventions directed toward these factors are minuscule. Similarly, the primary cause of America's relatively poor health outcomes, in comparison with other developed nations, as well as the most likely source for further health gains in the United States, resides in the huge and increasing gaps among racial and ethnic groups. The public health system, from national to state and local levels, must recognize these circumstances and move beyond them to advocate and build constituencies aggressively for efforts that target the most important of the traditional health risk factors and that promote social policies that will both minimize and equalize risks throughout the population. The task is as simple as following the golden rule and doing for others what we want done for ourselves because efforts to improve the health of others make everyone healthier. This does not constitute a new job description for public health in the United States, but rather a recommitment to an old, reasonably successful, and absolutely necessary one.

REFERENCES

1. Centers for Disease Control and Prevention. *Addressing Emerging Infectious Disease Threats: A Prevention Strategy for the United States.* Atlanta, GA: U.S. Public Health Service; 1994.
2. U.S. Department of Health and Human Services. *Healthy People 2020.* Accessible at www.healthypeople.gov. Accessed June 15, 2014.
3. McKinlay JB, Marceau LD. To boldly go …. *Am J Public Health.* 2000; *90*: 25–33.
4. Institute of Medicine. *The Future of Public Health.* Washington, DC: National Academy Press; 1988.
5. Institute of Medicine. *The Future of the Public's Health in the 21st Century.* Washington, DC: National Academy Press; 2003.
6. Institute of Medicine. *Who Will Keep the Public Healthy? Educating Public Health Professionals for the 21st Century.* Washington, DC: National Academy Press; 2003.
7. Fee E, Brown TM. The unfulfilled promise of public health: déjà vu all over again. *Health Aff.* 2002; *21*: 31–43.

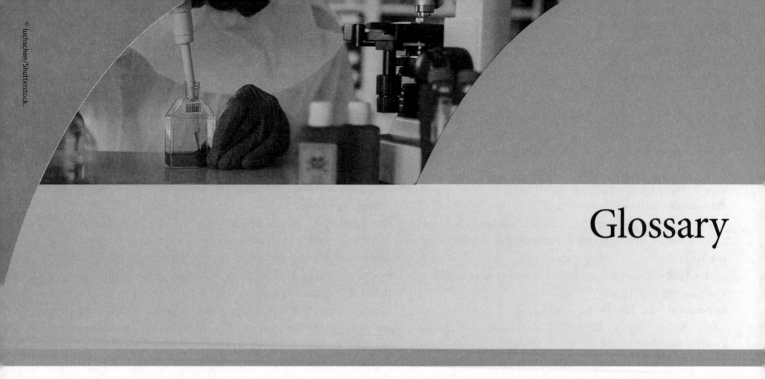

Glossary

TERM DEFINITION (NOTE: Some definitions are quoted from other sources; refer to text for citations.)

Access—The potential for or actual entry of a population into the health system. Entry is dependent on the wants, resources, and needs that individuals bring to the care-seeking process. Ability to obtain wanted or needed services may be influenced by many factors, including travel distance, waiting time, available financial resources, and availability of a regular source of care.

Accreditation—For public health agencies, accreditation is a process that measures the performance of the organization against a set of nationally recognized, practice-focused and evidence-based standards. The Public Health Accreditation Board recognizes (i.e., accredits) public health agencies that meet these standards.

Actual Cause of Death—A primary determinant or risk factor associated with a pathologic or diagnosed cause of death. For example, tobacco use would be the actual cause for deaths from many lung cancers.

Adjusted Rate—The adjustment or standardization of rates is a statistical procedure that removes the effect of differences in the composition of populations. Because of its marked effect on mortality and morbidity, age is the variable for adjustment used most commonly. For example, an age-adjusted death rate for any cause permits a better comparison between different populations and at different times because it accounts for differences in the distribution of age.

Administrative Law—Rules and regulations promulgated by administrative agencies within the executive branch of government that carry the force of law. Administrative law represents a unique situation in which legislative, executive, and judicial powers are carried out by one agency in the development, implementation, and enforcement of rules and regulations.

Age-Adjusted Mortality Rate—The expected number of deaths that would occur if a population had the same age distribution as a standard population, expressed in terms of deaths per 1,000 or 100,000 persons.

Affordable Care Act—The common name for the Patient Protection and Affordable Care Act of 2010 (Public Law 111-148), which is the federal statute incorporating many health reform provisions affecting health insurance policies, coverage, cost, and quality of care. This legislation is also known as "Obamacare," as it was proposed by the Obama Administration and signed into law by the President.

Appropriateness—Health interventions for which the expected health benefit exceeds the expected negative consequences by a wide enough margin to justify the intervention.

Assessment—One of public health's three core functions. Assessment calls for regularly and systematically collecting, analyzing, and making available information on the health of a community, including statistics on health status, community health needs, and epidemiologic and other studies of health problems.

Assets—Resources available to achieve a specific end, such as community resources that can contribute to community health improvement efforts or emergency response resources, including human, to respond to a public health emergency.

Association—The relationship between two or more events or variables. Events are said to be associated when they occur more frequently together than one would expect by chance. Association does not necessarily imply a causal relationship.

Assurance—One of public health's three core functions. It involves assuring constituents that services necessary to achieve agreed-upon goals are provided by encouraging actions on the part of others, by requiring action through regulation, or by providing services directly.

Attributable Risk—The theoretical reduction in the rate or number of cases of an adverse outcome that can be achieved by elimination of a risk factor. For example, if tobacco use is responsible for 75% of all lung cancers, the elimination of tobacco use will reduce lung cancer mortality rates by 75% in a population over time.

Behavioral Risk Factors Surveillance System—A national data collection system funded by the Centers for Disease Control and Prevention (CDC) to assess the prevalence of behaviors that affect health status. Through individual state efforts, CDC staff coordinate the collection, analysis, and distribution of survey data on seat belt use, hypertension, physical activity, smoking, weight control, alcohol use, mammography screening, cervical cancer screening, and AIDS, as well as other health-related information.

Biosurveillance—The process of gathering, integrating, interpreting, and communicating essential information that might relate to disease activity and threats to human, animal, or plant health. For public health workers, biosurveillance activities range from standard epidemiological practices to advanced technological systems, utilizing complex algorithms.

Bioterrorism—The threatened or intentional release of biologic agents (viruses, bacteria, or their toxins) for the purpose of influencing the conduct of government or intimidating or coercing a civilian population to further political or social objectives. These agents can be released by way of the air (as aerosols), food, water, or insects.

Capacity—The capability to carry out the core functions of public health. Also see infrastructure.

Capitation—A method of payment for health services in which a provider is paid a fixed amount for each person served, without regard to the actual number or nature of services provided to each person in a set period of time. Capitation is the characteristic payment method in health maintenance organizations.

Case Definition—Standardized criteria for determining whether a person has a particular disease or health-related condition. Criteria often include clinical and laboratory findings, as well as personal characteristics (e.g., age, sex, location, time period). Case definitions are often used in investigations and for comparing potential cases.

Case Management—The monitoring and coordinating of services rendered to individuals with specific problems or who require high-cost or extensive services.

Casualty—Any person suffering physical and/or psychological damage that leads to death, injury, or material loss.

Causality—The relationship of causes to the effects they produce; several types of causes can be distinguished. A cause is termed necessary when a particular variable must always precede an effect. This effect need not be the sole result of the one variable. A cause is termed sufficient when a particular variable inevitably initiates or produces an effect. Any given cause may be necessary, sufficient, neither, or both.

Cause of Death—For the purpose of national mortality statistics, every death is attributed to one underlying condition, based on the information reported on the death certificate and utilizing the international rules for selecting the underlying cause of death from the reported conditions.

Centers for Disease Control and Prevention (CDC)—The Centers for Disease Control and Prevention, based in Atlanta, Georgia, is the federal agency charged with protecting the nation's public health by providing direction in the prevention and control of communicable and other diseases and responding to public health emergencies. CDC's responsibilities as the nation's prevention agency have expanded over the years and will continue to evolve as the agency addresses contemporary threats to health, such as injury, environmental and occupational hazards, behavioral risks, and chronic diseases; and emerging communicable diseases, such as the Ebola virus.

Certification—A process by which an agency or association grants recognition to another party who has met certain predetermined qualifications specified by the agency or association.

Chronic Disease—A disease that has one or more of the following characteristics: (1) it is permanent, (2) it leaves residual disability, (3) it is caused by a nonreversible pathologic alteration, (4) it requires special training of the patient for rehabilitation, or (5) it may be expected to require a long period of supervision, observation, or care.

Clinical Practice Guidelines—Systematically developed statements that assist practitioner and patient decisions about appropriate health services for specific clinical conditions.

Clinical Preventive Services—Clinical services provided to patients to reduce or prevent disease, injury, or disability. These are preventive measures (including screening tests, immunizations, counseling, and periodic physical examinations) provided by a health professional to an individual patient.

Community—A group of people who have common characteristics; communities can be defined by location, race, ethnicity, age, occupation, interest in particular problems or outcomes, or other common bonds. Ideally, there should be available assets and resources, as well as collective discussion, decision making, and action.

Community Health Improvement Process—A systematic effort that assesses community needs and assets, prioritizes health-related problems and issues, analyzes problems for their causative factors, develops evidence-based intervention strategies based on those analyses, links stakeholders to implementation efforts through performance monitoring, and evaluates the effect of interventions in the community.

Community Health Needs Assessment—A formal approach to identifying health needs and health problems in the community. A variety of tools or instruments may be used; the essential ingredient is community engagement and collaborative participation.

Community Preventive Services—Population-based interventions to reduce or prevent disease, injury, or disability. These are preventive interventions targeting the entire population rather than individuals.

Comprehensive Emergency Management—A broad style of emergency management, encompassing prevention, preparedness, response, and recovery.

Condition—A health condition is a departure from a state of physical or mental well-being. An impairment is a health condition that includes chronic or permanent health defects resulting from disease, injury, or congenital malformations. All health conditions except impairments are coded according to an international classification system. Based on duration, there are two types of conditions—acute and chronic.

Consequence Management—An emergency management function that includes measures to protect public health and safety, restore essential government services, and provide emergency relief to governments in the event of terrorism.

Contamination—An accidental release of hazardous chemicals or nuclear materials that pollute the environment and place humans at risk.

Contributing Factor—A risk factor (causative factor) that is associated with the level of a determinant. Direct contributing factors are linked with the level of determinants; indirect contributing factors are linked with the level of direct contributing factors.

Core Functions—Three basic roles for public health for assuring conditions in which people can be healthy. As identified in the Institute of Medicine's landmark report, The Future of Public Health, these are assessment, policy development, and assurance.

Cost-Benefit Analysis—An economic analysis in which all costs and benefits are converted into monetary (dollar) values, and results are expressed as dollars of benefit per dollars expended.

Cost-Effectiveness Analysis—An economic analysis assessed as a health outcome per cost expended.

Cost-Utility Analysis—An economic analysis assessed as a quality-adjusted outcome per net cost expended.

Countermeasures—A measure or action that is taken to counter or offset another measure. Countermeasures are designed or selected for their precision and specificity in preventing undesired outcomes from occurring.

Covert Releases—For biologic agents, an unannounced release of a biologic agent that causes illness or other effects. If undetected, a covert release has the potential to spread widely before it is detected.

Crisis Management—Administrative measures that identify, acquire, and plan the use of resources needed to anticipate, prevent, and/or resolve a threat to public safety (such as terrorism).

Crude Mortality Rate—The total number of deaths per unit of population reported during a given time interval, often expressed as the number of deaths per 1,000 or 100,000 persons.

Cultural Competence—The ability to communicate with and provide services to an individual or a group with full respect for the culturally associated values, preferences, language, and experiences of the group.

Decision Analysis—An analytic technique in which probability theory is used to obtain a quantitative approach to decision making.

Decontamination—The removal of hazardous chemicals or nuclear substances from the skin and/or mucous membranes by showering or washing the affected area with water or by rinsing with a sterile solution.

Demographics—Characteristic data, such as size, growth, density, distribution, and vital statistics, which are used to study human populations.

Demonstration Settings—A population-based or clinic-based environment in which prevention strategies are field-tested.

Determinant—A primary risk factor (causative factor) associated with the level of health problem (i.e., the level of the determinant influences the level of the health problem).

Disability Limitation—An intervention strategy that seeks to arrest or eradicate disease and/or limit disability and prevent death.

Disaster—Any event, typically occurring suddenly, that causes damage, ecologic disruption, loss of human life, or deterioration of health and health services and that exceeds the capacity of the affected community on a scale sufficient to require outside assistance.

Disaster Severity Scale—A scale that classifies disasters by the following parameters: (1) the radius of the disaster site, (2) the number of dead, (3) the number of wounded, (4) the average severity of the injuries sustained, (5) the impact time, and (6) the rescue time. By attributing a numeric score to each of the variables from 0 to 2, with 0 being the least severe and 2 the most severe, a scale with a range of 0 to 18 can be created.

Discounting—A method for adjusting the value of future costs and benefits. Expressed as a present dollar value, discounting is based on the time value of money (i.e., a dollar today is worth more than it will be a year from now, even if inflation is not considered).

Distributional Effects—The manner in which the costs and benefits of a strategy affect different groups of people in terms of demographics, geographic location, and other descriptive factors.

Early Case Finding and Treatment—An intervention strategy that seeks to identify disease or illness at an early stage so that prompt treatment will reduce the effects of the process.

Effectiveness—The improvement in health outcome that a strategy can produce in typical community-based settings. Also, the degree to which objectives are achieved.

Efficacy—The improvement in health outcome effect that a strategy can produce in expert hands under ideal circumstances.

Emergency—Any natural or human-made situation that results in severe injury, harm, or loss to humans or property.

Emergency Management Agency—The agency, under the authority of the governor's office, that coordinates the efforts of the state's health department, housing and social service agencies, and public safety agencies (such as state police) during an emergency or disaster. The emergency management agency also coordinates federal resources made available to the states, such as the National Guard, Centers for Disease Control and Prevention, and the Public Health Service.

Emergency Medical Services (EMS) System—The coordination of the prehospital system (including public access, 911 dispatch, paramedics, and ambulance services) and the in-hospital system (including emergency departments, hospitals, and other definitive care facilities and personnel) to provide emergency medical care.

Emergency Operations Center (EOC)—The site from which civil governmental officials (such as municipal, county, state, or federal) direct emergency operations in a disaster.

Epidemic—The occurrence of a disease or condition at higher than normal levels in a population.

Epidemiology—The study of the distribution of determinants and antecedents of health and disease in human populations, the ultimate goal of which is to identify the underlying causes of a disease, then apply findings to disease prevention and health promotion.

Escherichia coli (E. coli) O57:H7—A bacterial pathogen that can infect humans and cause severe bloody diarrhea (hemorrhagic colitis) and serious renal disease (hemolytic uremic syndrome).

Essential Public Health Services—A formulation of the processes used in public health to prevent epidemics and injuries, protect against environmental hazards, promote healthy behaviors, respond to disasters, and ensure quality and accessibility of health services. Ten essential services have been identified:

1. Monitoring health status to identify community health problems
2. Diagnosing and investigating health problems and health hazards in the community
3. Informing, educating, and empowering people about health issues
4. Mobilizing community partnerships to identify and solve health problems
5. Developing policies and plans that support individual and community health efforts
6. Enforcing laws and regulations that protect health and ensure safety
7. Linking people to needed personal health services and ensuring the provision of health care when otherwise unavailable
8. Ensuring a competent public health and personal healthcare workforce
9. Evaluating effectiveness, accessibility, and quality of personal and population-based health services
10. Conducting research for new insights and innovative solutions to health problems

Evacuation—The organized removal of civilians from a dangerous or potentially dangerous area.

Evidence-Based Public Health—Key components of evidence-based public health include making decisions on the basis of the best available scientific evidence, using data and information systems systematically, applying program-planning frameworks, engaging the community in decision making, conducting sound evaluation, and disseminating what is learned. Three types of evidence have been presented on the causes of diseases and the magnitude of risk factors, the relative impact of specific interventions, and how and under which contextual conditions interventions were implemented.

Federal Response Plan—The plan that coordinates federal resources in disaster and emergency situations in order to address the consequences when there is need for federal assistance under the authorities of the Stafford Disaster Relief and Emergency Assistance Act.

Federally Funded Community Health Center—An ambulatory healthcare program (defined under Section 330 of the Public Health Service Act), usually serving a catchment area that has scarce or nonexistent health services or a population with special health needs; sometimes known as a neighborhood health center. Community health centers attempt to coordinate federal, state, and local resources in a single organization capable of delivering both health and related social services to a defined population. Although such a center may not directly provide all types of health care, it usually takes responsibility to arrange all medical services for its patient population.

Field Model—A framework for identifying factors that influence health status in populations. Initially, four fields were identified: (1) biology, (2) lifestyle, (3) environment, and (4) health services. Extensions of this approach have also identified genetic, social, and cultural factors and have related these factors to a variety of outcomes, including disease, normal functioning, well-being, and prosperity.

Foodborne Illness—Illness caused by the transfer of disease organisms or toxins from food to humans.

General Welfare Provisions—Specific language in the Constitution of the United States that empowers the federal government to provide for the general welfare of the population. Over time, these provisions have been used as a basis for federal health policies and programs.

Goals—For public health programs, general statements expressing a program's aspirations or intended effect on one or more health problems, often stated without time limits.

Governmental Presence at the Local Level—A concept that calls for the assurance that necessary services and minimum standards are provided to address priority community health problems. This responsibility ultimately falls to local government, which may utilize local public health agencies or other means for its execution.

Harm Reduction—A set of practical strategies reflecting individual and community needs that meet individuals with risk behaviors where they are to help them reduce any harms associated with their risk behaviors.

Hazard—A possible source of harm or injury.

Hazard Vulnerability Analysis—A systematic approach to recognizing hazards that may affect a population, community, or organization. The risks associated with each hazard are analyzed to prioritize planning, mitigation, response, and recovery activities. A hazard vulnerability analysis serves as a needs assessment for emergency preparedness and response activities.

Health—The state of complete physical, mental, and social well-being and not merely the absence of disease or infirmity. It is recognized, however, that health has many dimensions (anatomic, physiologic, and mental) and is largely culturally defined. The relative importance of various disabilities will differ, depending on the cultural milieu and on the role of the affected individual in that culture. Most attempts at measurement have been assessed in terms of morbidity and mortality.

Health Disparity—Difference in health status between two groups, such as the health disparity in mortality between men and women, or the health disparity in infant mortality between African American and white infants.

Health Education—Any combination of learning opportunities designed to facilitate voluntary adaptations of behavior (in individuals, groups, or communities) conducive to good health. Health education encourages positive health behavior.

Health Impact Assessment—A systematic process that uses an array of data sources and analytic methods, and considers input from stakeholders to determine the potential effects of a proposed policy, plan, program, or project on the health of a population and the distribution of those effects within the population. Health impact assessments provide recommendations on monitoring and managing those effects.

Health Maintenance Organizations—Entities that manage both the financing and provision of health services to enrolled members. Fees are generally based on capitation, and health providers are managed to reduce costs through controls on utilization of covered services.

Health Planning—Planning concerned with improving health, whether undertaken comprehensively for an entire community or for a particular population, type of health services, institution, or health program. The components of health planning include data assembly and analysis, goal determination, action recommendation, and implementation strategy.

Health Policy—Social policy concerned with the process whereby public health agencies evaluate and determine health needs and the best ways to address them, including the identification of appropriate resources and funding mechanisms.

Health Problem—A situation or condition of people (expressed in health outcome measures such as mortality, morbidity, or disability) that is considered undesirable and is likely to exist in the future.

Health Problem Analysis—A framework for analyzing health problems to identify their determinants and contributing factors so that interventions can be targeted rationally toward those factors most likely to reduce the level of the health problem.

Health Promotion—An intervention strategy that seeks to eliminate or reduce exposures to harmful factors by modifying human behaviors. Any combination of health education and related organizational, political, and economic interventions designed to facilitate behavioral and environmental adaptations that will improve or protect health. This process enables individuals and communities to control and improve their own health. Health promotion approaches provide opportunities for people to identify problems, develop solutions, and work in partnerships that build on existing skills and strengths.

Health Protection—An intervention strategy that seeks to provide individuals with resistance to harmful factors, often by modifying the environment to decrease potentially harmful interactions. Those population-based services and programs control and reduce the exposure of the population to environmental or personal hazards, conditions, or factors that may cause disease, disability, injury, or death. Health protection also includes programs that ensure that public health services are available on a 24-hour basis to respond to public health emergencies and coordinate responses of local, state, and federal organizations.

Health Regulation—Monitoring and maintaining the quality of public health services through licensing and discipline of health professionals, licensing of health facilities, and enforcement of standards and regulations.

Health Status Indicators—Measurements of the state of health of a specified individual, group, or population. Health status may be measured by proxies such as people's subjective assessments of their health; by one or more indicators of mortality and morbidity in the population, such as longevity or maternal and infant mortality; or by the incidence or prevalence of major diseases (communicable, chronic, or nutritional). Conceptually, health status is the proper outcome measure for the effectiveness of a specific population's health system, although attempts to relate effects of available medical care to variations in health status have proved difficult.

Health System—As used in this text, the sum total of the strategies designed to prevent or treat disease, injury, and other health problems. The health system includes population-based preventive services, clinical preventive and other primary medical care services, and all levels of more sophisticated treatment and chronic care services.

Healthy Communities—A framework for developing and tailoring community health objectives so that these can be tracked as part of the initiative to achieve the national health objectives included in *Healthy People 2020*.

Healthy People 2020—The national disease prevention and health promotion agenda that includes the national health objectives to be achieved by the year 2020, addressing improved health status, risk reduction, and utilization of preventive health services.

Incidence—A measure of the disease or injury in the population, generally the number of new cases occurring during a specified time period.

Incident Command System (ICS)—The model for command, control, and coordination of a response to an emergency providing the means to coordinate the efforts of multiple agencies and organizations.

Indicator—A measure of health status or a health outcome.

Infant Mortality Rate—The number of live-born infants who die before their first birthday per 1,000 live births; often broken into two components, neonatal mortality (deaths before 28 days per 1,000 live births) and postneonatal mortality (deaths from 28 days through the rest of the first year of life per 1,000 live births).

Infectious Disease—A disease caused by the entrance into the body of organisms (such as bacteria, protozoans, fungi, or viruses) that then grow and multiply there (often used synonymously with communicable disease).

Infrastructure—The systems, competencies, relationships, and resources that enable performance of public health's core functions and essential services in every community. Categories include human, organizational, informational, and fiscal resources.

Inputs—Human resources, fiscal and physical resources, information resources, and system organizational resources necessary to carry out the core functions of public health (sometimes referred to as capacities).

Intervention—A generic term used in public health to describe a program or policy designed to have an impact on a health problem. For example, a mandatory seat belt law is an intervention designed to reduce the incidence of automobile-related fatalities. Five categories of heath interventions are: (1) health promotion, (2) specific protection, (3) early case finding and prompt treatment, (4) disability limitation, and (5) rehabilitation.

Leading Causes of Death—Those diagnostic classifications of disease that are most frequently responsible for deaths (often used in conjunction with the top 10 causes of death).

Leading Health Indicators—A panel of health-related measures that reflect the major public health concerns in the United States. They were selected to track progress toward achievement of Healthy People goals and objectives. They address 10 public health concerns: (1) physical activity, (2) overweight and obesity, (3) tobacco use, (4) substance abuse, (5) responsible sexual behavior, (6) mental health, (7) injury and violence, (8) environmental quality, (9) immunizations, and (10) access to health care.

Life Expectancy—The number of additional years of life expected at a specified point in time, such as at birth or at age 45.

Local Health Department (LHD)—Functionally, a local (county, multicounty, municipal, town, other) health agency, operated by local government, often with oversight and direction from a local board of health, that carries out public health's core functions throughout a defined geographic area. A more traditional definition is an agency serving less than an entire state that carries some responsibility for health and has at least one full-time employee and a specific budget.

Local Health Jurisdiction (LHJ)—A unit of local government (county, multicounty, municipal, town, other), often with oversight and direction from a local board of health and with an identifiable local health department, that carries out public health's core functions throughout a defined geographic area.

Local Public Health Authority—The agency charged with responsibility for meeting the health needs of the community. Usually this is the policy/governing body and its administrative arm, the local health department. The authority may rest with the policy/governing body, may be a city/county/regional authority, or may consist of a legislative mandate from the state. Some local public health authorities have independence from all other governmental entities, whereas others do not.

Local Public Health System—The collection of public and private organizations having a stake in and contributing to public health at the local level. It involves far more than the local public health agency.

Managed Care—A system of administrative controls intended to reduce costs through managing the utilization of services. Managed care can also mean an integrated system of health insurance, financing, and service delivery that focuses on the appropriate and cost-effective use of health services delivered through defined networks of providers and with allocation of financial risk.

Measure—An indicator of health status or a health outcome, used synonymously with indicator in this text.

Medicaid—A federally aided, state-operated and administered program that provides basic medical services to eligible low-income populations, established through amendments as Title XIX of the Social Security Act in 1965. It does not cover all of the poor, however, but only persons who meet specified eligibility criteria. Subject to broad federal guidelines, states determine the benefits covered, program eligibility, rates of payment for providers, and methods of administering the program.

Medical Reserve Corps—Locally based teams of health professionals and other personnel who provide surge capacity for emergencies.

Medicare—A national health insurance program for elderly persons established through amendments to the Social Security Act in 1965 that were included in Title XVIII of that act.

Midlevel Practitioners—Non-physician healthcare providers, such as nurse practitioners and physician assistants.

Mission—For public health, ensuring conditions in which people can be healthy.

Mitigation—Measures taken to reduce the harmful effects of a disaster or emergency by attempting to limit the impact on human health and economic infrastructure.

Mobilizing for Action through Planning and Partnerships (MAPP)—A voluntary process for organizational and community self-assessment, planned improvements, and continuing evaluation and reassessment. The process focuses on community-wide public health practice, including a health department's role in its community and the community's actual and perceived problems. It provides for a community health improvement process to assess health needs, sets priorities, develops policy, and ensures that health needs are met.

Morbidity—A measure of disease incidence or prevalence in a given population, location, or other grouping of interest.

Mortality—Expresses the number of deaths in a population within a prescribed time. Mortality rates may be expressed as crude death rates (total deaths in relation to total population during a year) or as death rates specific for diseases and sometimes for age, sex, or other attributes (e.g., the number of deaths from cancer in white males in relation to the white male population during a given year).

National Health Expenditures—The amount spent for all health services and supplies and health-related research and construction activities in the United States during the calendar year.

Obamacare—See Affordable Care Act.

Objectives—Targets for achievement through interventions. Objectives are time-limited and measurable in all cases. Various levels of objectives for an intervention include outcome, impact, and process objectives.

Outcomes—Indicators of health status, risk reduction, and quality-of-life enhancement (sometimes referred to as results of the health system). Outcomes are long-term objectives that define optimal, measurable future levels of health status; maximum acceptable levels of disease, injury, or dysfunction; or prevalence of risk factors.

Outputs—Health programs and services intended to prevent death, disease, and disability, and to promote quality of life.

Personal Health Services—Diagnosis and treatment of disease or provision of clinical preventive services to individuals or families in order to improve individual health status.

Police Power—A basic power of government that allows for restriction of individual rights to protect the safety and interests of the entire population.

Policy Development—One of public health's three core functions. Policy development involves serving the public interest by leading in developing comprehensive public health policy and promoting the use of the scientific knowledge base in decision making.

Population-Based Public Health Services—Interventions aimed at disease prevention and health promotion that affect an entire population and extend beyond medical treatment by targeting underlying risks, such as tobacco, drug, and alcohol use; diet and sedentary lifestyles; and environmental factors.

Postponement—A form of prevention in which the time of onset of a disease or injury is delayed to reduce the prevalence of a condition in the population.

Preparedness—All measures and policies taken before an event occurs that allow for prevention, mitigation, and readiness.

Prevalence—A measure of the burden of disease or injury in a population, generally the number of cases of a disease or injury at a particular point in time or during a specified time period. Prevalence is affected by both the incidence and the duration of disease in a population.

Prevented Fraction—The proportion of an adverse health outcome that has been eliminated as a result of a prevention strategy.

Prevention—Anticipatory action taken to prevent the occurrence of an event or to minimize its effects after it has occurred. Prevention aims to minimize the occurrence of disease or its consequences. It includes actions that reduce susceptibility or exposure to health threats (primary prevention), detect and treat disease in early stages (secondary prevention), and alleviate the effects of disease and injury (tertiary prevention). Examples of prevention include immunizations, emergency response to epidemics, health education, modification of risk-prone behavior and physical hazards, safety training, workplace hazard elimination, and industrial process change.

Preventive Strategies—Frameworks for categorizing prevention programs, based on how the prevention technology is delivered—provider to patient (clinical preventive services), individual responsibility (behavioral prevention), or

alteration in an individual's surroundings (environmental prevention)—or on the stage of the natural history of a disease or injury (primary, secondary, tertiary).

Primary Medical Care—Clinical preventive services, first-contact treatment services, and ongoing care for commonly encountered medical conditions. Basic or general health care focuses on the point at which a patient ideally seeks assistance from the medical care system. Primary care is considered comprehensive when the primary provider takes responsibility for the overall coordination of the care of the patient's health problems, whether these are medical, behavioral, or social. The appropriate use of consultants and community resources is an important part of effective primary health care. Such care is generally provided by physicians but can also be provided by other personnel, such as nurse practitioners or physician assistants.

Primary Prevention—Prevention strategies that seek to prevent the occurrence of disease or injury, generally through reducing exposure or risk factor levels. These strategies can reduce or eliminate causative risk factors (risk reduction).

Public Health—Activities that society undertakes to ensure the conditions in which people can be healthy. These include organized community efforts to prevent, identify, and counter threats to the health of the public.

Public Health Accreditation Board—The organization that establishes performance standards for public health agencies and coordinates the process of measuring those standards and recognizing (i.e., accrediting) those agencies that meet these standards. Also see accreditation.

Public Health Agency—A unit of government (federal, state, local, or regional) charged with preserving, protecting, and promoting the health of the population through ensuring delivery of essential public health services.

Public Health in America—A document developed by the Core Functions Project that characterizes the vision, mission, outcome aspirations, and essential services of public health. Also see essential public health services.

Public Health Organization—A nongovernmental entity (e.g., not-for-profit agency, association, corporation) participating in activities designed to improve the health status of a community or population.

Public Health Practice—The development and application of preventive strategies and interventions to promote and protect the health of populations.

Public Health Practice Guidelines—Systematically developed statements that assist public health practitioner decisions about interventions at the community level.

Public Health Processes—Those collective practices or processes that are necessary and sufficient to ensure that the core functions and essential services of public health are being carried out effectively, including the key processes that identify and address health problems and their causative factors and the interventions intended to prevent death, disease, and disability, and to promote quality of life.

Public Health Service—U.S. Public Health Service, as reorganized in 1996, which now includes the Office of Public Health and Science (which is headed by the Assistant Secretary for Health and includes the Office of the Surgeon General), eight operating agencies (Health Resources and Services Administration; Indian Health Service; Centers for Disease Control and Prevention; National Institutes of Health; Food and Drug Administration; Substance Abuse and Mental Health Services Administration; Agency for Toxic Substances and Disease Registry; and Agency for Healthcare Research and Quality); and the Regional Health Administrators for the 10 federal regions of the country.

Public Health System—That part of the larger health system that seeks to ensure conditions in which people can be healthy by carrying out public health's three core functions. The system can be further described by its inputs, practices, outputs, and outcomes.

Public Health Workforce—The public health workforce includes individuals

- Employed by an organization engaged in an organized effort to promote, protect, and preserve the health of a defined population group. The group may be public or private, and the effort may be secondary or subsidiary to the principal objectives of the organization
- Performing work made up of one or more specific public health services or activities
- Occupying positions that conventionally require at least 1 year of postsecondary specialized public health training and that are (or can be) assigned a professional occupational title

Quality-Adjusted Life Years (QALYs)—A measure of health status that assigns to each period of time a weight, ranging from 0 to 1, corresponding to the health-related quality of life during that period. These are then summed across time periods to calculate QALYs. For each period, a weight of 1 corresponds to optimal health, and a weight of 0 corresponds to a health state equivalent to death.

Quality of Care—The degree to which health services for individuals increase the likelihood of desired health outcomes and are consistent with established professional standards and judgments of value to the consumer. Quality also may be seen as the degree to which actions taken or not taken maximize the probability of beneficial health outcomes and minimize risk and other undesired outcomes, given the existing state of medical science and art.

Rapid Needs Assessment—A variety of epidemiologic, statistic, anthropologic techniques designed to provide information about an affected community's needs following a disaster or other public health emergency.

Rate—A mathematical expression for the relation between the numerator (e.g., number of deaths, diseases, disabilities, services) and denominator (population at risk), together with specification of time. Rates make possible a comparison of the number of events between populations and at different times. Rates may be crude, specific, or adjusted.

Recovery—Actions of responders, government, and victims that help return an affected community to normal by stimulating community cohesiveness and governmental involvement. The recovery period falls between the onset of an emergency and the reconstruction period.

Rehabilitation—An intervention strategy that seeks to return individuals to the maximum level of functioning possible.

Response—The phase in a disaster or public health emergency when relief, recovery, and rehabilitation occur.

Risk—The probability that exposure to a hazard will lead to a negative consequence.

Risk Assessment—A determination of the likelihood of adverse health effects to a population after exposure to a hazard.

Risk Factor—A behavior or condition that, on the basis of scientific evidence or theory, is thought to influence susceptibility to a specific health problem.

Risk Ratio/Relative Risk—The ratio of the risk or likelihood of the occurrence of specific health outcomes or events in one group to that of another. Risk ratios provide a measure of the relative difference in risk between the two groups. Relative risk is an example of a risk ratio in which the incidence of disease in the exposed group is divided by the incidence of disease in an unexposed group.

Screening—The use of technology and procedures to differentiate those individuals with signs or symptoms of disease from those less likely to have the disease. Then, if necessary, further diagnosis and, if indicated, early intervention and treatment can be provided.

Secondary Medical Care—Specialized attention and ongoing management for common and less frequently encountered medical conditions, including support services for people with special challenges because of chronic or long-term conditions. Services are provided by medical specialists who generally do not have their first contact with patients (e.g., cardiologists, urologists, dermatologists). In the United

States, however, there has been a trend toward self-referral by patients for these services rather than referral by primary care providers.

Secondary Prevention—Prevention strategies that seek to identify and control disease processes in their early stages before signs and symptoms develop (screening and treatment).

Span of Healthy Life—A measure of health status that combines life expectancy with self-reported health status and functional disabilities to calculate the number of years in which an individual is likely to function normally.

Specific Rate—Rates vary greatly by race, sex, and age. A rate can be made specific for sex, age, race, cause of death, or a combination of these.

State Health Agency—The unit of state government that has leading responsibility for identifying and meeting the health needs of the state's citizens. State health agencies can be freestanding or units of multipurpose health and human service agencies.

Strategic National Stockpile—A collection of pharmaceuticals, medical supplies, and equipment that can be immediately deployed to meet state and local needs during a public health emergency (formerly known as the National Pharmaceutical Stockpile).

Strategic Planning—A disciplined process aimed at producing fundamental decisions and actions that will shape and guide what an organization is, what it does, and why it does what it does. The process involves assessing a changing environment to create a vision of the future; determining how the organization fits into the anticipated environment, based on its mission, strengths, and weaknesses; and then setting in motion a plan of action to position the organization.

Surveillance—Systematic monitoring of the health status of a population through collection, analysis, and interpretation of health data in order to plan, implement, and evaluate public health programs, including determining the need for public health action.

Tertiary Medical Care—Subspecialty referral care requiring highly specialized personnel and facilities. Services are provided by highly specialized providers (e.g., neurologists, neurosurgeons, thoracic surgeons, intensive care units). Such services frequently require highly sophisticated equipment and support facilities. The development of these services has largely been a function of diagnostic and therapeutic advances attained through basic and clinical biomedical research.

Tertiary Prevention—Prevention strategies that prevent disability by restoring individuals to their optimal level of functioning after a disease or injury is established and damage is done.

Triage—The selection and categorization of victims of a disaster or other public health emergency as to their need for medical treatment according to the degree of severity of illness or injury as well as the availability of medical and transport facilities.

Vulnerability—The susceptibility of a population to a specific type of event, generally associated with the degree of possible or potential loss from a risk that results from a hazard at a given intensity. Vulnerability can be influenced by demographics, the age and resilience of the environment, technology, social differentiation and diversity, as well as regional and global economics and politics.

Weapons of Mass Destruction—Any device, material, or substance used in a manner, in a quantity or type, or under circumstances evidencing intent to cause death or serious injury to persons or significant damage of property.

Years of Potential Life Lost (YPLL)—A measure of the impact of disease or injury in a population that calculates years of life lost before a specific age (often age 65 or age 75). This approach places additional value on deaths that occur at earlier ages.

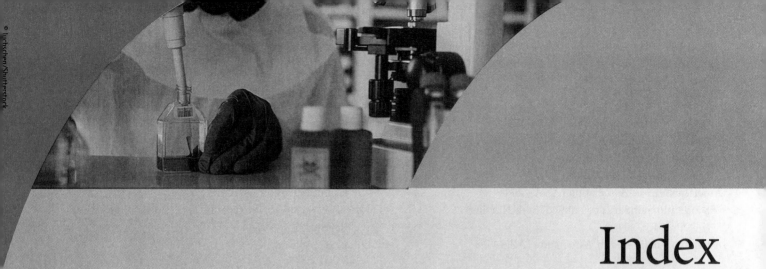

Index

Note: Page numbers followed by *f*, or *t* indicates materials in figures, or tables respectively.

RNs. *See* registered nurses

Robert T. Stafford Disaster Relief and Emergency Assistance Act, 124*t*

Robert Wood Johnson Foundation, 112, 114

rural areas, job opportunities for healthcare workers in, 158

S

Safe Drinking Water Act, 86

safety in the workplace, improvements and remaining challenges with, 256

salaries

for behavioral and mental health workers, 235

for environmental and occupational workers, 190–192, 190*t*, 191*t*

for epidemiology and disease control professionals, 215–217

mean, for full-time equivalent workers of state and local health agencies, 1998–2012, U.S., 151*f*

for medical and health administrators, 175–176

for nutritionists and dietitians, 237

for public health education and information professionals, 226–227

for public health laboratory specialists, 238

for public health laboratory technologists, 240

for public health nurses, 202–203, 202*t*, 203*t*

for public health workers, 152, 157

Salk vaccine, against polio, 16

SAMHSA. *See* Substance Abuse and Mental Health Services Administration

sanitary movement, 4, 5

Satcher, David, 6

school lunch programs, 237

schools of public health, training activities for public health workers and, 147

science, public health grounded in, 14–15

scope, of public health, 12

screenings, health care and, 47

seat belt use, 256

secondary building blocks, 111

secondary medical care, 50, 50*t*

secondary prevention

comprehensive model of chronic disease prevention and control, 49*f*

defined, 48

effects of, 47*f*

health services pyramid, 51*f*

Secretary of Homeland Security, responsibilities of, 124–125

September 11, 2001 terrorist attacks, 12

septicemia, as leading cause of death, 2000, 22, 23*f*

severe acute respiratory syndrome, 251

sexual behaviors, risky, 256

sexually transmitted diseases (STDs), state statutes and legal frameworks relative to, 76

SHAs. *See* state health agencies

Shattuck, Lemuel, 4

Sixteenth Amendment, 5

Snow, John, 3

cholera outbreak (1854) investigated by, 207

SNS. *See* Strategic National Stockpile

social enterprise, public health as, 6, 8

social justice philosophy, in public health, 11–12

societal benefits, 11

Society for Epidemiologic Research, 218

Society of Public Health Educators, 228

sociology, 14

special emergency powers, 119

stakeholders, in health system, 64

standard occupational categories (SOCs), 144, 148*t*–149*t*, 152

state agencies

health responsibilities of, 82

key activities performed by, 82

for public emergency preparedness and services, 126–127

state constitutions/statutes

local governments and, 73

role of, 74

state government health agencies, full-time equivalent (FTE) workers in, U.S., 1995–2012, 142, 142*t*

state governments, environmental health programs and, 86

state health agencies (SHAs), 72–73

selected characteristics, 2012, 85*f*

selected organizational responsibilities of, 2005, 83*f*

vital statistics for, 84*t*

state health departments, 126

state health expenditures, 86

state legal systems, 74

state legislatures, 73

state public health activities, in U.S., growth of, 4

statisticians

number and salary profile for federal and state/local workers, 2013, 216*t*

number of, in 2013, and projected for 2022 and number of positions to be filled, 2012–2022 for all industries and government, 216*t*

salaries for, 215–217

statutory-based laws, governmental policy choices and, 74